PAEDIATRIC RESPIRATORY CARE

A guide for physiotherapists and health professionals

Edited by

S. Ammani Prasad

Superintendent Physiotherapist, Respiratory Unit,
Great Ormond Street Hospital for Children NHS Trust, London, UK

and

Juliette Hussey

Lecturer in Physiotherapy, School of Physiotherapy,
Faculty of Health Sciences, Trinity College, Dublin, Republic of Ireland

Jo Campling

Commissioning Editorial Consultant

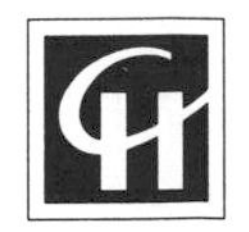

CHAPMAN & HALL

London · Glasgow · Weinheim · New York · Tokyo · Melbourne · Madras

Published by Chapman & Hall, 2–6 Boundary Row, London SE1 8HN, UK

Chapman & Hall, 2–6 Boundary Row, London SE1 8HN, UK

Blackie Academic & Professional, Wester Cleddens Road, Bishopbriggs, Glasgow G64 2NZ, UK

Chapman & Hall GmbH, Pappelallee 3, 69469 Weinheim, Germany

Chapman & Hall USA, One Penn Plaza, 41st Floor, New York NY 10119, USA

Chapman & Hall Japan, ITP-Japan, Kyowa Building, 3F, 2-2-1 Hirakawacho, Chiyoda-ku, Tokyo 102, Japan

Chapman & Hall Australia, Thomas Nelson Australia, 102 Dodds Street, South Melbourne, Victoria 3205, Australia

Chapman & Hall India, R. Seshadri, 32 Second Main Road, CIT East, Madras 600 035, India

Distributed in the USA and Canada by Singular Publishing Group Inc., 4284 41st Street, San Diego, California 92105

First edition 1995

Typeset in 10/12 Palatino by Mew Photosetting, Beckenham, Kent
Printed in Great Britain by Clays Ltd, St Ives plc

ISBN 0 412 55000 8 1 56593 292 7 (USA)

A catalogue record for this book is available from the British Library

Library of Congress Catalog Card Number: 94-72639

∞ Printed on permanent acid-free text paper, manufactured in accordance with the proposed ANSI/NISO Z39.48–1992 and ANSI/NISO Z39.48–1984 (Permanence of Paper).

PAEDIATRIC RESPIRATORY CARE

To Guy and Ella, Garry and Robert with love

CONTENTS

CONTRIBUTORS

Dr Robert Dinwiddie MB, FRCP
Consultant Paediatrician,
Respiratory Unit,
Great Ormond Street Hospital for
Children NHS Trust, London.

Mr Martin Elliott MD, FRCS
Consultant Cardiothoracic Surgeon,
Great Ormond Street Hospital for
Children NHS Trust, London.

Dr Christopher D. George FRCS, FRCR
Consultant Radiologist,
Department of Diagnostic Radiology,
Epsom District Hospital, Epsom.

Dr Isky Gordon FRCR
Consultant Radiologist,
Department of Diagnostic Radiology,
Great Ormond Street Hospital for
Children NHS Trust, London.

Professor Anne Greenough MD, FRCP, DCH
Professor of Clinical Respiratory
Physiology,
Department of Child Health,
King's College Hospital, London.

Mrs Annette Parker MCSP, SRP
Superintendent Physiotherapist,
Department of Child Health,
King's College Hospital, London.

Dr Robert C. Tasker MA, MB, MRCP
Consultant in Paediatric Critical Care
Medicine,
Great Ormond Street Hospital for
Children NHS Trust, London.

FOREWORD

The last decade has witnessed many advances in our knowledge of and practice of health care. This has been accompanied by an increasing trend towards subspecialization, both in clinical medicine and its allied professions. This has certainly been true in paediatric practice, particularly with the current development of paediatric intensive care as a speciality in its own right. Paediatric pulmonology has been established for a somewhat longer period and in many respects is a major stimulus to the development of paediatric intensive care.

Physiotherapy is an integral and important part of the management of the respiratory problems that are seen so frequently in sick children, whether or not the primary problem is pulmonary. It too is becoming more specialized and it is highly appropriate that this new book is published at this time. The editors have merged the clinical input from experts in the most important areas of paediatric respiratory disorders with the principles of physiotherapy as discussed by very experienced paediatric physiotherapists. This amply illustrates both the importance of the physiological and clinical background to sound physiotherapy, and the importance of the team approach to the care of sick children.

Dr Ian G. James
Clinical Director
Paediatric Intensive Care Unit
Great Ormond Street Hospital for
Children NHS Trust,
London
UK

ACKNOWLEDGEMENTS

We are very grateful to the contributors who have taken time from their busy schedules to make this text possible. We are indebted to our physiotherapy colleagues Lindsey Hayward and Melanie Andrews, whose clinical expertise and friendship have contributed to this book in many ways. Our thanks are extended to Laura Irwin, Catherine Dunne and all the physiotherapy staff at Great Ormond Street Hospital for Children NHS Trust, whom we have been privileged to work with, and to Mrs Jeeva-Mutucumarana for her support. Mention must be made of the nursing staff on the paediatric intensive care unit, the respiratory unit and the cardiothoracic unit whose dedication and expertise have been an inspiration over many years.

We express our gratitude to medical colleagues who have always been available to provide support and encouragement in all aspects of our work, particularly Robert Dinwiddie, Ian James, Robert Tasker, Kathy Wilkinson, Martin Elliott and Duncan Macrae. Special thanks also to Su Madge and to the staff of the respiratory laboratory at Great Ormond Street.

The expertise of Sylvia Prasad and of the Department of Medical Illustrations at the hospital is acknowledged.

Peter Yung and colleagues at the School of Physiotherapy, Faculty of Health Sciences, Trinity College, Dublin are thanked for their help and encouragement.

S.A.P.
J.M.H.

GROWTH AND DEVELOPMENT OF THE CARDIORESPIRATORY SYSTEM 1

S. Ammani Prasad

DEVELOPMENT OF THE LUNGS

Fetal lung development begins at approximately three weeks' gestation and is a complex process rarely complete before 34 weeks' gestation. Classically, four stages of human fetal lung development have been described (Inselman and Mellins, 1981): the embryonic stage (3rd–5th week), the pseudoglandular stage (6th–16th week), the cannalicular stage (17th–24th week) and the terminal sac stage (25th week–term) (Figure 1.1).

STAGES OF LUNG DEVELOPMENT

Embryonic stage

During the embryonic period the lung arises as an outgrowth of the foregut. The lining of the whole respiratory system arises from this endodermal bud. As it separates from the foregut the respiratory bud grows in a caudal direction, forming a midline tubular structure, the trachea and two lateral lung buds. This process is usually complete by 28

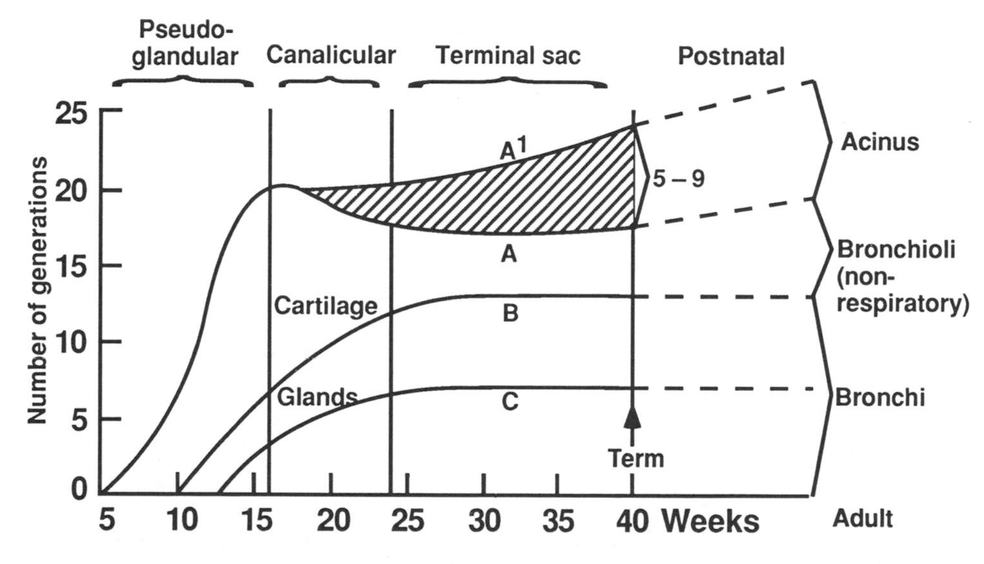

Figure 1.1 Fetal and postnatal development of the bronchial tree, showing the number of bronchial generations (line A), respiratory bronchioles and terminal sacs (area A–A^1), extent of cartilage along the bronchial tree (line B) and the extension of mucous glands (line C) during the four phases of lung development. Reproduced with permission from P.D. Phelan *et al. Respiratory Illness in Children*, Blackwell Scientific Publications, 1982.

days. The right lung bud subsequently divides into three branches and the left into two branches, the major bronchi. The lung buds continue to grow in a caudolateral direction penetrating the surrounding mesoderm, thereby filling the pericardio-peritoneal canals. The parietal and visceral pleura develop from mesoderm.

Pseudoglandular stage

During this ten week period the airways develop through dichotomous branching and become lined with either columnar or cuboidal epithelial cells, closely related to the adjacent mesenchyme. The latter subsequently differentiates from ten weeks into the surrounding cartilage, muscle, blood and lymphatic vessels and connective tissue (Avery and Fletcher, 1974; Yu, 1986). By the end of the pseudoglandular period all the branches of the conducting portion of the airway, from the trachea to the terminal bronchioles, are established. The conducting portion of the airway is known as the preacinus. Although these branches may increase in size with subsequent lung growth, no new branches are formed.

The pulmonary arteries arise from the sixth branchial arches (Langman, 1977). On the right the dorsal part of the artery, distal to the origin of its pulmonary branch, disappears leaving the right pulmonary artery unconnected with the systemic circulation. On the left, the pulmonary artery retains connection with the dorsal aorta by means of the ductus arteriosus which remains open until birth.

Cannalicular stage

This stage involves differentiation of the mesenchyme and maturation of the airways. The mesenchyme thins and a rich vascular circulation develops within it. There is considerable proliferation of the capillaries which become closely associated with and protrude into the airway epithelium, in particular with the respiratory bronchioles and alveolar ducts, thus preparing the lungs for their future role in gas exchange (Woods and Daulton, 1958). This distal portion of the lung, comprising the respiratory bronchioles, alveolar ducts and the alveoli themselves, is called the acinus (Figure 1.2).

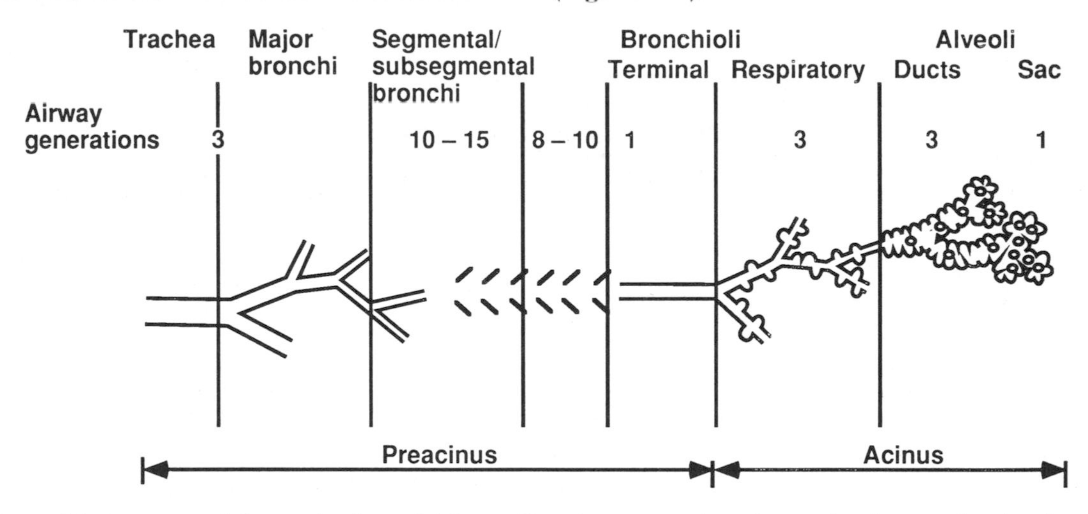

Figure 1.2 Anatomy of the tracheobronchial tree. Preacinus comprises the conducting portion (trachea, bronchi and bronchioli to terminal bronchiolus). Acinus comprises the gas exchanging unit (respiratory bronchioli, alveolar ducts and alveolar sacs). Reproduced with permission from R. Dinwiddie, *The Diagnosis and Management of Paediatric Respiratory Disease,* Churchill Livingstone, 1990.

Terminal sac stage

This final stage of lung differentiation lasts from 24 weeks until delivery. Some of the terminal bronchioles undergo further transformation into respiratory bronchioles, which then give off further subdivisions or saccules. Finally the saccules may subdivide to form the alveoli. Although termed alveoli, in utero these structures are larger and lack a smooth outline; they are, however, capable of effective gas exchange.

With advancing gestation the epithelial thickness decreases and the cells differentiate. At birth the distal airways are lined by flattened epithelium, the intermediate airways by cuboidal epithelium and the most proximal airways by pseudostratified columnar epithelium. The alveoli are lined by pneumocytes. Type I pneumocytes cover more than 95% of the alveolar surface and their principal function is to enhance gas exchange within the lung. Type II pneumocytes, up to ten times larger than type I cells, are principally responsible for the production of pulmonary surfactant.

THE DIAPHRAGM

The diaphragm is a dome-shaped septum dividing the abdominal and thoracic cavities. It is formed by the fusion of four different structures: (i) the septum transversum, (ii) the dorsal oesophageal mesentery, (iii) the pleuroperitoneal membrane, and (iv) the body wall (Gray and Skandalakis, 1972; Moore, 1982; Snell, 1983). The septum transversum is a mesodermal structure giving rise to the central tendon of the diaphragm. The medial part of the diaphragm originates from the dorsal oesophageal mesentery. The pleuroperitoneal membranes initially provide a relatively large segment of the embryonic diaphragm, closing the pleuroperitoneal cavity. However, their contribution to the developed diaphragm is relatively small, as is that of the body wall which provides a narrow peripheral segment. Although the diaphragm is completely formed by the eighth week of gestation, modelling continues throughout gestation.

FETAL LUNG LIQUID

During lung development fluid-filled spaces appear after the tracheal buds have formed and grown laterally into the mesenchyme. These represent primitive air spaces. The fluid these spaces contain is not aspirated amniotic fluid. There is a net outflow of fluid from the trachea that increases in volume with gestational age (Dawes and Patrick, 1985). The site of secretion of this lung fluid has not been established, but it is thought to originate from the epithelial lining. The volume produced is similar to the functional residual capacity of a neonate (approximately 30 ml/kg body weight). The function of this fluid is in helping to determine the shape and volume of the peripheral lung units. Animal studies have shown that chronic drainage of this fluid results in pulmonary hypoplasia (Alcorn *et al.*, 1977). In the human fetus laryngeal atresia results in lung fluid retention and consequent lung hypertrophy (Wigglesworth *et al.*, 1987).

SURFACTANT

Pulmonary surfactant is a complex mixture of lipids and protein, characterized by high surface activity, which is absorbed as a monolayer at the alveolar air–liquid interface to promote alveolar stability on deflation (Morely, 1992). It has also been suggested that surfactant may have a role in pulmonary defence mechanisms and fluid movement (Ballard, 1986).

Gas exchange in the lung occurs through an air–liquid interface within a spherical structure of small radius. Such a structure would collapse unless the surface tension is reduced. It is now well documented that pulmonary surfactant prevents alveolar collapse by progressively reducing surface tension during expiration. As early as 1959 investigators (Avery and Mead) established that hyaline membrane disease, or respiratory distress syndrome (RDS), is primarily a disease of surfactant deficiency. Surfactant is a product of type II alveolar pneumocytes and is stored in characteristic lamellar bodies which are discharged into the alveolar space via the cell surface. Small quantities of surfactant may be detected in the fetal lung as early as 23 weeks' gestation, but it is not usually found in physiological amounts until at least 30 weeks (Gluck and Kulovich, 1973). Surfactant production is accelerated during labour and following initiation of respiration (Gluck *et al.*, 1967).

INITIATION OF RESPIRATION

Using antenatal ultrasound scanning fetal breathing movements are seen as paradoxical motions of the fetal chest and abdomen. These movements appear to be the result of diaphragmatic contraction, retracting the chest wall and distending the abdomen. Appropriate amniotic fluid volume together with fetal breathing movements appear to be essential for normal lung development. The association between fetal breathing movements and subsequent neonatal respiratory function in pregnancies complicated by reduced amniotic fluid volume (oligohydramnios) is uncertain (Blott *et al.*, 1987; Moissinger *et al.*, 1987).

The onset of breathing at birth is initiated by the interaction of a variety of stimuli (Walters and Olver, 1978; Yu, 1986). Amongst these temperature change, relative hypoxia and hypercapnoea are the strongest. Other factors include pain, tactile stimuli and the release of catecholamines. For effective gas exchange to occur the fetal lung fluid must be removed and replaced by air. During the final stages of a vaginal delivery the chest is compressed and this aids the expression of a considerable quantity of fluid. Subsequent recoil of the chest wall produces a small passive inspiration of air. A significant negative pressure of up to 25 cmH_2O must be generated by the muscles of respiration to encourage alveolar expansion. The volume of the first inspiration is 12–16 ml, some 30% of which remains following expiration, helping to form the functional residual capacity (FRC). Until recently it was generally believed that some lung fluid was rapidly removed, perhaps by lymphatic drainage. However, it is now apparent that the fluid may be lost slowly, the residual fluid helping to form the surfactant bubbles that maintain alveolar stability (Scarpelli, 1976) and establish the FRC.

POSTNATAL DEVELOPMENT

At birth the structure and branching pattern of the respiratory airways is complete. There are no major changes in the number of generations or structure of the airways postnatally. Lung growth is characterized by the formation of true alveoli, maturation of lung structures and the secretion of various substances within the lung. At birth the alveoli are multilocular and in postnatal life these increase in size and number. Thus in the newborn human lung there are approximately 150 million alveoli and the adult number of 300–400 million is reached by four years of age (Hislop *et al.*, 1986). Most of the alveoli develop in the first year of life and up to three years of age the increase in lung size is mainly due to alveolar multiplication, there being little change in alveolar size. Thereafter the alveoli continue to increase in size and number up to the age of seven years. From eight years the alveoli increase in size only, until the chest wall stops growing. The average diameter of an adult alveolus is 250–300 μm as compared to 150–180 μm at two months of age (Dunhill, 1962).

The smaller alveolar size of the infant predisposes it to alveolar collapse. Until five years of age distal airway growth lags behind that of the proximal airways. This gives rise to a high peripheral airways resistance in the young. Since resistance to flow is inversely related to the fourth power of the radius (Poiseuille's law) a small decrease in an infant's airway diameter (e.g. caused by inflammation or oedema) significantly increases the peripheral airway resistance and therefore the work of breathing (Figure 1.3).

In the first few years of infancy the large airways increase in diameter (Hislop and Reid, 1974). Following the final alveolar budding the lung continues to increase in size until physical growth is complete. The alveolar surface area therefore increases from 4 m^2 at birth to 75 m^2 in the adult (Hislop *et al.*, 1986; Dunhill, 1962). There is a linear relationship between the increase in air–tissue interface and body surface area. Cartilaginous support stabilizes the conducting airways down to the level of the segmental bronchi. It is present from the twelfth week of gestation but increases in total area throughout childhood (Thurlbeck, 1975; Sinclair-Smith *et al.*, 1976); thus infants have a relatively weak cartilagenous support compared to adults. This may explain the dynamic compression of the trachea associated with high expiratory flow rates and increased airway resistance associated with certain disease states (e.g. bronchiolitis).

In adults anatomical collateral ventilatory channels allow ventilation distal to an obstructed airway. These channels may be interbronchiolar (channel of Martin), bronchiole-alveolar (canals of Lambert) and interalveolar (pores of Kohn). These pathways have not been identified in neonates and are generally assumed to develop after infancy. Pores of Kohn have been identified between the first and second year of life and canals of Lambert by six years of age. Without collateral ventilatory pathways infants and young children are at increased risk of atelectasis and hyperinflation associated with infection.

The angle of insertion of the diaphragm in the child is almost horizontal, whereas in

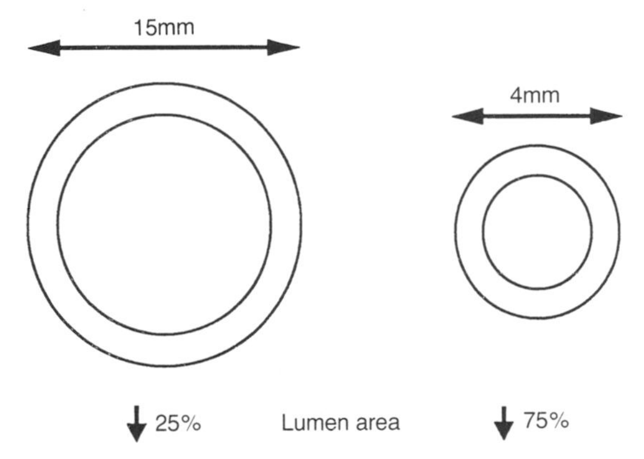

Figure 1.3 Adult and infant airway diameters, showing the effect of lumen size in the presence of a 1 mm cuff of oedema. In the infant there is a 75% reduction in the lumen area, significantly increasing airway resistance and therefore the work of breathing.

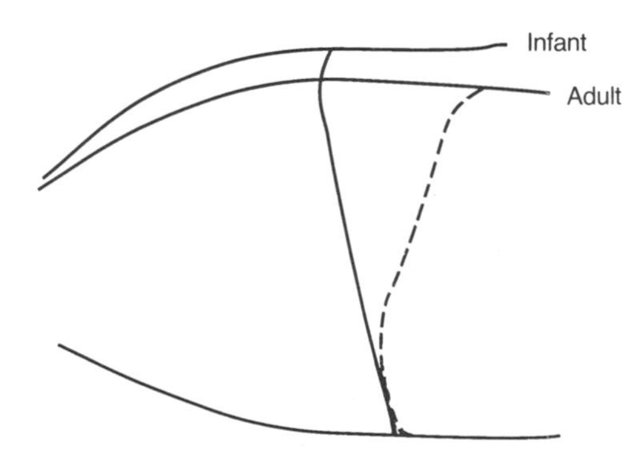

Figure 1.4 Angle of insertion of the diaphragm, showing the more oblique insertion of the adult (dotted line) compared to the horizontal insertion in the infant (continuous line). Modified from N.L. Muller and A.C. Bryan, Chest wall mechanics and respiratory muscles in infants, *Pediatric Clinics of North America*, 1979.

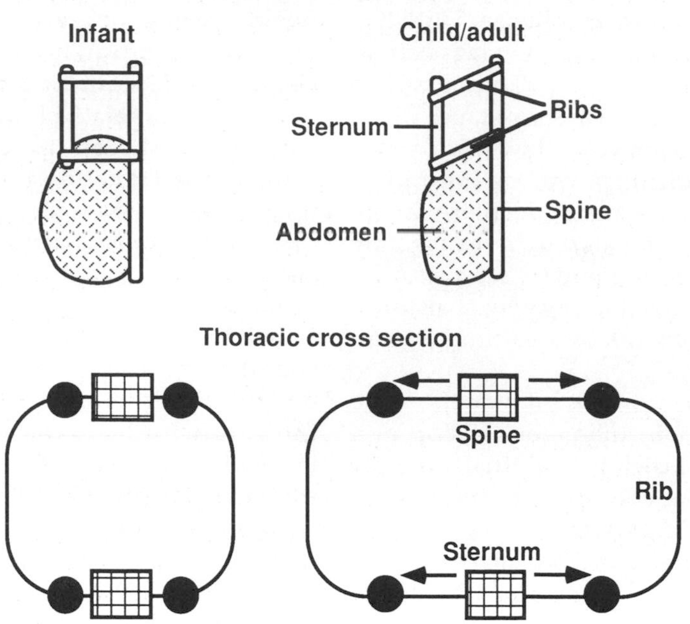

Figure 1.5 Rib cage configuration in the adult (above right) compared to the infant (above left). Rib growth at costochondral junctions and posterior rib angles as a possible explanation to changes in thoracic cross-sectional shape (below left and right). Reproduced with permission from P. Oppenshaw *et al.*, Changes in rib cage geometry during childhood, *Thorax*, 1984.

the adult it is oblique. This results in a decreased efficiency of contraction. In addition contraction of the diaphragm may tend to distort the rib cage inward (Muller and Bryan, 1979) (Figure 1.4). The configuration of the rib cage of the infant differs from that of the adult in that the ribs lie horizontally. In the horizontal plane the rib cage of an infant is circular, whereas that of an adult is ellipsoid (Figure 1.5). Therefore in the infant anteroposterior and transverse diameter expansion is reduced, limiting the potential increase in lung volume. The development of the adult ovoid pattern is associated with the adoption of an upright posture and occurs at approximately 2–3 years of age (Oppenshaw *et al.*, 1984).

ABNORMALITIES OF LUNG GROWTH AND DEVELOPMENT

Pulmonary agenesis results from failure of normal embryological development of the endodermal tracheal bud or from an abnormal interaction between the bud and the surrounding mesenchyme. Left sided agenesis is more common than right sided agenesis and has a better prognosis (Avery *et al.*, 1981). This condition may be associated with congenital cardiovascular or thoracic cage abnormalities. In the normal situation lung development is dependent on the interaction of several hormones including glucocorticosteroids (Liggins and Howie, 1973) thyroid hormone, prolactin and oestradiol (Ballard, 1984). In addition normal lung development is also dependent on an adequate thoracic space for growth, normal fetal breathing movements, appropriate amniotic fluid volume and adequate nutrition.

Pulmonary hypoplasia occurs when there are lesions that diminish the intrathoracic space available for lung growth: congenital diaphragmatic hernia (Areechon and Reid, 1963), cystic adenomatoid malformation (Yu, 1986), pleural effusions (Barr and Burdi, 1975), enlarged thymus (Balcom *et al.*, 1985) and skeletal dysplasias (Davis and Reid, 1971). It may also occur secondary to oligohydramnios. Oligohydramnios may be a consequence of premature rupture of the placental membranes, fetal renal tract malformation (e.g. renal agenesis) or severe intrauterine growth retardation.

Congenital diaphragmatic hernia is most often caused by a failure of the pleuroperitoneal membranes to close the pericardioperitoneal canals. This allows abdominal viscera (usually the stomach) to enter the thoracic cavity. Consequently the lungs are compressed and may become hypoplastic. Cystic adenomatoid malformation is a hamartoma of the lung characterized by overgrowth of the terminal bronchioles at the expense of the saccular spaces. The disease generally affects one lobe and may be macro or microcystic in nature. The abnormal lung tissue displaces the heart and may compress the normal lung, impairing its normal development. Several fetal abnormalities may give rise to intrauterine pleural effusions (e.g. congenital heart disease). Irrespective of the aetiology of the effusion pulmonary hypoplasia may result from compression and displacement of normal lung tissue. The value of antenatal pleural shunting for this condition is not fully established (Nicolaides and Azar, 1990).

Respiratory distress syndrome is the most common neonatal respiratory disorder, occurring in up to 15% of infants under 2.5 kg with an associated neonatal mortality of 3–4%. It is a disease primarily of the preterm infant and is a consequence of a deficiency in surfactant. Male infants and infants of diabetic mothers are at an increased risk of developing this condition. Normal postnatal development of the lungs may be impaired due to complications resulting from mechanical ventilation that may be required to treat respiratory distress syndrome or other neonatal respiratory disorders (see Chapter 7, p. 107).

DEVELOPMENT OF THE CARDIOVASCULAR SYSTEM

DEVELOPMENT OF THE HEART

Development of the heart begins on the 18th to 19th postconceptual day. Two endothelial tubes meet in the midline and form a single heart tube lying within the pericardial cavity. This tube is suspended from the dorsal wall of the cavity by a dorsal mesocardium. A process of elongation, dilatation and constriction eventually results in a four-chambered structure. The heart begins to contract at 22 days. Initially there are six cardiac chambers which are, from the caudal to cranial ends, the sinus venosus, the atrium, the atrioventricular canal, the ventricle, the bulbus cordis and the truncus arteriosus (Figure 1.6). The sinus venosus is a dilatation consisting of left and right sinus horns, each of which receives the principal venous channels on the ipsilateral side. The atrium is another dilatation which is separated from the sinus venosus by a sinuatrial opening guarded by a pair of flimsy venous valves. The atrioventricular canal is a narrow segment of tube leading cranially from the atrium and containing a pair of subendocardial cushions. The primitive ventricle is a dilatation following the canal and leading to the bulbus cordis. This structure is also a dilated chamber and a slight constriction demarcates it from the ventricle. The truncus arteriosus

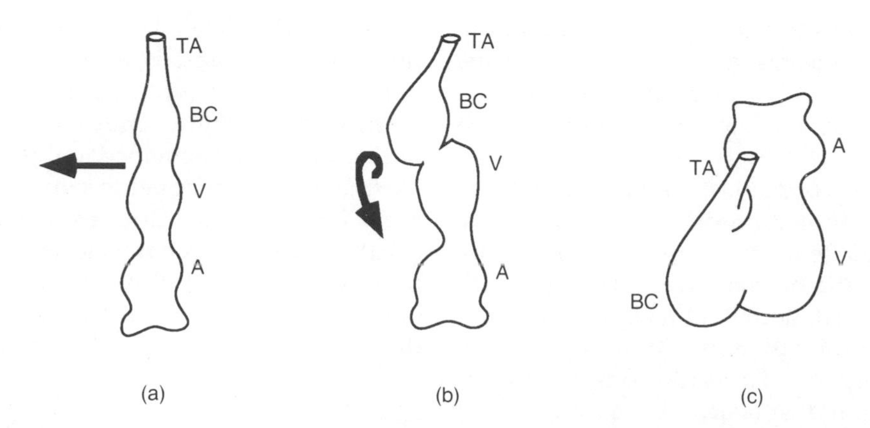

Figure 1.6 Growth and development of the embryonic heart. Initially there is a linear sequence of chambers, the truncus arteriosus (TA) lying cranially (a), later (b) the bulbus cordis (BC) bends to lie on the right side of the ventricle (V) and then (c) the bulbus cordis and ventricle move caudally to the atrium (A).

is the most cranial part of the heart and is another narrowed segment.

The intrapericardial part of the heart consists of the future bulboventricular portion. The atrial portion and the sinus venosus are paired and remain outside the pericardium, in the mesenchyme of the septum transversum. The initially longitudinal arrangement of the heart chambers is of no disadvantage because the embryo does not possess a double circulation. However, a pulmonary circulation must eventually be incorporated and therefore the cardiac chambers undergo realignment. This occurs during the 4th and 5th weeks of gestation, whilst the internal processes of partition of the heart continue into the second month of gestation. This is the time of greatest risk to teratogenic influences. The bulboventricular portion of the heart tube grows much more rapidly than the pericardial space and because its two ends are fixed outside the pericardial cavity, further elongation of the tube cannot be achieved without it bending. The bulboventricular loop is shifted to the right, ventrally and caudally. As a consequence of this bending and torsion, the atrioventricular junction comes to lie on the left side of the pericardial cavity.

The developmental processes, whereby the heart is partitioned into left and right streams, are associated with the appearance of the lung buds and the development of the primitive pulmonary circulation. The principal embryonic veins entering the sinus venosus are the cardinal, vitelline and umbilical veins, of which the latter two cross the septum transversum. As the septum transversum is invaded by the developing liver, the vitelline and umbilical veins are interrupted and contribute to the hepatic sinusoidal network. Of the posthepatic channels only the right vitelline vein persists to form the inferior vena cava. The two vitelline veins become linked and form the hepatic portal vein, receiving blood from the gut and liver. The right umbilical vein disappears and oxygenated blood is carried by the left umbilical vein. Most of this blood enters the hepatic sinusoids, but 25% is diverted past the liver in the ductus venosus. Eventually the left sinus horn of the sinus venosus receives three tributaries: (1) the posthepatic segment of the right vitelline vein (inferior vena cava), (2) the right common cardinal vein (superior vena cava) and (3) the attenuated left sinus horn (coronary sinus).

The atrial chamber is partitioned by two septa, the septum primum and septum secundum, which appear in that order. A small gap remains in utero between the septum primum and the atrioventricular cushions, termed the foramen ovale. This structure allows oxygented blood to pass from the right side to the left. The two ventricles are separated from each other by a downgrowth from the atrioventricular cushions (Navaratnam, 1975).

DEVELOPMENT OF THE GREAT VESSELS

The major intraembryonic vessels are represented by dorsal aortas which form as continuations of the endocardial heart tubes. As a result of rotation and fusion of the heart tubes, the dorsal aortas become arched. Six pairs of aortic arches form as a consequence of the development of the pharyngeal arches. The first and second arch arteries involute. The third arch arteries give rise to the common carotid and internal carotid arteries. The fourth arch on the left persists as the dorsal aorta. The fifth aortic arches are transient and never well developed. The sixth aortic arches on the right supply branches to the lung buds forming the right pulmonary artery and on the left the distal part persists as the ductus arteriosus (Langman, 1977).

The pulmonary arteries develop alongside the airways during the psuedoglandular and cannalicular periods of lung development. With each airway division the arteries branch forming the preacinar vessels. By 16 weeks' gestation this development is complete. The preacinar arteries give rise to as many as four branches that supply the adjacent lung tissue. After 16 weeks intra-acinar arteries develop alongside the respiratory bronchioles and saccules. This vascular development continues during childhood as new alveolar ducts and alveoli arise.

THE FETAL CIRCULATION

The essential features of the fetal circulation are: (i) the umbilical arteries and vein

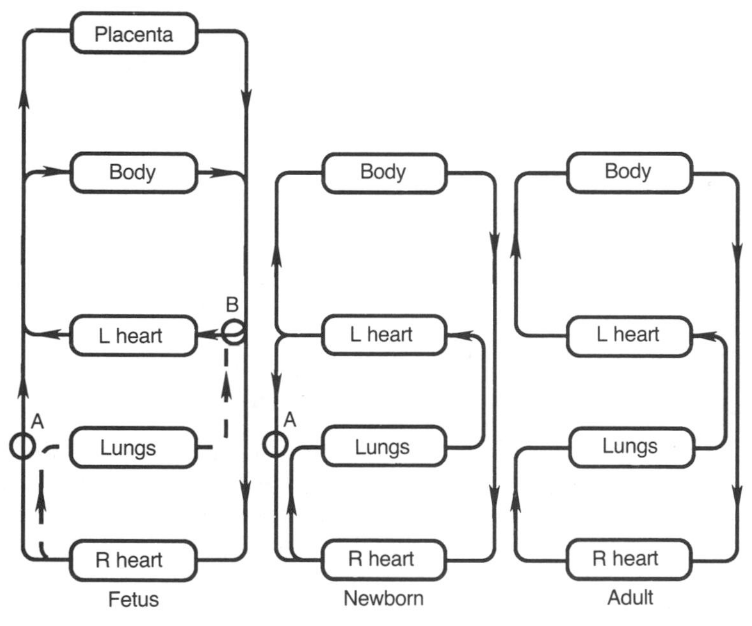

Figure 1.7 Changes in the fetal circulation, to circulation in the neonate and the adult. (A, ductus arteriosus; B, foramen ovale)

supplying and draining the placenta, (ii) a shunt from the right to the left atrium (foramen ovale) and (iii) a shunt from the pulmonary artery to the aorta (ductus arteriosus) (Figure 1.7). The umbilical artery initially arises as a branch of the dorsal aorta but by term has become a branch of the internal iliac artery. Its purpose is to carry deoxygenated blood and waste products to the placenta. The umbilical vein runs through the liver to the inferior vena cava carrying oxygenated blood to the fetal heart. The foramen ovale streamlines oxygenated blood arriving in the right atrium into the left atrium and thence to the left ventricle. Poorly oxygenated blood from the superior vena cava is directed into the right ventricle. The left ventricle pumps oxygenated blood into the aorta and thence to the brain and upper limbs. The right ventricle ejects poorly oxygenated blood towards the pulmonary trunk. However, in fetal life a high vascular resistance exists in the pulmonary circulation and the blood flow is diverted through the ductus arteriosus into the aorta. The ductus joins the aorta distal to those branches supplying the brain and upper limbs and its blood flow is therefore principally to the distal organs.

POSTNATAL CHANGES

At birth there are major cardiovascular changes as gas exchange is transferred from the placenta to the lungs (Figure 1.7). A few minutes after birth the umbilical arteries cease to pulsate due to touch and cold stimuli. The umbilical vein may remain open for up to 30 minutes and a substantial volume of blood is thereby returned from the placenta to the baby. With cessation of umbilical blood flow there is a marked decrease in deoxygenated blood returning to the heart and a significant increase in systemic vascular resistance. After birth and the onset of ventilation, pulmonary vascular resistance falls rapidly from 70–75 mmHg to 30 mmHg within the first 24 hours. There is a rapid tenfold increase in pulmonary blood flow. Pulmonary vascular resistance continues to fall gradually for up to six weeks postnatally, eventually reaching adult values (9 mmHg). The changes in pulmonary resistance are induced by local effects and sustained by humoral changes. The fetal lungs, fluid filled in utero, rapidly fill with gas and the alveoli expand. As the pulmonary vascular resistance falls the pulmonary arterioles dilate (Cassin *et al.*, 1964). Increasing fetal oxygenation causes pulmonary vasodilation and increased blood flow (Heymann and Hoffman, 1979).

Closure of the ductus arteriosus occurs in two stages, initial functional closure followed by permanent closure with connective tissue formation. The increase in postnatal oxygen concentration appears to be the most potent stimulus for this change. Other stimuli may include acetylcholine and catecholamines (Heymann and Rudolph, 1975). Eventually the ductus fibroses to become the ligamentum arteriosum attaching the left pulmonary artery to the aortic arch. After birth the left atrial pressure increases due to increased pulmonary blood flow and the right atrial pressure falls, as a result of cessation of umbilical blood flow and reduced inferior vena caval return. These changes represent a reversal of the fetal circulation and the foramen ovale is obliterated some six to eight months after delivery by connective tissue growth.

ABNORMALITIES OF CARDIOVASCULAR DEVELOPMENT

Abnormalities of cardiovascular structure and function are relatively common in the fetus and newborn. Congenital heart disease may occur in 7–8 per 1000 live births and is more common in stillbirths. There are several possible aetiologies. In some cases there appears to be a familial component as certain specific problems may be more common in twins and specific families. All types of chromosomal abnormalities (e.g. Down's syndrome) are associated with congenital heart disease. Several drugs (e.g. phenytoin and lithium) may be teratogenic particularly when exposure occurs in the early developmental phases. Infective causes such as rubella are also well recognized (Best and Banatvala, 1990).

Embryological abnormalities of cardiac development fall into six groups. Abnormalities of the atrial septum may give rise to a single atrial chamber or premature closure of the foramen ovale. Failure of normal development of the endocardial cushions give rise to atrioventricular canal defects, e.g. failure of the cushions to fuse results in a persistent atrioventricular canal. Abnormalities of the interventricular septum will lead to defects of varying sizes affecting the membranous septum. The severity of such a lesion would depend on its size, but at its worst may present as a single common ventricle. Failure of normal development of the truncus is classically associated with tetralogy of Fallot. Defects of the semilunar valves may give rise to stenosis or regurgitation. If fusion of the valve leaves is complete valvular atresia results and may be secondarily associated with hypoplastic development of the musculature. Finally the heart may not be positioned correctly within the thorax; the most frequently seen anomaly is dextrocardia where the heart is located in the right chest.

REFERENCES

Alcorn, D., Adamson, T.M., Lambert, T.F. *et al.* (1977) Morphological effects of chronic tracheal ligation and drainage in the fetal lamb lung. *Journal of Anatomy*, **123**, 649–60.

Areechon, N. and Reid, L. (1963) Hypoplasia of lung with congenital diaphragmatic hernia. *British Medical Journal*, **1**, 230–3.

Avery, M.E. and Fletcher, B.D. (1974) Lung development, in *The Lung and its Disorders in the Newborn Infant*, (eds M.E. Avery and B.D. Fletcher), W.B. Saunders, Philadelphia, pp. 1–21.

Avery, M.E., Fletcher, B.D. and Williams, R.A. (1981) *Lung and its Disorders in the Newborn Infant*, 2nd edn, W.B. Saunders, Philadelphia, pp. 171–2, 290–6.

Avery, M.E. and Mead, J. (1959) Surface properties in relation to atelectasis and hyaline membrane disease. *American Journal of Diseases of Childhood*, **97**, 517.

Balcom, R.J., Hakanson, D.O., Werner, A. and Gordon, L. (1985) Massive thymic hyperplasia in an infant with Beckwith–Wiedemann syndrome. *Archives of Pathological Laboratory Medicine*, **109**, 153–5.

Ballard, P.L. (1984) Combined hormonal treatment and lung maturation. *Seminars in Perinatology*, **8**, 283–92.

Ballard, P.L. (1986) Lung development, in *Hormones and Lung Maturation*, (ed. P.L. Ballard), Springer Verlag, Berlin, pp. 1–23.

Barr, M. and Burdi, A.R. (1975) Spontaneous pleural effusion in the human fetus. *Teratology*, **11**, 139–42.

Best, J.M. and Banatvala, J.E. (1990) Rubella, in *Principles of Bacteriology, Virology and Immunity*, 8th edn, (eds L. Collier and M. Timbury), Edward Arnold, London, pp. 501–31.

Blott, M., Greenough, A., Nicolaides, K.H. *et al.* (1987) Fetal breathing movements as predictor of favourable pregnancy outcome after oligohydramnios due to membrane rupture in the second trimester. *Lancet*, **2**, 129–31.

Cassin, S., Dawes, G.S., Mott, J.C. *et al.* (1964) The vascular resistance of the fetal and newly ventilated lung of the lamb. *Journal of Physiology*, **171**, 61–79.

Davis, G. and Reid, L. (1971) Effect of scoliosis on growth of alveoli and pulmonary arteries and on right ventricle. *Archives of Diseases of Childhood*, **46**, 623–32.

Dawes, G.S. and Patrick, J.E. (1985) Fetal breathing activity, in *Pulmonary Development*, (ed. G.H. Nelson), Marcel Dekker, New York, p. 93.

Dunhill, M.S. (1962) Postnatal growth of the lung. *Thorax*, **17**, 329–33.

Gluck, L. and Kulovich, M.V. (1973) L/S ratios in amniotic fluid and abnormal pregnancies. *American Journal of Obstetrics and Gynecology*, **115**, 539–52.

Gluck, L., Motoyama, E.K., Smits, H.L. and Kulovich, M.V. (1967) The biochemical development of the surface activity in the mammalian lung 1. *Pediatric Research*, **1**, 237–46.

Gray, S.W. and Skandalakis, J.E. (1972) The diaphragm, in *Embryology for Surgeons: the Embryological Basis for the Treatment of Congenital Defects*, (eds S.W. Gray and J.E. Skandalakis), W.B. Saunders, Philadelphia, pp. 359–85.

Heymann, M.A. and Hoffmann, J.I. (1979) Pulmonary circulation in the perinatal period, in *Neonatal Pulmonary Care*, (eds D.W. Thibeault and G.A. Gregory), Addison Wesley, Menlo Park, p. 70.

Heymann, M.A. and Rudolph, A.M. (1975) Control of the ductus arteriosus. *Physiology Reviews*, **55**, 62–78.

Hislop, A. and Reid, L. (1974) Development of the acinus in the human lung. *Thorax*, **29**, 90–4.

Hislop, A., Wigglesworth, J.S. and Desai, R. (1986) Alveolar development in the human fetus and infant. *Early Human Development*, **13**, 1–11.

Inselman, L.S. and Mellins, R.B. (1981) Growth and development of the lung. *Journal of Pediatrics*, **98**, 1–15.

Langman, J. (1977) *Medical Embryology*, Williams and Wilkins, Baltimore, pp. 201–24, 233–51.

Liggins, G.C. and Howie, R. (1973) A controlled trial of antipartum glucocorticoid treatment for prevention of the respiratory distress syndrome in premature infants. *Pediatrics*, **50**, 515–25.

Moissinger, A.C., Fox, H.E., Higgins, A. *et al.* (1987) Fetal breathing movements are not a reliable predictor of continued lung development in pregnancies complicated by oligohydramnios. *Lancet*, **2**, 1297–9.

Moore, K.L. (1982) The developing human, in *Clinically Oriented Embryology*, (ed. K.L. Moore), W.B. Saunders, Philadelphia, pp. 172–5.

Morely, C.J. (1992) Surfactant, in *Textbook of Neonatology*, 2nd edn, (ed. N.C.R. Roberton), Churchill Livingstone, Edinburgh, pp. 369–83.

Muller, N.L. and Bryan, A.C. (1979) Chest wall mechanics and respiratory muscles in infants. *Pediatric Clinics of North America*, **26**, 503–16.

Navaratnam, V. (1975) *The Human Heart and Circulation*, Academic Press, London.

Nicolaides, K.H. and Azar, G.B. (1990) Thoraco-amniotic shunting. *Fetal Diagnosis and Therapy*, **5**, 153–64.

Oppenshaw, P., Edwards, S. and Helms, P. (1984) Changes in rib cage geometry during childhood. *Thorax*, **39**, 624–7.

Scarpelli, E.M. (1976) Fetal pulmonary fluid, in *Reviews in Perinatal Medicine*, (eds E.M. Scarpelli and E.V. Cosmi), University Park Press, Baltimore, pp. 49–107.

Sinclair-Smith, C.C., Emery, J.L., Gadson, D., Linsdale, F. and Baddeley, J. (1976) Cartilage in children's lungs: a quantitative assessment using the right middle lobe. *Thorax*, **31**, 40.

Snell, R.S. (1983) *Clinical Embryology for Medical Students*, Little, Brown, Boston, pp. 177–94.

Thurlbeck, W.M. (1975) Postnatal growth and development of the lung. *American Review of Respiratory Disease*, **111**, 803.

Walters, D.V. and Olver, R.E. (1978) The role of catecholamines in lung liquid absorption at birth. *Pediatric Research*, **12**, 239–42.

Wigglesworth, J.S., Desai, R. and Hislop, A.A. (1987) Fetal lung growth in congenital laryngeal atresia. *Pediatric Pathology*, **7**, 515–25.

Woods, de G.L. and Daulton, A.J. (1958) The ultrastructure of lung tissue for newborn and embryo mice. *Journal of Ultrastructure Research*, **2**, 28–54.

Yu, V.Y.H. (1986) Development of the lung, in *Respiratory Disorders of the Newborn*, (ed. V.Y.H. Yu), Churchill Livingstone, Edinburgh, pp. 1–17.

PHYSIOLOGY OF THE CARDIORESPIRATORY SYSTEM

2

Juliette Hussey

THE RESPIRATORY SYSTEM

The primary function of the respiratory system is to allow oxygen (O_2) to move from the air into the venous blood and carbon dioxide (CO_2) to move out. Oxygen and carbon dioxide pass between air and blood by simple diffusion across the alveolar–capillary membrane. The basic concepts of cardiorespiratory physiology and the differences that exist between adults and infants will be discussed in this chapter.

MECHANICS OF VENTILATION

Chest wall and respiratory muscle function

During spontaneous respiration a pressure gradient develops between the mouth and alveoli. This is achieved by the contraction of the respiratory muscles, which increases the intrathoracic volume and lowers the pleural pressure to subatmospheric levels. Compliance is the volume change per unit of pressure. Total lung compliance is a function of the lung tissue, the surface characteristics and volume. The chest wall of the infant is cartilaginous, soft and pliable (and therefore facilitates easy passage through the birth canal) and this means that it is very compliant compared to adult lungs. The floppy chest wall of the infant is unable to counteract the elastic recoil of the lungs, resulting in a low functional residual capacity (FRC). With increasing age the thorax becomes relatively stiffer and gains a greater amount of outward recoil, i.e. the thoracic compliance decreases. This is due to increasing calcification of the ribs, connective tissue changes and growth of the chest wall relative to the lungs. Once the upright posture has been assumed and the abdomen has grown, abdominal contents shift away from the upper abdomen thus creating a more negative pressure under the diaphragm, favouring outward recoil of the chest wall. The chest wall of the adult has a similar compliance to that of the lungs and so is better able to oppose the action of the diaphragm. The principal muscle of respiration is the diaphragm. An adult diaphragm has 55% of slow twitch, high oxidative fibres, whereas a term infant has only 25% and a preterm may only have 10% of these fatigue resistant fibres (Muller and Bryan, 1979). Inspiration is initiated by the diaphragm and intercostal muscles. When an adult diaphragm contracts the dome descends and aids the elevation of the lower ribs. In the upright posture the adult rib cage and diaphragm contribute equal amounts to the volume change during quiet tidal volume breathing whereas in the supine position, 70% of the volume change is abdominal (Konno and Mead, 1967). Contraction of the intercostal muscles elevates the anterior end of each rib and therefore increases thoracic volume during inspiration. The intercostal spaces become tense and stabilize the rib cage during the diaphragmatic descent.

In the neonate nearly all the volume change is abdominal and the circular rather than oblique lie of the ribs in the horizontal plane does not allow such increases in lung volume. The accessory muscles of respiration (sternocleidomastoid and scalene) are not used during quiet tidal volume breathing but are recruited during times of respiratory embarrassment. Expiration is passive and is facilitated by the elastic properties of the lungs.

Clinical implications

There are many clinical implications in the mechanical differences between developing and mature chest walls. In the range of normal breathing the thorax of the infant is highly compliant. This becomes functionally significant in the presence of lung disease, when the greater negative pressure and therefore respiratory effort required to inflate the lungs can 'suck' in the chest wall. This results in less effective gas exchange and a further increase in the work of breathing.

The very low elastic recoil pressure of the newborn chest wall is one of the factors which predisposes the infant to lung collapse. In order to achieve an adequate tidal volume the infant has to generate comparatively greater pressures than an adult, because the contraction of the diaphragm produces a negative pleural pressure which tends to distort the compliant rib cage. In times of respiratory distress the infant may show signs of intercostal, subcostal and sternal recession. With severe distress the rib cage will actually move inward as the abdomen moves outward during inspiration, causing a 'see-saw' effect.

The infant's muscles of respiration will fatigue at a relatively quicker rate than an adult's (due to the difference in fibre composition). When confronted with the need to increase their work of breathing to maintain ventilation (e.g. during times of respiratory distress) the muscles can fatigue to such an extent that the baby may become apnoeic. During rapid eye movement (REM) sleep it is believed that tonic inhibition of intercostal muscles occurs, which may allow rib cage distortion during inspiration. This may have serious consequences as the premature infant spends as much as 50% of sleeping time in the REM sleep state and may during this time be less able to defend against an increase in inspiratory load.

The respiratory pump and control of ventilation

The respiratory pump is a feedback loop mechanism consisting of sensors (chemoreceptors, lung and airway receptors), controlling mechanisms (cerebrum, brainstem and spinal cord) and effectors (respiratory muscles) (Berger *et al.*, 1977). The respiratory muscles are described later in this chapter.

The peripheral chemoreceptors are located in the carotid bodies at the bifurcation of the common carotid arteries and they monitor the arterial oxygen tension (PaO_2) of blood perfusing the brain. A falling PaO_2 stimulates the carotid bodies, signalling the brainstem to increase ventilation. The central chemoreceptor lies in the medulla. When arterial carbon dioxide tension ($PaCO_2$) rises, the cerebral spinal fluid (CSF) surrounding the chemoreceptors becomes acidic and the increase in hydrogen ion (H^+) concentration (pH) also stimulates the brainstem to increase the ventilation.

Pulmonary receptors lie in the upper airways and they moderate breathing. Sensory input is received by the respiratory controller in the brainstem. This centre is divided into the pneumotaxic centre, apneustic centre and the medullary centre. The pneumotaxic centre tunes respiration by switching inspiration to expiration. The apneustic centre is responsible for cutting off inspiration but neither is absolutely essential. It is the medulla that is the site of the basic respiratory rhythm generator and its destruction leads to apnoea (Mitchell, 1963). The cerebral cortex connects with the brainstem respiratory centres and, together with the spinal cord, allows voluntary control of respiration. The spinal cord finally interprets the central nervous system (CNS) commands before relating them to the phrenic and intercostal nerves supplying the respiratory muscles.

The respiratory pump of the newborn and the preterm infant has impaired regulation of alveolar ventilation. There is a reduction of carbon dioxide responsiveness during hypoxaemia which is a response opposite to that found in adults (Rigatto, 1982). Preterm infants often breathe periodically and their breathing is marked by phases of periodic breathing (Pasterkamp, 1990). The more premature the infant the higher the incidence of such breathing patterns. There is an association between periodic breathing and true apnoea, defined as an absence of breathing for 20 seconds or more. The term infant has a higher oxygen demand per unit mass (VO_2/kg) than the adult. To meet these higher requirements the newborn has a greater minute ventilation (MV) per unit mass.

AIRWAYS AND AIR SPACES

The airways are a series of dividing tubes which become narrower, shorter and greater in number as they branch from the trachea outward to the alveoli. Gas passes through these conducting airways from the nose and mouth to the respiratory alveoli where gas exchange occurs across the alveolar–capillary membrane.

Dead space

The vital process of gas exchange occurs in the terminal respiratory units. In order for this to occur efficiently the volume of gas arriving at the alveoli must be comparable to the volume of blood passing through the pulmonary capillary bed. The alveolar–capillary membrane then permits the transfer of gases between the inspired gas and the circulating blood, whilst at the same time restricting the movement of fluid from the pulmonary vasculature. Not all the gas entering the respiratory system takes part in gas exchange and the volume of this 'wasted' gas is termed dead space. Total dead space within the respiratory system is known as 'physiological dead space' and this is then divided into 'anatomical dead space' (gas within the conducting part of the respiratory system) and the 'alveolar dead space' (gas which has reached the terminal lung units but does not take part in exchange).

Airway resistance

When air flows through a tube, a difference in pressure exists between the ends. A major component of airflow is airway resistance and this is measured by relating flow to the pressure drop from the alveolus to the mouth. Resistance to gas flow along a tube depends on whether the flow is laminar or turbulent. Low gas flow within a straight wide tube is termed laminar, i.e. the gas moves in a series of concentric cylinders with the innermost moving the fastest. When gas travels at high velocities through tubes there is a high resistance to flow and the stream lines become disorganized and local eddy currents may develop. This is termed turbulent flow. In the respiratory system, the velocity of airflow increases from small to large airways (O'Brodovich and Hadad, 1990) and in terms of type of flow the situation is complex. True turbulent flow may be seen in the trachea but in general flow is transitional, i.e. with eddy formation at the branches (West, 1992). Poiseuille's law describes the pressure gradient required to maintain laminar flow through a tube:

$$P = v\left(\frac{8l\,\eta}{\pi r^4}\right)$$

P = pressure
v = flow
l = length
r = tube radius
η = gas viscosity

Because resistance is equal to pressure divided by flow, it is the radius of the tube which is the most important determinant of resistance. If the radius is halved the resistance is increased 16-fold. In the infant the small peripheral airways may contribute to up to 50% of the total airway resistance and this proportion does not decrease until the age of approximately five years (Hogg *et al.*, 1970).

Alveoli

After birth there is a dramatic increase in the number of alveoli, from 20 million alveolar saccules at birth to 300 million by the age of eight years (Dunhill, 1962). Although alveolar multiplication is the predominant mechanism for lung growth, the size increase of individual alveoli is also important. The large expansion in alveolar size and number results in an increase in alveolar surface from 2.8 m^2 at birth to 32 m^2 by the age of eight years. Therefore the diffusing capacity of oxygen across the alveolar–capillary membrane increases. The small alveolar size of the infant is a liability because it predisposes the infant to alveolar collapse.

Collateral ventilation

The adult lung develops channels which allow ventilation to an obstructed airway by 'collateral' flow. Three types of pathway have been described: pores of Kohn (intra-alveolar), canals of Lambert (bronchiole-alveolar) and channels of Martin (interbronchiolar) (Figure 2.1) and have been previously discussed in Chapter 1, p. 5.

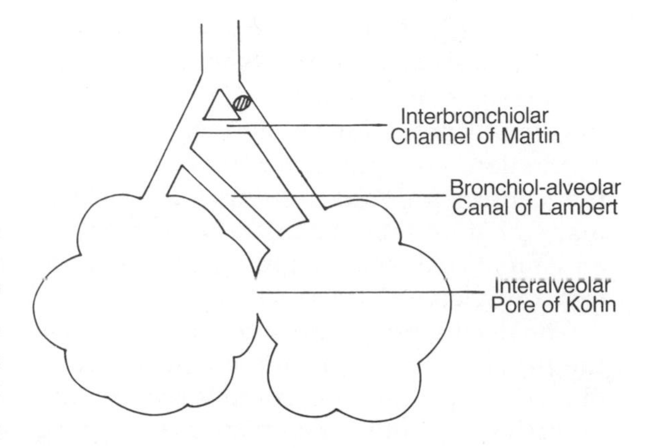

Figure 2.1 Pathways of collateral ventilation.

Interdependence

Without surfactant smaller alveoli would tend to empty into larger alveoli in accordance with the Laplace relationship which relates pressure across a surface (P) to surface tension (T) and the radius of curvature (r): $P=2T/r$. The smaller the radius, the greater the tendency to collapse. However, individual lung units are effectively connecting bubbles, i.e. the inside wall of one alveolus is the outside wall of an adjacent alveolus. The interdependence model of the lung demonstrates how any decrease in size of one alveolus is stabilized by adjacent alveoli. Deep breathing techniques and breath holds use the concept of interdependence in order to try and increase alveolar expansion.

Clinical implications

Adults differ from children in the site of the main contribution to the total airway resistance. The upper airway, particularly the nose, accounts for the major proportion of total resistance in the adult. Up to five years of age the peripheral airway resistance is approximately four times greater than that of the older child/adult. This, together with the late development of collateral ventilation, probably explains the high incidence of lower obstructive airways disease in young children. Pores of Kohn and canals of Lambert may be found in the infant lung, but are probably not sufficiently large to allow air drift (Wohl and Mead, 1990). The infant and small child is therefore at greater risk of developing atelectasis and consequent ventilation/perfusion mismatching. However, despite the several factors which may appear as a handicap to respiratory function in the infant, one distinct gain is that of continuing alveolar development due to the ability of the alveoli to increase in number, expand in size and participate in gas exchange following disease induced lung damage.

LUNG VOLUMES AND LUNG COMPLIANCE

Static volumes of the lungs at various stages of respiration offer valuable measurements which help in the assessment of lung function. These lung volumes are represented in Figure 2.2 where the subject initially breathes normally at his own comfortable rate and then takes a maximal inspiration followed by maximal expiration. The amount of gas moved during normal quiet respiration is termed the tidal volume (TV). Functional residual capacity (FRC) represents the volume of gas remaining in the lungs at the end of a quiet expiration during tidal breathing. Following a maximal inspiration to total lung capacity (TLC), the gas exhaled with a maximal expiration is known as the vital capacity (VC). The residual volume (RV) is the air that remains in the lung after maximal expiration. The FRC (comprising the expiratory reserve volume (ERV) and the RV) serves as a source of oxygen during expiration until the lungs are reinflated with the next breath; thus major changes in PaO_2 are buffered.

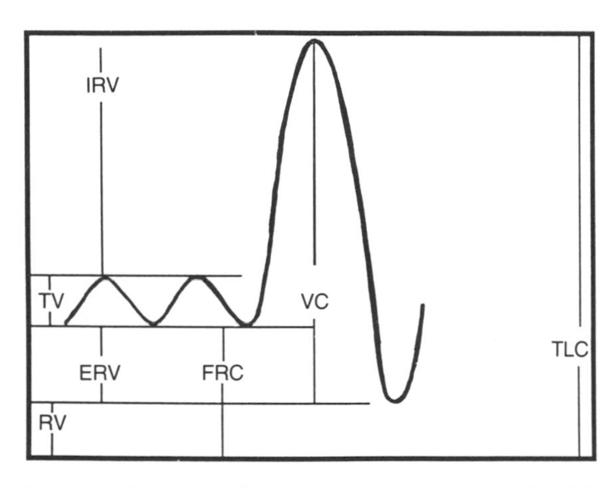

Figure 2.2 Lung volumes representing normal tidal volume breathing followed by maximum inspiration and full expiration. TV = tidal volume, FRC = functional residual capacity, TLC = total lung capacity, VC = vital capacity, RV = residual volume, ERV = expiratory reserve volume, IRV = inspiratory reserve volume.

Another useful volume measurement is that of the FEV1 which represents the volume of air expired in the first second of a forced expiration from TLC. Most of these volumes are measured using simple spirometric techniques but measurement of FRC and RV requires more sophisticated techniques such as the helium dilution method (see Chapter 5, p. 60). The peak expiratory flow rate (PEFR) is a measurement of the maximal flow (litres/minute) achieved during a forced expiration from TLC and is easily measured using a peak flow meter.

Closing volume (CV) is the volume at which small airways close. The closing capacity is defined as the sum of the CV and the RV. When the closing capacity exceeds the FRC some lung segments are closed during tidal breathing and as a result the ventilation/perfusion (V/Q) ratio falls. It is the relationship between FRC and the closing capacity that to a large extent determines the matching of ventilation and perfusion.

Children under six years of age and adults over 40 have a closing capacity which is greater than FRC when in the supine position (Mansell *et al.*, 1972). The relatively high closing capacity in the child is due to the reduced elastic recoil of the lung and the high compliance of the thoracic cage. When the closing capacity exceeds FRC and TV some lung segments will be closed during both the inspiratory and expiratory phase of tidal breathing. This represents complete atelectasis of these segments.

Clinical implications

The very low elastic recoil of the newborn chest wall raises the risk of lung collapse. The majority of tidal breathing in the infant takes place in the range of the closing capacity. When lung volumes are reduced below FRC (e.g. postoperatively) and closing capacity exceeds FRC, small alveoli and airways in dependent regions of the lung are closed, resulting in atelectasis and impairment of ventilation. The use of positive pressure (positive end expiratory pressure or continuous positive airway pressure) to increase FRC above closing capacity in disease states associated with alveolar collapse is common practice.

As the chest wall of the newborn is very compliant, lung volume in the completely relaxed state is 10–15% of TLC compared to 30–35% in the adult. However, the FRC of a full term infant can be maintained at a higher volume by a mechanism of expiratory breaking (grunting), where upper airway resistance is increased during expiration thus increasing end expiratory lung volume (Helfaer *et al.*, 1992). Grunting therefore, is produced by adducting the vocal cords, a mechanism premature infants may lack.

The equal pressure point

During inspiration the bronchial diameter increases and the elastic forces of the lung parenchyma produce traction on the exterior of the bronchial walls. Expiration is by means of passive recoil. During forced expiration the expiratory muscles are active and the intrathoracic pressure is greatly increased. The external surface of the bronchi are then submitted to a higher intrathoracic pressure. In a forced expiration the point at which the extrabronchial and intrabronchial pressures are equal is termed the equal pressure point (EPP). The concept of the equal pressure point allows the airway to be divided into two segments; the upstream segment from the EPP to the alveoli and the downstream segment from the EPP to the mouth (Figure 2.3). During a forced expiratory manoeuvre the EPP first develops in the trachea and as the intrathoracic pressure becomes sufficiently positive it travels upstream as the airflow increases and then reaches the bronchi. The point of equal pressure therefore moves peripherally as expiration progresses. This occurs because the resistance of the airways rises as lung volume falls and the pressure within the airways falls more rapidly with distance from the alveoli. The dynamic bronchial compression is an indispensable part of the mechanism of an effective cough (Gaultier,

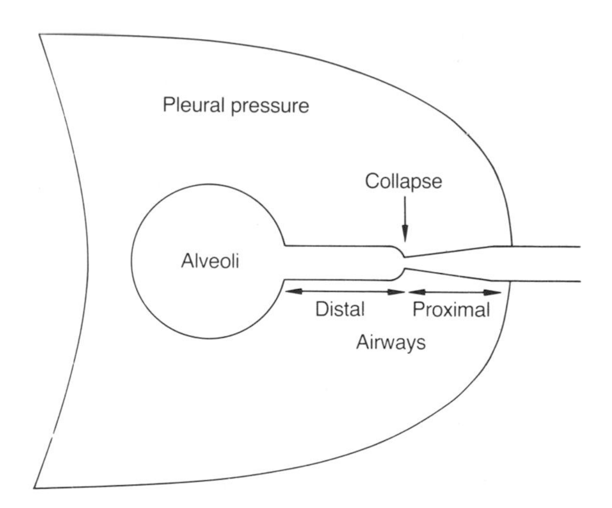

Figure 2.3 The equal pressure point, showing compression of the airways at the point where airway pressure equals pleural pressure. Reproduced with permission from J.B. West, *Pulmonary Pathophysiology*, Williams and Wilkins, 1987.

1982; West, 1992). Forced expiration manoeuvres using the concept of the EPP which moves peripherally during the course of a forced expiratory manoeuvre are used to enhance bronchial clearance from peripheral lung regions (Pryor, 1991).

DISTRIBUTION OF VENTILATION

Inspired gas is not evenly distributed throughout the lungs. During normal quiet breathing in the upright position the bases of the lungs receive about 50% more ventilation than the apices. The differences in ventilation between areas of the lungs are due to gravity and to variations in airway size and elastic properties. In the upright position at FRC the alveoli in the apex of the lung are more distended than those at the base. This is due to the pleural pressure being more negative at the top of the pleural cavity. Alveoli at the apex are more distended than those at the bases, they are less yielding and therefore less air enters the apices than the bases.

The distribution of ventilation is also related to the resistance of the airways and compliance of the air spaces. The product of flow resistance and compliance is known as the time constant. Each branch of the lung has a time constant so the distribution of gas within a lung depends on all its various time constants. In disease there may be local increases in resistance which lengthen the time constant to such an extent that complete expansion of alveoli does not occur during inspiration.

In the adult there is a considerably greater load (from the abdominal viscera) on the dependent hemidiaphragm when the subject is in the side lying position (Davies *et al.*, 1985). In the infant the difference in preload on the dependent as compared to the uppermost diaphragm is much smaller as the abdomen is smaller and narrower. Therefore there is little difference in the contractility between the hemidiaphragms and as a result less discrepancy between the lungs in terms of gravitational ventilation.

Bronchospirometric and radioisotope studies of regional ventilation in adults have shown that ventilation is preferentially distributed toward dependent lung regions (Zack *et al.*, 1974). However, due to differences in chest wall mechanics and diaphragmatic function the reverse situation is observed in infants where ventilation is preferentially distributed toward the uppermost parts of the lungs. This has been demonstrated by the use of krypton 81 m ventilation scans (Davies *et al.*, 1985). This observation reinforces the finding that children with unilateral lung pathology have a higher arterial oxygen tension when positioned with their unaffected lung uppermost (Heaf *et al.*, 1983). The effects of gravity on perfusion are however, similar in children and adults and this imbalance may have clinical importance (Bhuyan *et al.*, 1989).

Clinical implications

Children with airway disease will have an increase in airway resistance (caused by factors such as oedema and accumulation of secretions). This will lead to an increased time constant, incomplete expansion and therefore impaired ventilation. Children with unilateral lung pathology (particularly critically ill infants) should be nursed with their affected lung dependent in order to achieve optimum ventilation/perfusion matching and therefore maximum PaO_2.

TRANSPORT OF OXYGEN IN THE BLOOD

While in utero the lungs are fluid filled and gas exchange takes place across the placenta. Fetal haemoglobin has a higher affinity for oxygen than adult haemoglobin, i.e. the blood leaving the placenta with a PaO_2 of 4 kPa is 68% saturated whereas the oxygen saturation (SaO_2) of the mother's blood at this tension is 6.8% lower. Fetal haemoglobin has a high haemoglobin concentration which results in an increase in oxygen carrying capacity (Strang, 1977). When the fetal blood gives up carbon dioxide the change this produces in acidity (pH) increases its oxygen affinity.

Oxygen molecules are transported in the blood in two ways. The vast majority of oxygen in the blood is combined with haemoglobin (Hb). When the blood is fully saturated 1 g of Hb carries 1.34 ml of oxygen. A small proportion of the oxygen is dissolved in the plasma and water of the red blood cell. The oxyhaemoglobin dissociation curve (Figure 2.4) shows that Hb is nearly 95% saturated at a PaO_2 of 10.7 kPa. The steep portion of the curve indicates that at this level large amounts of oxygen can be removed from haemoglobin resulting in only small changes of PaO_2. Under normal circumstances inspiring 100% oxygen will only increase the amount of oxygen carried by the blood by a small amount, because at a PaO_2 of 13.3 kPa Hb is already 97.5% saturated.

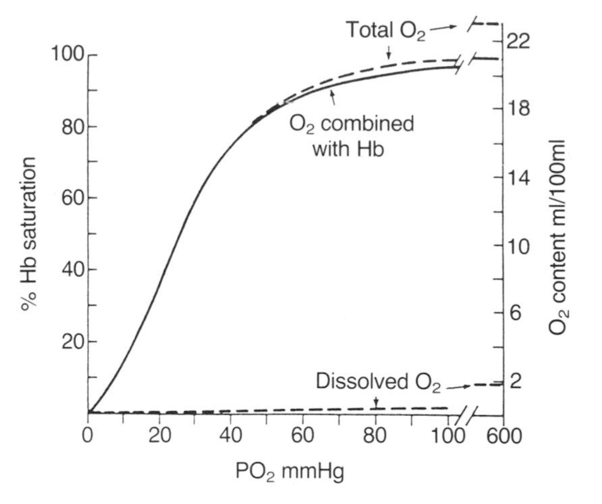

Figure 2.4 Oxygen dissociation curve. The solid line represents oxygen combined with haemoglobin, the broken line represents total blood oxygen content. Reproduced from J.B. West, *Respiratory Physiology*, Williams and Wilkins, 1984.

The oxyhaemoglobin dissociation curve is affected by changes in pH, $PaCO_2$ and temperature. A decrease in pH, an increase in $PaCO_2$ or an increase in temperature shifts the curve to the right. Thus for a given PaO_2 the saturation percentage is less under acidotic or hypercapnoeic conditions. The fetal oxyhaemoglobin dissociation curve lies to the left of that of the adult at a similar pH. Thus at a given PaO_2 fetal haemoglobin contains more oxygen than adult haemoglobin. This ensures that maximal oxygen reaches fetal tissues, since the fetus in utero has a PaO_2 of approximately 4 kPa. Fetal haemoglobin disappears from the circulation shortly after birth and at two months of age only 2% of the total haemoglobin is fetal in origin.

OXYGEN DELIVERY TO THE TISSUES

The cardiopulmonary system must transport oxygenated blood to the systemic tissues. The total oxygen delivery to the tissues is determined by the PaO_2, the amount of saturated haemoglobin, the left ventricular output and the patency of the vessels. Therefore three ways in which oxygenation can be improved are to increase haemoglobin saturation, increase haemoglobin concentration and to augment cardiac output. Cyanosis is one clinical sign of inadequate oxygenation of systemic tissues. The degree of visible cyanosis depends on the amount of unsaturated haemoglobin present in the blood perfusing the superficial vessels. An anaemic patient may be inadequately oxygenated without appearing cyanotic. The opposite is true for a patient with polycythaemia. Therefore the most reliable estimate of the oxygen content of the blood requires sampling and direct measurement.

CARBON DIOXIDE TRANSPORT

Arterial carbon dioxide ($PaCO_2$) is also a reflection of lung function and a measure of gas exchange at alveolar level. Any rise in $PaCO_2$ is an acute stimulant to breathing in the normal child and results in a compensatory increase in respiratory rate and tidal volume. Elevated $PaCO_2$ levels are indicative of ventilatory failure which can be due to reduced lung function or loss of the central control of breathing. Increased $PaCO_2$ causes cerebral vasodilation, whilst reduced $PaCO_2$ results in cerebral vasoconstriction and a resulting decrease in cerebral blood flow.

THE PULMONARY CIRCULATION

The development of the pulmonary vasculature closely follows the development of the airways. During development there is remodelling of the muscular wall of the pulmonary arterial tree. Muscular arteries reach the pleural surface in the adult, but in the fetus and the newborn extend only to the level of the terminal bronchiole. During childhood these gradually extend to reach alveolar level. Pulmonary vascular thickness is a function of gestational age and blood flow. Children with longstanding pulmonary hypertension, e.g. as a result of congenital heart disease, have a significant increase in smooth muscle in their pulmonary arteries. Premature infants have less well developed vascular smooth muscle which regress more quickly after birth than that of the term infant. Incomplete development and earlier regression of this smooth muscle produces an earlier drop in pulmonary vascular resistance (PVR) in the preterm infant following birth.

Posture is a major determinant of pulmonary blood volume, which is increased in the supine position due to a shift of blood from dependent portions of the body to the central circulation (Hirasuna and Gorin, 1981). Pulmonary perfusion is distributed according to the forces of gravity so most blood travels to the dependent regions. The upright lung can schematically be divided into three regions (Figure 2.5). In zone 1 the

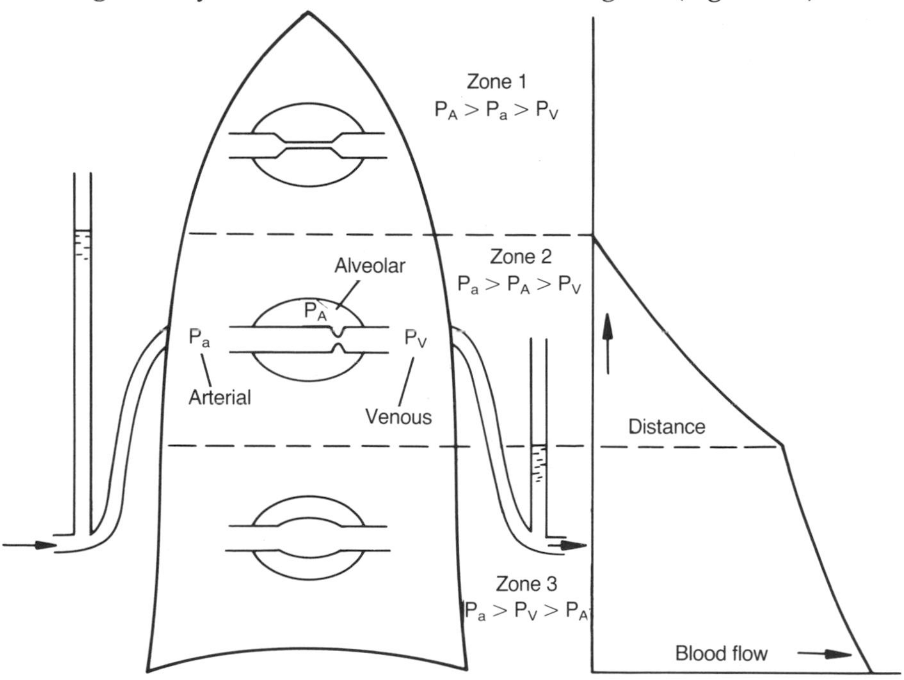

Figure 2.5 Distribution of blood flow in the lung based on pressures affecting the capillaries. Reproduced with permission from J.B. West *et al.*, *Journal of Applied Physiology*, 1964.

alveolar pressure (PA) is greater than the pulmonary artery presure (Pa) and much greater than the pulmonary venous pressure (PV). Therefore pulmonary vessels collapse and pulmonary blood flow and gas exchange stops. In zone 2 blood flows once Pa exceeds PA. Flow rates increase linearly as the gradient between Pa and PA increases down the lung until pulmonary venous pressure and alveolar pressure are equal. In the third zone Pa and PV are both greater than PA. The driving pressure Pa–PV is constant throughout this lower dependent zone because gravity produces equal increases in Pa and PV. The transmural pressures Pa–pleural pressure (PPL) and PV–PPL are increased in the dependent regions and therefore the vessels are dilated and the flow is increased. This explanation pertains to a model of the upright lung; it is assumed that in infants lying supine the gravity related differences in distribution of flow are less pronounced.

THE CARDIAC SYSTEM

The cardiac cycle is a sequence of contraction and relaxation of the heart muscle. At rest a preloaded right ventricular pressure of about 40 mmHg exists. The tricuspid valve closes as isovolumic contraction begins before the pulmonary valve opens. Contraction continues after the pulmonary valve opens and the blood rushes into the pulmonary circuit until the pulmonary valve closes. The cardiac muscle then relaxes and the pressure falls rapidly. Right ventricular pressure approaches zero, the tricuspid valve opens and the right ventricular volume reaccumulates. This cycle is then repeated. The same occurs on the left side of the heart with the mitral and aortic valves, but the pressures generated are much greater.

THE FRANK-STARLING RELATIONSHIP

The energy of contraction is proportional to the initial length of the cardiac muscle fibre. In the heart the length of the muscle fibre is proportional to the end diastolic volume. This correlation is known as the Frank–Starling relationship. It is present in infants but is incomplete, with a narrow range over which stroke volume increases with increasing end-diastolic pressure. The ability of heart muscle to generate greater contractility with volume increases is believed to be a function of the fundamental properties of actin-myosin mechanics. The relationship of muscle fibres to adjacent fibres in the heart may also be a contributory factor. There are many muscular bridges between the muscle fibres in the myocardium which at rest are mainly perpendicular to the main vector of muscle fibre contraction. With stretching from an increase in volume these bridges may become parallel to the predominant fibres and then may contribute more effectively to the overall strength of contraction (Parker and Case, 1979).

TRANSITIONAL CIRCULATION

The fetal circulation and the circulatory adjustments made after birth are fully described in Chapter 1. The placenta allows transport of oxygen from the mother to the fetus and carbon dioxide transport in the opposite direction. It allows the passage of nourishment and the excretion of fetal waste. Blood enters the placenta from the umbilical arteries and returns through the umbilical vein. Oxygen is transferred by diffusion and the fetal venous PaO_2 is always less than the maternal PaO_2. Blood returning to the fetus has a PaO_2 of 4–4.7 kPa (30–35 mmHg) and passes through the liver. By midterm 60% of the umbilical venous blood bypasses the hepatic circulation through the ductus venosus to enter the inferior caval vein. Following closure of the duct after birth all portal venous blood passes into the capillary system of the liver before entering the inferior vena cava

(IVC) via the hepatic veins. Therefore blood of a relatively high oxygen content enters the right atrium from the IVC and one third of this blood is directed into the left atrium through the foramen ovale. The highly saturated left atrial blood enters the left ventricle and is pumped into the ascending aorta.

The mature infant usually passes through the transitional circulation without any problems. Delay is usually due to hypoxia and therefore pulmonary vasoconstriction and dilation of the duct. A mild hypoxic stimulus can stimulate an increase in pulmonary vascular response. A vicious cycle can ensue if hypoxia remains untreated. Pulmonary artery pressure remains elevated, the duct remains open and there may be right to left shunting of blood through the foramen ovale. The respiratory rate increases and myocardial function may be impaired. This situation is termed persistent fetal circulation (PFC) and is discussed further in Chapter 8. Significant cardiac malformations, e.g. transposition of the great arteries, pulmonary stenosis and septal defects, may also disturb normal transitional circulation.

CARDIAC OUTPUT

In fetal life one third of the cardiac output (CO) enters the ascending aorta and two thirds enters the pulmonary artery. Only 8% of blood entering the pulmonary artery enters the lungs and the remainder passes through the ductus arteriosus to the descending aorta. There is a greater cardiac output per kilogram (kg) of body weight in the fetus and newborn infant than in the adult. The infant has a resting cardiac output per kg of body weight of 2–3 times that in the adult (Dawes, 1968).

CIRCULATORY CONTROL

Baroreceptor and chemoreceptor functions are present in the fetus. Fetal cardiac output is controlled almost completely by changes in fetal heart rate as the fetal heart has little ability to alter its stroke volume. There is a lag in sympathetic innervation of the heart compared to that of the parasympathetic system. The distribution of blood flow to fetal tissue is controlled by changes in local vascular resistance. Under conditions of stress, e.g. fetal growth retardation, fetal cardiac output favours the maintenance of umbilical flow and support of the myocardium and brain probably due to chemoreceptor reflexes (Benson and Freedom, 1991).

REFERENCES

Benson, L.N. and Freedom, R.M. (1991) The transitional circulation, in *Neonatal Heart Disease*, (eds R. Freedom, L.N. Benson and J.F. Smallhorn), Springer Verlag, London, pp. 149–62.

Berger, A.J., Mitchell, R.A. and Severinghaus, J.W. (1977) Regulation of respiration. *New England Journal of Medicine*, **297**, 92–7.

Bhuyan, U., Peters, A.M., Gordon, I. and Helms, P. (1989) Effect of posture on the distribution of pulmonary ventilation and perfusion in children and adults. *Thorax*, **44**, 480–4.

Davies, H., Kitchman, R., Gordon, I., and Helms, P. (1985) Regional ventilation in infancy. *New England Journal of Medicine*, **313**, 1626–8.

Dawes, G.S. (1968) *Foetal and Neonatal Physiology*. Year Book Medical, Chicago, pp. 141–59.

Dunhill, M.S. (1962) Postnatal growth of the lung. *Thorax*, **17**, 329.

Gaultier, C. (1982) Physiology of respiration: application of functional exploration of the lungs in infants and children, in *Paediatric Respiratory Disease*, 2nd edn, (eds J. Gerbeaux, J. Couvrer and G. Tournier), John Wiley & Sons, New York, pp. 17–59.

Heaf, D.P., Helms, P., Gordon, I. and Turner, H.M. (1983) Postural effects on gas exchange in infants. *New England Journal of Medicine*, **303**, 1505–8.

Helfaer, M.A., Nichols, D.G. and Rogers, M.C. (1992) Developmental physiology of the respiratory system, in *Textbook of Pediatric Intensive Care*, 2nd edn, (ed. M.C. Rogers), Williams and Wilkins, Baltimore, p. 104.

Hirasuna, J.O. and Gorin, A.B. (1981) Effect of prolonged recumbancy on pulmonary blood volume in normal humans. *Journal of Applied Physiology*, **50**, 950–5.

Hogg, J.C., Williams, J., Richardson, J.B. *et al.* (1970) Age as a factor in the distribution of lower airway conductance and in the pathologic anatomy of obstructive lung disease. *New England Journal of Medicine*, **282**, 1283–7.

Konno, K. and Mead, J. (1967) Measurement of the separate volume changes of rib cage and abdomen during breathing. *Journal of Applied Physiology*, **22**, 407–22.

Mansell, A., Bryan, C. and Levison, H. (1972) Airway closure in children. *Journal of Applied Physiology*, **33**, 711.

Mitchell, R.A. (1963) Respiratory responses mediated through superficial chemosensitive areas on the medulla. *Journal of Applied Physiology*, **18**, 523.

Muller, N.L. and Bryan, A.C. (1979) Chest wall mechanics and respiratory muscles in infants. *Pediatric Clinics of North America*, **26**, 503–16.

O'Brodovich, H.M. and Haddad, G.G. (1990) The functional basis of respiratory physiology, in *Kendigs Disorders of the Respiratory Tract in Children*, 5th edn, (ed. V. Chernick), W.B. Saunders, Philadelphia, pp. 3–47.

Parker, J.O. and Case, R.B. (1979) Normal left ventricular function. *Circulation*, **60**, 4–12.

Pasterkamp, H. (1990) The history and physical examination, in *Kendigs Disorders of the Respiratory Tract in Children*, 5th edn, (ed. V. Chernick), W.B. Saunders, Philadelphia, pp. 56–77.

Pryor, J.A. (1991) The forced expiration technique, in *Respiratory Care*, (ed. J.A. Pryor), Churchill Livingstone, Edinburgh, pp. 79–100.

Rigatto, H. (1982) Apnea. *Pediatric Clinics of North America*, **29**, 1105–66.

Strang, L.B. (1977) Oxygen transport in the blood, in *Neonatal Respiration*, (ed. L.B. Strang), Blackwell Scientific Publications, Oxford, pp. 138–60.

West, J.B. (1992) Ventilation, in *Pulmonary Pathophysiology*, 4th edn, (ed. J.B. West), Williams and Wilkins, Baltimore, pp. 3–18.

Wohl, M.E.B. and Mead, J. (1990) Age as a factor in respiratory disease, in *Kendigs Disorders of the Respiratory Tract in Children*, 5th edn, (ed. V. Chernick), W.B. Saunders, Philadelphia, pp. 175–82.

Zack, M.B., Pontoppidan, H. and Kazemi, H. (1974) The effect of lateral positons on gas exchange in pulmonary disease. *American Review of Respiratory Diseases*, **110**, 49–55.

IMAGING THE PAEDIATRIC CHEST 3

Christopher D. George and Isky Gordon

INTRODUCTION

Despite the advent of new imaging modalities, such as ultrasound, computed tomography (CT), magnetic resonance imaging (MRI) and ventilation/perfusion lung scans (V/Q scan), the plain chest radiograph remains the mainstay of paediatric chest imaging. In most circumstances the clinical history and examination will be augmented by a chest radiograph before a working diagnosis is made and treatment or further investigations planned.

This chapter aims to provide a concise and practical introduction to imaging the paediatric chest, emphasizing the importance of the plain chest radiograph but also indicating where other modalities provide additional information or allow the same information to be acquired with less use of ionizing radiation. The first section provides an overview of imaging modalities currently available, the second reviews important radiological signs commonly seen in paediatric chest radiographs and the final section discusses common paediatric chest problems and their radiological signs.

The text has not been referenced extensively; however, a number of selected general references suitable for further reading are given at the end of the chapter.

MODALITIES IN PAEDIATRIC CHEST IMAGING

PLAIN CHEST RADIOGRAPHS AND FLUOROSCOPY

Chest radiographs may be taken in the erect posteroanterior (PA) or anteroposterior (AP) position or in the supine AP position. In some circumstances, such as on the neonatal unit (NNU), where patient handling is minimized all films are obtained in the supine AP projection. Up to the age of three years any of the projections may be used depending on the policy of the department. Over the age of three most units obtain erect PA films. It is important that within any given unit techniques are standardized and films clearly labelled as the appearances of some radiological signs, particularly those of pleural fluid and pneumothorax, are profoundly different in the erect and supine positions. These changes will be discussed in greater detail in the next section. Frontal chest radiographs should be obtained in inspiration, using a short exposure time and with attention to technical factors so as to minimize the radiation exposure to the patient and attendants.

The lateral chest radiograph necessitates a significantly higher exposure than the frontal and is not required routinely. It is usually obtained during the follow-up of patients with cystic fibrosis, malignant disease likely to metastasize to the chest and in the assessment of recurrent chest infections. A lateral view may also be performed to clarify an abnormality seen on the frontal projection.

Coned, AP plain radiographs using a high kV technique and filtration to give an optimal exposure are used to demonstrate the anatomy and calibre of the major airways.

One of the disadvantages of conventional radiographs is that it is difficult to adequately demonstrate all soft tissue and bony structures using the same exposure factors. Two major recent developments have attempted to overcome these disadvantages. The first is digital chest radiography in which a phosphor plate is used for the exposure. The plate is then scanned with a laser beam which reads the information and stores it in digital form. The information can then be reconstructed as the 'chest X-ray' on a computer screen and manipulated to allow optimal visualization of areas of interest. Hard copies of the images can be printed on a laser imager. The advantages of this technique in paediatric radiology are the uniformity of image that can be maintained from day to day, the facility for image manipulation and a reduction in radiation dose.

The second technique, scanning equalization radiography (SER), uses a beam of X-rays which scans the patient. The exposure is continuously changing according to the tissues within the beam at any given time. This results in a more even exposure and a more uniform image.

Fluoroscopy remains a useful technique for assessing diaphragmatic movements and for detecting changes in airway calibre during respiration in conditions like tracheomalacia.

BRONCHOGRAPHY AND TOMOGRAPHY

Since CT and MRI have become widely available conventional tomography is no longer used and bronchography is only rarely undertaken to demonstrate focal bronchial narrowing.

ULTRASOUND

Ultrasound is useful for examining the pleural space for fluid (Figure 3.1). Effusions and empyemas can be located, measured and drained under ultrasound control. Because the ultrasound beam is strongly reflected by the aerated lung, ultrasound is less useful for assessing lung lesions unless they are peripheral, lie against the chest wall and consist of either solid or fluid. The movement and integrity of the hemidiaphragms can be assessed using ultrasound. The disadvantage is that each hemidiaphragm can only be assessed independently and not in relationship to each other. This is important in mild hemidiaphragm paresis. Cardiac ultrasound is an extremely accurate non-invasive way of assessing congenital heart disease.

COMPUTED TOMOGRAPHY (CT) AND MAGNETIC RESONANCE IMAGING (MRI)

In many ways these techniques are complementary and will be discussed together. Both techniques require the patient to remain still for the duration of the scan and this is particularly important in MRI. Neonates and young infants may be examined if asleep after a feed but older infants and children usually require sedation or general anaesthesia.

CT uses a narrow beam of X-rays to image the patient in 'slices'. The thickness of the slice may be varied from 1.5 mm to 1 cm and slices may be taken with or without gaps between them depending on the region being examined and the likely pathology. Assessment of the mediastinum and of vascular structures is facilitated by using intravascular contrast medium. High resolution

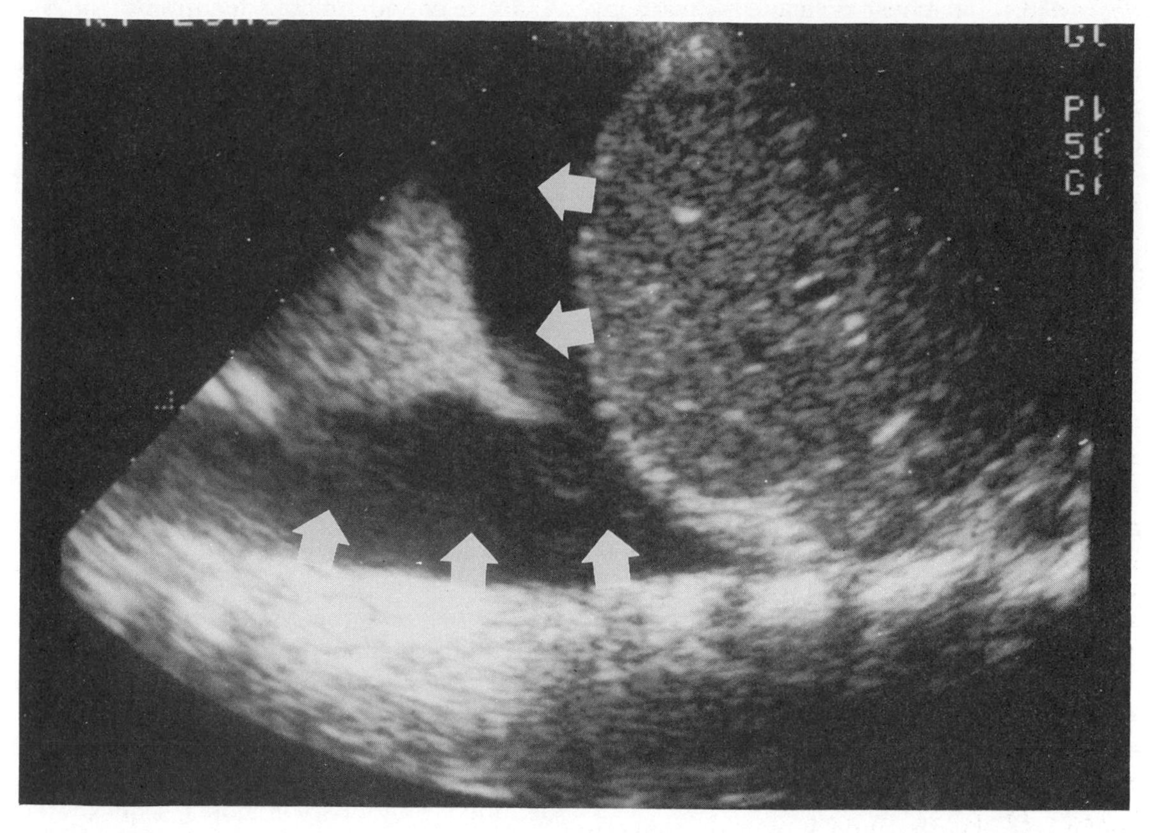

Figure 3.1 Sagittal ultrasound of a large pleural effusion which is poorly echogenic and appears black (white arrows). The patient's back is seen at the bottom of the image and the liver lies to the right. The effusion surrounds the partly collapsed, triangular lower lobe.

computed tomography (HRCT) uses a thin slice thickness and special software to demonstrate the lung parenchyma. HRCT is used in the diagnosis of diffuse parenchymal disease and bronchiectasis.

In MRI the patient lies within a strong magnetic field and is exposed to pulses of radio frequency energy. This energy is absorbed by protons within the body. When the radio frequency pulses are stopped the protons return to their normal state but as they do so they release energy, the magnetic resonance signal, which can be detected by coils placed around the body. Magnetic resonance signals are different for different tissues and may be altered by disease. Intravascular contrast medium for MRI is available.

CT has better spatial resolution and can detect fine calcification which affords it an advantage in evaluating mediastinal masses and lymphadenopathy. Bone structure and in particular cortical changes are best imaged on CT. Currently lung pathology is best evaluated on CT using HRCT if necessary. Vascular structures are well demonstrated on CT if intravascular contrast is used and ultrafast CT scanners, which enable the entire chest to be scanned in a matter of seconds, facilitate the investigation of congenital vascular and cardiac abnormalities.

MRI of the chest is made difficult by cardiac and respiratory movements. These effects can be minimized by only taking images at the same point in each cardiac and respiratory cycle, a technique known as gating. MRI has three major advantages over CT: its superior soft tissue contrast, its ability to acquire images in any plane and the fact that it does not use ionizing radiation. Sagittal and coronal images are of immense value in assessing the extent of a mediastinal mass and in deciding whether a paraspinal mass extends into the spinal canal.

One of the most exciting branches of MRI is magnetic resonance angiography (MRA) which allows blood vessels and the heart to be imaged without the need for artery puncture or the injection of any contrast media.

ANGIOGRAPHY AND CARDIAC CATHETERIZATION

Cardiac ultrasound and the advent of MRA have reduced the indications for conventional angiography and cardiac catheterization to assess congenital anomalies of the aorta and pulmonary vessels and congenital arteriovenous malformations.

BARIUM STUDIES

These studies have a limited but very important role in the assessment of chest problems, specifically the barium swallow to evaluate extrinsic oesophageal compression by aberrent vessels or masses and the swallow/meal to assess intrinsic abnormalities such as incoordinated swallowing, abnormal oesophageal peristalsis or gastro-oesophageal reflux which can cause aspiration. If a tracheo-oesophageal fistula is suspected a tube oesophagogram must be performed in the prone position.

There is no reliable technique for the positive diagnosis of aspiration; this includes the barium swallow/meal as well as the isotope milk scan. Recurrent aspiration may be inferred when there is severe gastro-oesophageal reflux.

RADIONUCLIDE STUDIES

Radionuclide studies provide quantifiable functional information which complements the anatomical information provided by other imaging modalities. The ventilation/perfusion scan (V/Q scan) uses krypton (^{81m}Kr) gas for ventilation and technetium (^{99m}Tc) labelled macroaggregates for perfusion. The V/Q scan is the only method which will provide information on regional lung function. The radiation burden from the V scan is less than one fifth of a chest radiograph while the Q scan has a dose equal to less than 60 seconds of fluoroscopy.

Most ventilatory disturbances result in a corresponding reduction in perfusion whereas if the pulmonary artery to a region is occluded (pulmonary embolus, sequestrated segment or pulmonary artery disease) that region remains ventilated. Occasionally other radionuclide studies such as bone scans or milk scans are indicated in the assessment of chest pathology.

BASIC SIGNS ON THE PLAIN CHEST RADIOGRAPH

CONSOLIDATION

Replacement of air in the very distal airways and alveoli by fluid or solid is called consolidation. The cardinal signs of consolidation are an area of increased opacity which may have an irregular shape, irregular margins, a non-segmental distribution and contains an air bronchogram (Figure 3.2). The volume of the affected lung remains unchanged and consequently there are no signs of loss of volume. If an area of consolidation abuts the mediastinum, heart or diaphragm their clear silhouette, which is dependent upon the sharp radiological contrast between normally aerated lung (black) and solid structures (white), is lost (Figure 3.2). Similarly the presence of air bronchograms within an area of consolidation can be explained by the sharp contrast between air in the medium and large bronchi (black) and the surrounding non-aerated and 'solid' lung (white) (Figures 3.2 and 3.3).

A variant of infective consolidation frequently seen in infants and children is the 'round pneumonia'. This may mimic a mass lesion radiologically since it has well defined borders; however, the clinical picture points to an infective aetiology. While infection is the commonest cause of consolidation, it is also caused by any pathological process in which the alveoli are filled by fluid or solid.

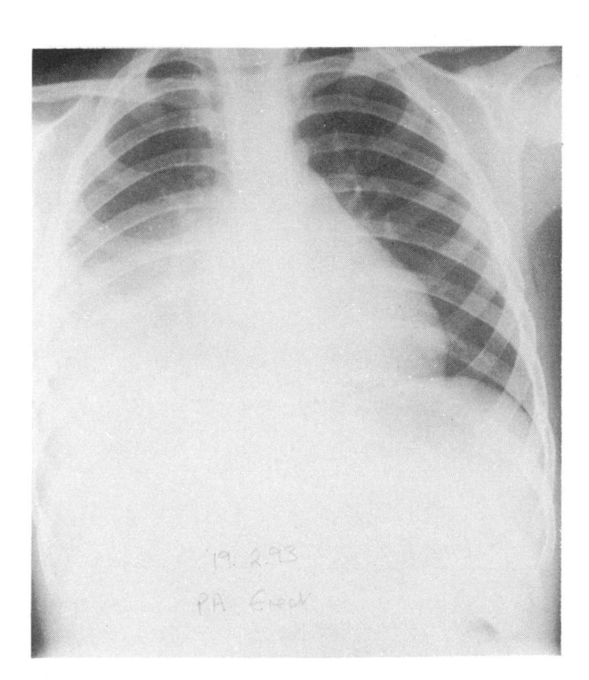

Figure 3.2 Right lower lobe consolidation caused by the bacterium *Streptococcus pneumoniae*. There is increased opacity in the right lower and mid zones, loss of the clear outline of the right hemidiaphragm and a proximal air bronchogram.

The commonest causes of consolidation are listed in Table 3.1.

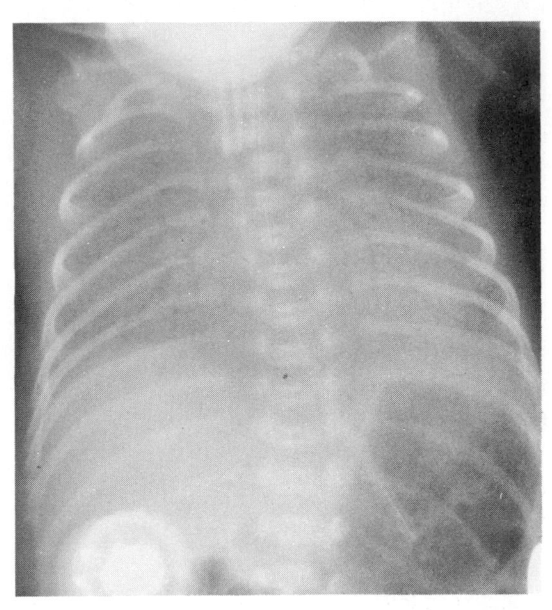

Figure 3.3 AP supine radiograph of a premature neonate with respiratory distress syndrome (RDS). The lungs show generalized opacity due to consolidation and a prominent air bronchogram.

Table 3.1 Common causes of consolidation

Pulmonary oedema
Cardiogenic
Non-cardiogenic
Respiratory distress syndrome
Aspiration
Pulmonary exudate
Infection
Blood
Traumatic contusion
Infarction
Aspiration
Other rare causes
Alveolar proteinosis
Alveolar microlithiasis
Lymphoma
Sarcoidosis

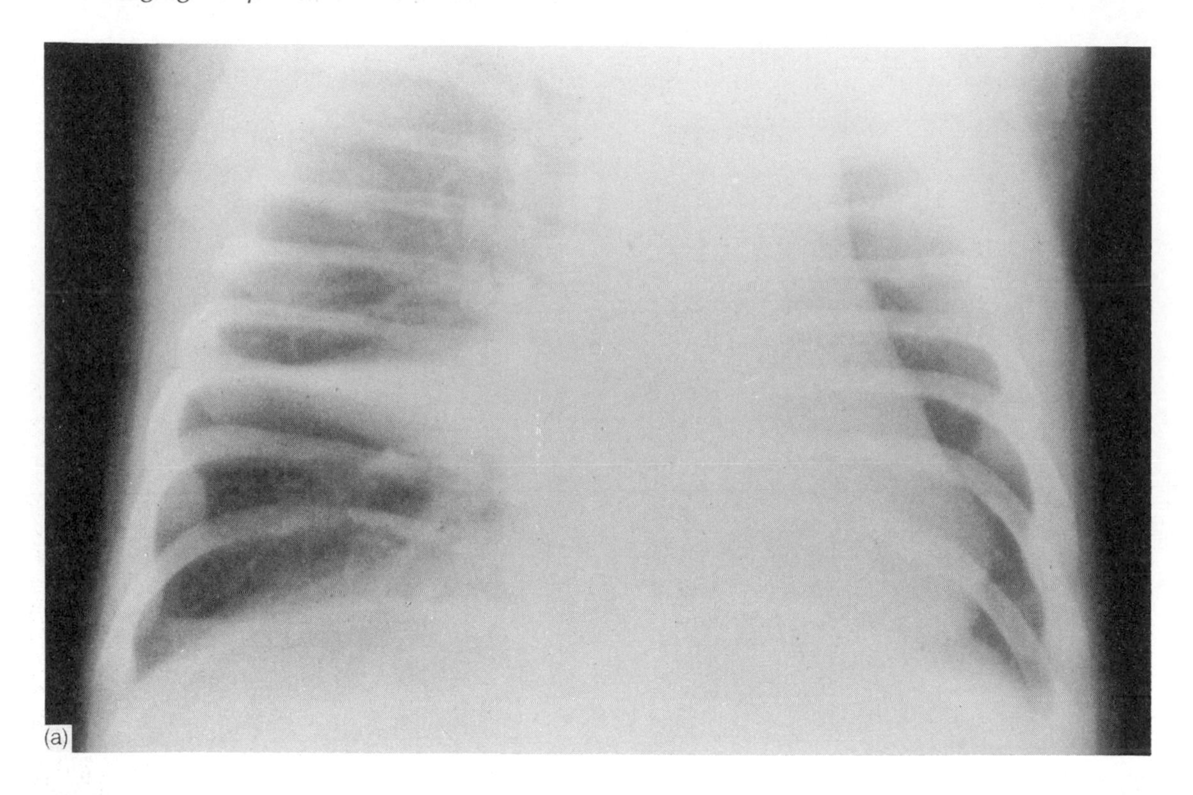

COLLAPSE

Collapse means loss of lung volume and this may affect a lung, lobe or segment. This is manifest on the radiograph by shift of the normal fissures and crowding of airways in the collapsed lung (Figures 3.4a,b and 3.5a,b). If the volume loss is large there may also be mediastinal shift towards the affected side, elevation of the ipsilateral hemidiaphragm, ipsilateral rib crowding and alteration in hilar positon. The collapsed lobe

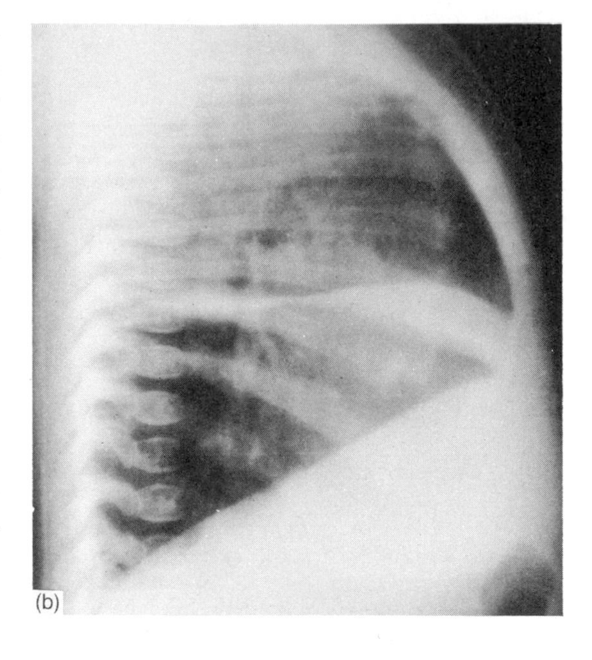

Figure 3.4 (a) AP radiograph taken in a lordotic projection to show the bandlike opacity of middle lobe collapse. Part of the right heart silhouette is lost where the collapsed lobe abuts the heart. (b) Lateral radiograph showing the collapsed middle lobe and displaced fissures. In addition the lungs show generalized overinflation with some flattening of the diaphragm.

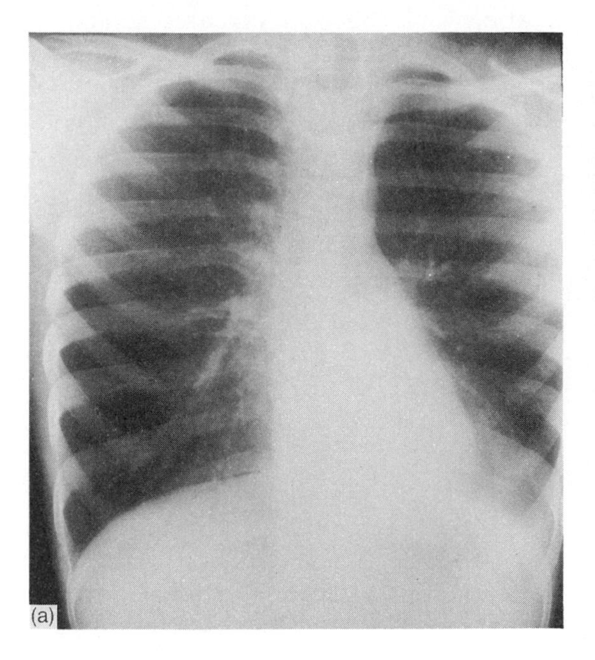

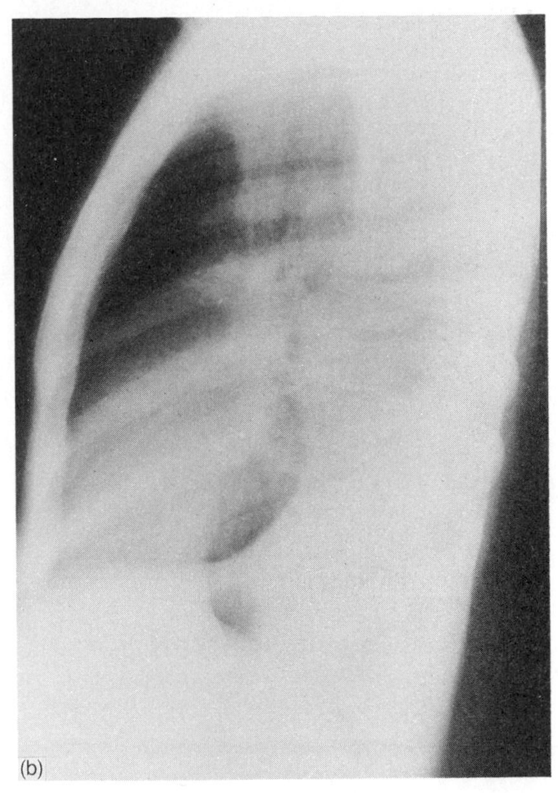

Figure 3.5 (a) Frontal radiograph of a patient with asthma and a left lower lobe collapse caused by a mucus plug. Generalized overinflation, increased opacity in the left cardiac region and loss of clarity of the outline of the medial left hemidiaphragm. (b) The lateral radiograph shows the collapsed left lower lobe as a wedge-shaped opacity in the lower chest posteriorly.

may or may not cause increased radio-opacity and there may be compensatory hyperinflation of unaffected lobes. If the collapsed lobe abuts on part of the diaphragm or cardiomediastinal silhouette the clear outline of these may be lost on the radiograph as in consolidation (Figures 3.4a,b and 3.5a,b). Collapse is most often due to obstruction of a large airway by foreign body, mucous plug, tumor or extrinsic compression. Less commonly it occurs secondary to poor ventilation.

PLEURAL FLUID

The radiological appearance of plural fluid is largely determined by the position of the patient. In the erect position the fluid collects at the bases and initially causes blunting to the costophrenic angles. Larger effusions cause a homogeneous opacity with a concave upper border higher laterally than medially, the meniscus. Very large effusions may cause mediastinal shift to the opposite side.

In the supine position, often used for neonatal and infant radiographs, an effusion causes reduced transradiancy (whiter hemithorax) of the affected side and may collect around the apex of the lung. In larger effusions a peripheral band of soft tissue density appears between the chest wall and the lung; on the right this band has a characteristic step at the position of the horizontal fissure (Figures 3.1 and 3.6). Pleural fluid may collect and loculate within fissures or between the inferior surface of the lung and the diaphragm, the 'subpulmonic' effusion.

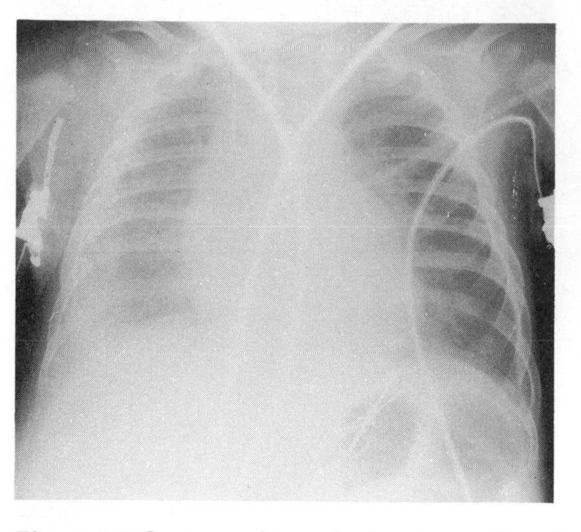

Figure 3.6 Supine radiograph showing a pleural effusion. There is reduced transradiancy on the right and a peripheral band of soft tissue density paralleling the chest wall with a 'step' at the position of the horizontal fissure.

PNEUMOTHORAX

In the erect positon pleural air collects at the apex causing increased apical transradiancy (darker apex) and absent lung markings beyond a visible lung edge. In the supine position air collects initially in the anteroinferior chest causing quite different and often subtle signs. These include small slivers of air at the apex, around the heart and between the lung and the diaphragm. Where free air as opposed to aerated lung abuts part of the cardiomediastinal or diaphragmatic silhouette the clarity of that border is especially sharp, this being the opposite of the effect seen in consolidation (see above). A large pneumothorax in neonates and infants when supine may collect anteriorly and cause an increased ipsilateral transradiancy (darker hemithorax) and increased sharpness of the cardiomediastinal silhouette (Figure 3.7).

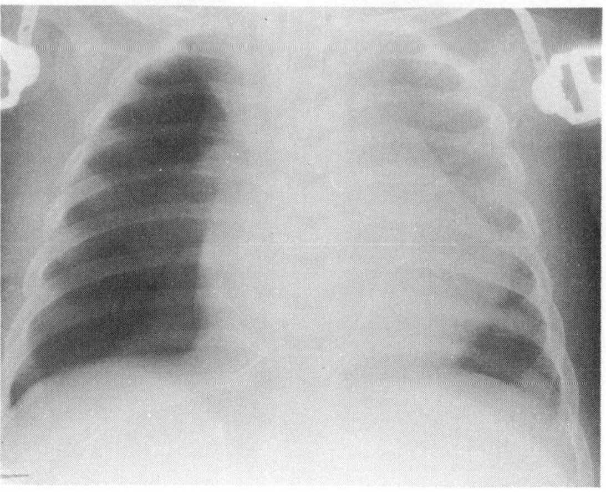

Figure 3.7 Supine radiograph showing a postoperative right pneumothorax. There is increased transradiancy of the right hemithorax. The right heart border is very clearly defined and the right lung edge is visible.

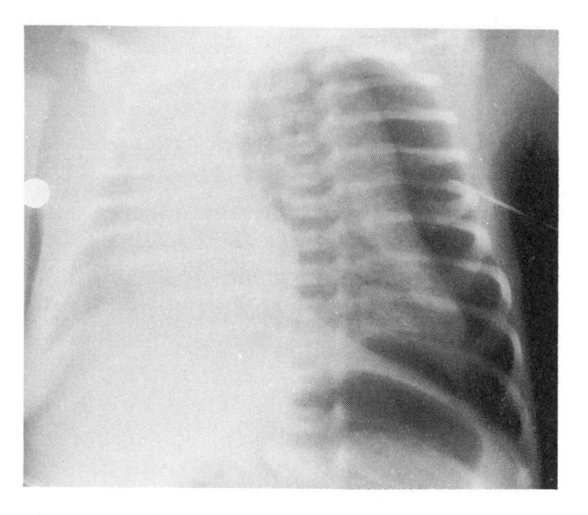

Figure 3.8 Supine radiograph of a patient with RDS. There is a left tension pneumothorax causing flattening of the hemidiaphragm and mediastinal shift to the right. The pneumothorax is seen surrounding a consolidated left lung. A needle drain has been inserted.

A tension pneumothorax occurs when a pleural tear acts as a one-way flap valve, allowing air into the pleural space but preventing egress. The pressure within the hemithorax rises and may remain positive for much of the respiratory cycle causing mediastinal shift to the contralateral side and flattening, or even eversion, of the ipsilateral hemidiaphragm (Figure 3.8).

COMMON PAEDIATRIC CHEST PROBLEMS

CONGENITAL ABNORMALITIES OF THE CHEST

Congenital diaphragmatic hernia

Large congenital diaphragmatic hernias frequently present as neonatal respiratory distress although many are now diagnosed antenatally on routine antenatal ultrasound examination. Many are associated with other congenital anomalies. Most hernias are left sided, situated posteriorly and large. Abdominal organs are sited in the chest and appear on the radiograph as a cystic/solid mass. The mediastinum is shifted to the contralateral side and one or both lungs may be hypoplastic (Figure 3.9). When large the condition carries a high mortality.

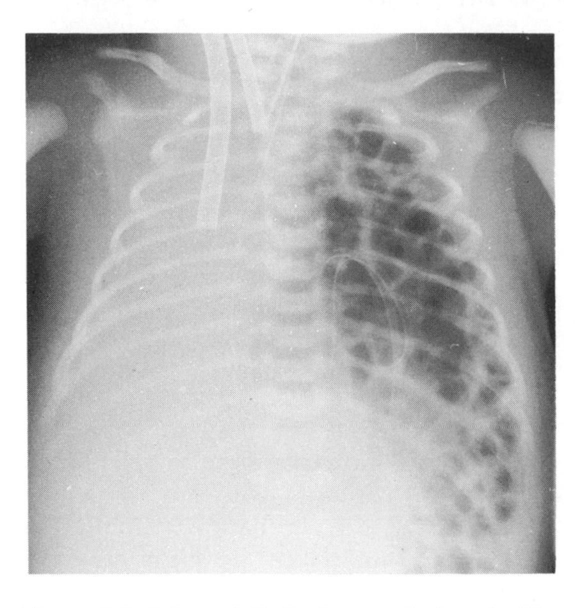

Figure 3.9 A large left diaphragmatic hernia. The left hemithorax contains the stomach (nasogastric tube) and loops of small bowel. The mediastinum is shifted to the right. The right lung is airless and opaque because the patient is on an extracorporeal membrane oxygenator (ECMO).

Hiatus hernia

A sliding hiatus hernia exists when the lower oesophageal sphincter and part of the stomach are situated in the thorax, above the diaphragm. This condition is usually associated with incompetence of the sphincter and may result in feeding problems, gastro-oesophageal reflux and aspiration.

Congenital lobar emphysema

A focal abnormality of a lobar bronchus leads to a ball valve effect causing air trapping and overinflation of the affected lobe. The left upper, right middle and right upper lobes are most frequently affected. Initial radiographs in the first few hours of life may show an opaque mass in the region of the affected lobe. As fluid clears the appearances are those of an overinflated lobe with compression of normal surrounding lung and mediastinal shift to the contralateral side (Figure 3.10). Treatment is surgical excision of the affected lobe if the neonate is in respiratory distress; if found in the older infant conservative management is advocated.

Cystic adenomatoid malformation

This condition, caused by a disorganized and usually cystic mass of pulmonary tissue, can mimic both congenital diaphragmatic hernia and congenital lobar emphysema. The hamartomatous mass can affect any lobe, although the middle lobe is rarely affected and in one fifth of cases more than one lobe

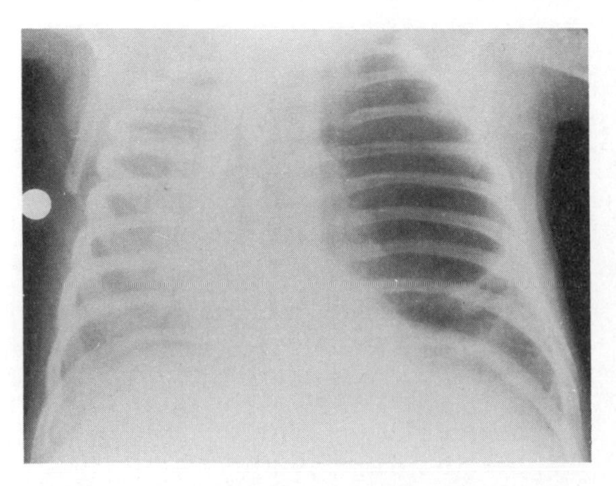

Figure 3.10 Congenital lobar emphysema of the left upper lobe. The lower lobe is compressed and the mediastinum is shifted to the right.

is affected. The radiograph shows a well defined cystic mass which may be large, compressing adjacent lung and causing mediastinal shift.

NEONATAL CHEST PROBLEMS

Respiratory distress syndrome (RDS)

Immature surfactant produced in premature infants, infants of diabetic mothers and infants who experience perinatal asphyxia fails to reduce the alveolar surface tension sufficiently to prevent alveolar collapse. This is the commonest cause of respiratory distress in premature neonates and causes tachypnoea, cyanosis, expiratory grunting and chest wall retraction. The radiograph shows bilateral symmetrical hypoaeration, small volume lungs, ground glass granularity of the pulmonary parenchyma and well defined air bronchograms extending from the hilum into the peripheral lung (Figure 3.3).

These neonates frequently require intermittent positive pressure ventilation which may give rise to specific complications of pulmonary interstitial emphysema (PIE) (Figure 3.11), pneumothorax (Figures 3.8 and 3.11), pneumomediastinum and bronchopulmonary dysplasia (BPD) (Figure 3.12).

Pulmonary interstitial emphysema is caused by gas leaking from overdistended alveoli and tracking along bronchovascular sheaths. The radiographic appearance is that of a branching pattern of gas with associated bubbles affecting all or part of the lung (Figure 3.11).

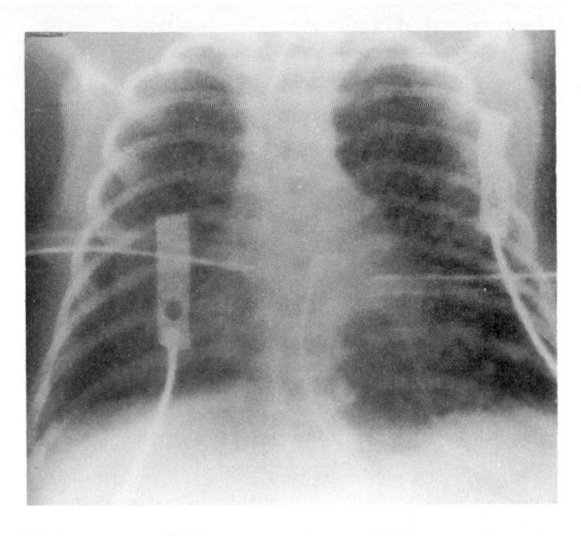

Figure 3.11 Pulmonary interstitial emphysema (PIE) complicating RDS. There is a branching pattern of gas with associated small bubbles. Bilateral chest drains and persistent right pneumothorax.

Bronchopulmonary dysplasia is seen exclusively in infants who have been on positive pressure ventilation, usually for RDS. The combination of high pressure trauma and oxygen toxicity results in lung damage. The lung passes through a number of radiological stages during the evolution of BPD. There is a RDS pattern which progresses to almost complete opacification and then to a coarse pattern of linear

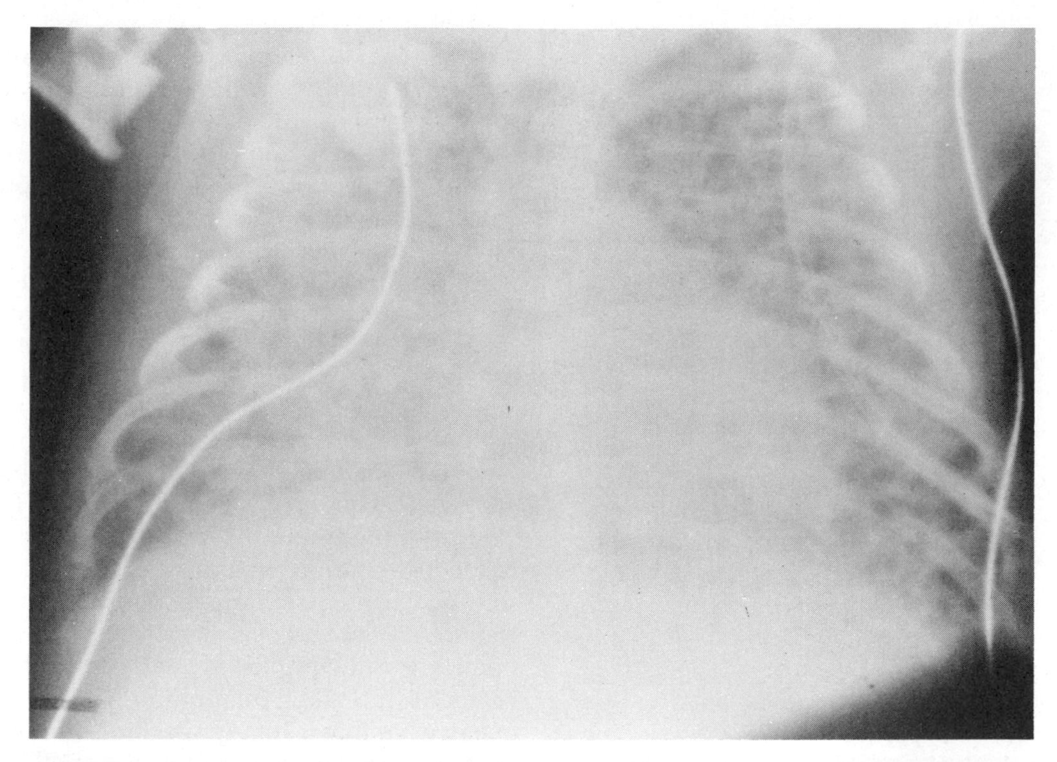

Figure 3.12 Bronchopulmonary dysplasia. A coarse pattern of linear opacities and cystic lucencies.

opacities and cystic lucencies (Figure 3.12). The lack of adequate oxygenation in RDS may result in failure of the ductus arteriosus to close. The consequent left-to-right shunt may progress to frank plethora and heart failure.

Meconium aspiration syndrome

This is the commonest cause of respiratory distress in full or post-term neonates. The aspirated meconium causes a chemical pneumonitis and bronchial obstruction. The radiographic picture is of bilateral diffuse patchy collapse with other areas of overinflation (Figure 3.13). Spontaneous pneumothorax, pneumomediastinum and small effusions are common but air bronchograms are rare.

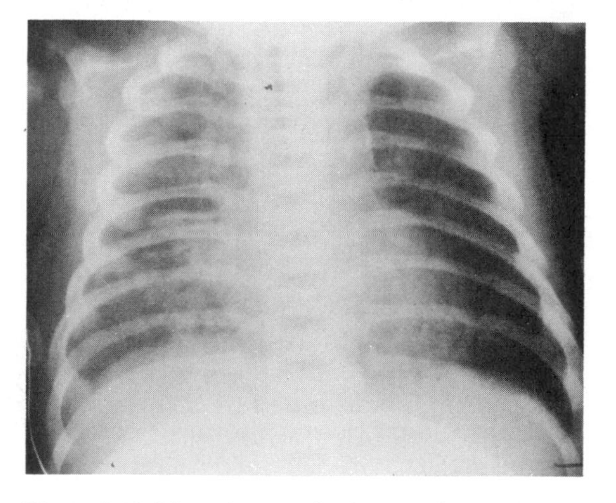

Figure 3.13 Meconium aspiration syndrome. Areas of patchy collapse with other areas of overinflation. The right lung is most affected.

RESPIRATORY TRACT INFECTIONS

Viral infections

Viral infections generally affect the bronchi and peribronchial tissues and this is reflected in the radiological signs: symmetrical parahilar, peribronchial streaky shadowing radiating for a variable distance into the lung periphery, hilar lymphadenopathy, occasionally reticulonodular shadowing, segmental/lobar collapse and generalized overinflation secondary to narrowing of the bronchi (Figure 3.14). Effusions are rare. Organisms commonly encountered are the respiratory syncytial virus (RSV), influenza and parainfluenza viruses, adenovirus and rhinovirus.

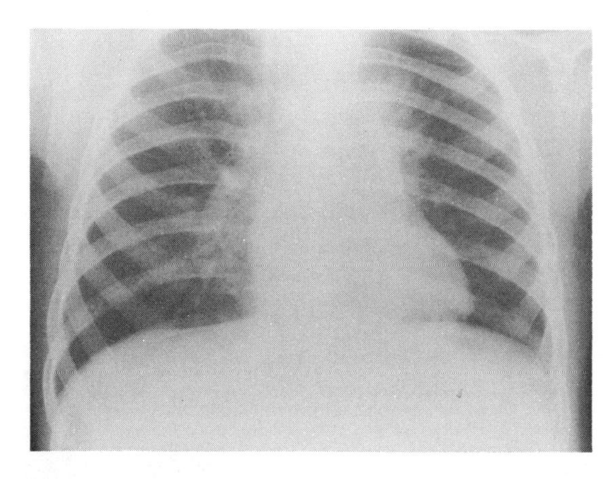

Figure 3.14 Viral pneumonia caused by the respiratory syncytial virus (RSV). There is symmetrical parahilar, peribronchial streaky shadowing and mild hilar lymphadenopathy.

Bacterial and mycoplasma infections

In the neonatal period the most common organisms are non-haemolytic streptococci, *Staphylococcus aureus* and *Escherichia coli*. Lobar consolidation is rare and more often the following signs are seen: radiating perihilar streakiness, coarse patchy parenchymal infiltrates, nodular or reticulonodular shadowing or diffuse hazy shadowing, most often basal. One important pattern to recognize is the diffuse bilateral granularity of group B haemolytic streptococcal pneumonia which so closely mimics RDS.

In infants bacterial infection is more often seen as lobar or patchy consolidations (Figure 3.2). The organisms are most commonly *Haemophilus influenzae*, *Streptococcus pneumoniae*, *Staphylococcus aureus* and *Mycoplasma pneumoniae*. Pleural effusions, empyemas, abscesses and pneumatocoeles are well recognized complications. The 'round pneumonia' is an area of infective consolidation which transiently has a rounded configuration and mimics a mass lesion. *Mycoplasma pneumoniae* infection can mimic the radiographic appearances of both bacterial and viral pneumonia. However, one pattern that is highly specific is unilobar reticulonodular infiltration especially if associated with hilar lymphadenopathy and/or a small pleural effusion.

Tuberculosis

Tuberculosis acquired in infancy is usually manifest by unilateral hilar or paratracheal lymphadenopathy and occasionally the primary or Ghon focus is seen as an area of consolidation in the periphery of the ipsilateral lung (Figure 3.15). Collapse is seen, usually due to compression of a bronchus by lymph nodes. Bronchopneumonic spread, with widespread areas of consolidation, occurs if either an infected node discharges into a bronchus or when host resistance is very low facilitating spread through the airways. Miliary tuberculosis, with multiple small nodules, is caused by the haematogenous spread that occurs when an infected node discharges into the blood stream. Cavitation is unusual in children.

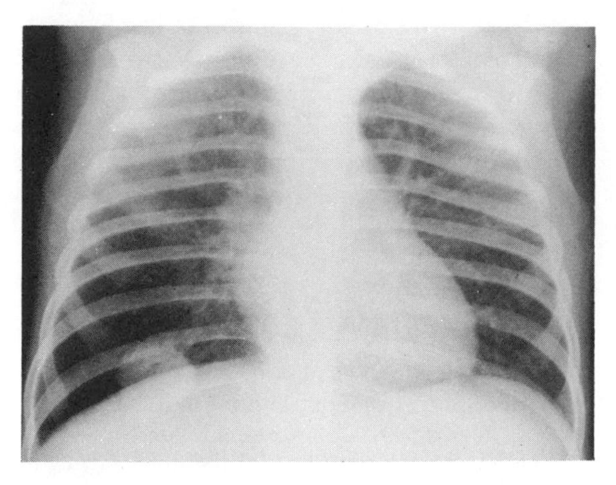

Figure 3.15 Primary tuberculous infection. Unilateral right hilar lymphadenopathy and an area of consolidation (Ghon focus) in the ipsilateral lower zone.

AIRWAY OBSTRUCTION

Asthma

The radiological features are rarely seen before the age of three. In chronic asthma there is generalized overinflation of the lungs with parahilar, peribronchial infiltrates but hilar lymphadenopathy is rare. Plugs of viscid mucus obstruct the airways and cause recurrent segmental or lobar collapse (Figure 3.5a,b). Pneumomediastinum is a common complication but rarely requires specific treatment; pneumothorax is seen less frequently.

Obstruction by foreign bodies

Aspirated foreign bodies most commonly lodge in the major bronchi and act like a ball valve causing a distal obstructive emphysema (Figure 3.16a,b). Radiographs are taken in inspiration and expiration to demonstrate the air trapping. Less commonly the lung distal to the obstruction collapses and may become infected.

CYSTIC FIBROSIS

This autosomal recessive condition causes excessively thick and viscid mucus. In the neonatal period bowel obstruction due to meconium ileus may draw attention to the condition. In the chest the earliest signs are

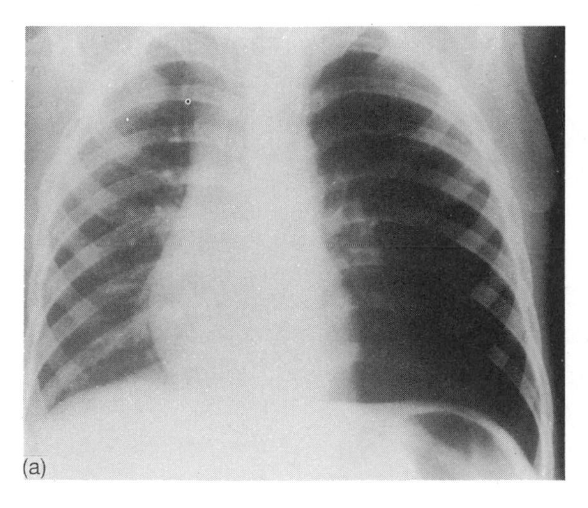

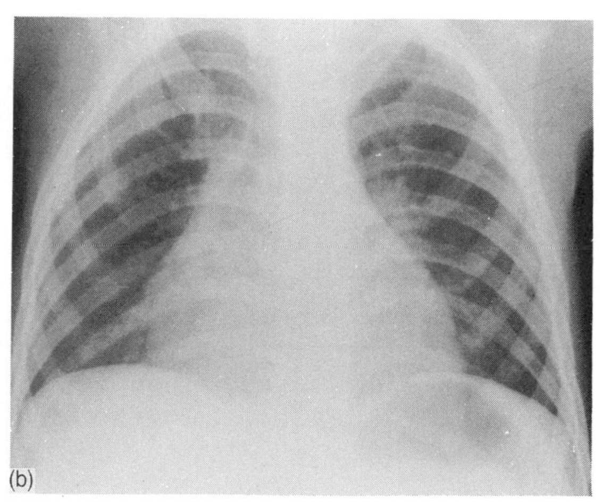

Figure 3.16 (a) Aspirated foreign body lodged in the left mainstem bronchus. Marked air trapping in the affected lung causing overinflation, increased transradiancy and mediastinal shift. (b) Same patient after bronchoscopic removal of the obstruction.

very similar to those of viral bronchiolitis; overinflation, focal collapse and parahilar, peribronchial infiltrates (Figure 3.17). Recurrent infections lead to bronchiectasis, fibrosis and generalized overinflation with segmental areas of collapse. Bronchial collaterals are recruited and when these become large haemoptysis may be a problem.

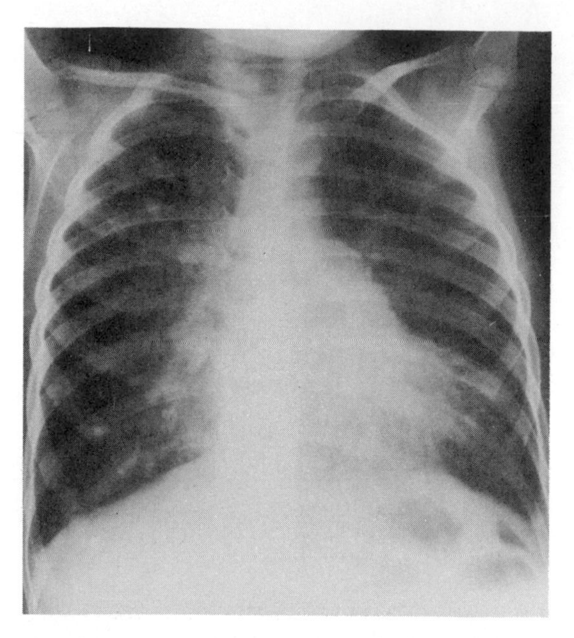

Figure 3.17 Cystic fibrosis. Overinflation, focal collapse and parahilar, peribronchial infiltrates.

ACKNOWLEDGEMENTS

We are most grateful to Dr B.J. Loveday at the Royal Surrey County Hospital, Guildford, and Dr D.B. Reiff at St George's Hospital, London, for allowing us to use their radiographs as illustrations. We wish to thank Mrs Hazel Cook, Mrs Mary Shoesmith and Mrs Susan Ranson of the Department of Diagnostic Radiology at the Royal Surrey County Hospital, Guildford, and the Department of Medical Illustration at the Great Ormond Street Hospital for Children NHS Trust, for their help in preparing the illustrations.

FURTHER READING

De Bruyn, R. (1993) Paediatric chest, in *Clinical Ultrasound: Abdominal and General Ultrasound*, vol. 2, (eds D. Cosgrove, H. Meire and K. Dewbury), Churchill Livingstone, London, pp. 983–8.

Edelman, R.L. and Warach, S. (1993) Magnetic resonance imaging (part 1). *New England Journal of Medicine*, **328**, 708–16.

Edelman, R.L. and Warach, S. (1993) Magnetic resonance imaging (part 2). *New England Journal of Medicine*, **328**, 785–91.

Gordon, I., Helms, P. and Fazio, F. (1981) Clinical applications of radionuclide lung scanning. *British Journal of Radiology*, **54**, 576–85.

Gordon, I., Matthew, D.J. and Dinwiddie, R. (1987) Respiratory system, in *Diagnostic Imaging in Paediatrics*, (ed. I. Gordon), Chapman & Hall, London, pp. 27–57.

Hayden, C.K. and Swischuk, L.E. (eds) (1992) *Pediatric Ultrasonography*, 2nd edn, Williams and Wilkins, Baltimore.

Newman, B. (1993) The pediatric chest. *Radiology Clinics of North America*, **31**, 453–719.

Piepsz, A., Gordon, I. and Hahn, K. (1991) Paediatric nuclear medicine. *European Journal of Nuclear Medicine*, **18**, 41–66.

Swischuk, L.E. (1989) *Imaging of the Newborn, Infant and Young Child*, 3rd edn, Williams and Wilkins, Baltimore.

Weinberger, E. and Brewer, D.K. (1992) Pediatric body imaging, in *Computed Tomography of the Body with Magnetic Resonance Imaging*, 3rd edn, (eds A.A. Moss, G. Gamsu and H.K. Genant), W.B. Saunders, Philadelphia, pp. 1267–96.

MANAGEMENT OF THE ACUTELY ILL CHILD IN RESPIRATORY FAILURE 4

Robert C. Tasker

INTRODUCTION

Many of the medical problems seen in acutely ill children have the potential for culminating in respiratory failure. The approach to managing such patients whilst requiring paediatric intensive care has largely 'evolved' over the past 20 years from an historical disease-orientated focus to a meticulous and coordinated multiorgan system of review (Rogers, 1987).

In children, the conditions that most commonly cause respiratory failure differ with age. In the newborn infant, prematurity, hyaline membrane disease, asphyxia and aspiration pneumonia are the most common aetiologies. Under two years of age, bronchopneumonia, bronchiolitis, croup, status asthmaticus, foreign body inhalation and congenital heart and airway anomalies are important, compared with asthma, accidental poisoning and central nervous system infection, trauma and hypoxia/ischaemia in the over two year olds. Whilst it is evident that the lung is the 'target organ' for many of these conditions, when respiratory failure ensues, there may be significant vital organ impairment resulting from reduced arterial blood gas tensions, acidosis and hypercarbia. The emphasis of this chapter will be an overview of respiratory supportive therapy in the context of managing the critically ill child.

RESPIRATORY MONITORING

The infant or child with obvious respiratory distress, consisting of decreased or absent breath sounds, severe intercostal recession, accessory muscle use during inspiration, a decreased level of consciousness and cyanosis, needs emergency assistance (Table 4.1). However, so do those patients with a less severe degree of respiratory failure, which may be more easily and more effectively treated. Over recent years technological developments in transcutaneous oxygen and carbon dioxide monitoring and pulse oximetry have been invaluable in enabling such an early recognition, particularly because of their sensitivity in detecting significant hypoxia and hypercarbia not recognizable by clinical examination.

Table 4.1 Clinical signs of Respiratory Failure

Respiratory	Cardiac
Tachypnoea	Tachycardia
Altered depth and pattern of breathing (deep, shallow, apnoea, irregular)	Hypertension Bradycardia Hypotension
Intercostal recession	Cardiac arrest
Nasal flaring	
Cyanosis	
Decreased or absent breath sounds	**Cerebral** Restlessness
Expiratory grunting	Irritability
Wheeze and/or prolonged expiration	Headache Mental confusion
General	Papilloedema
Fatigue	Seizures
Excessive sweating	Coma

Hypoxaemia is defined as a blood oxygen level that is less than normal, which may or may not be adequate to meet the body's metabolic demands. Hypoxia occurs when the oxygen requirements of the body's tissues are not met by the oxygen being delivered to the tissues by the circulating blood. In response to hypoxia, the body has several mechanisms to increase the systemic delivery of oxygen. These include: increased pulmonary gas exchange, increased pulmonary blood flow, improved matching of ventilation and pulmonary perfusion, increased haemoglobin affinity for oxygen, greater dissociation of oxygen from haemoglobin in the tissues, increased cardiac output and tissue perfusion.

Carbon dioxide, the end product of aerobic cellular metabolism, is carried by the blood in a manner similar to oxygen. After diffusing into the blood plasma most of the carbon dioxide enters the red blood cells and undergoes chemical transformation to carbonic acid. Ultimately hydrogen and bicarbonate ions are formed. The bicarbonate freely diffuses from the red blood cell into the plasma. Some of the hydrogen ions liberated in the red blood cell as a result of hypoxia are bound to and reduce the haemoglobin molecule. The presence of reduced haemoglobin promotes the loading of carbon dioxide, whereas the oxygenation that occurs in the pulmonary capillary promotes unloading. A rise in the arterial blood gas level of carbon dioxide causes a shift of the oxygen–haemoglobin dissociation curve to the right, facilitating the release of oxygen to the tissues (Figure 4.1). Carbon dioxide also stimulates the respiratory centres to increase ventilation, which results in carbon dioxide excretion and increased oxygen consumption. Finally, the autonomic effects associated with a high arterial carbon dioxide level, such as increased pulmonary vascular resistance, bronchoconstriction, increased cardiac output and increased ventilation, are in the main due to secondary pH changes.

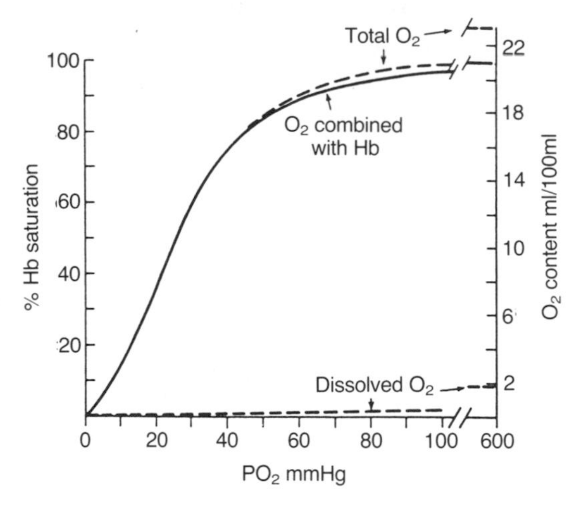

Figure 4.1 Oxygen–haemoglobin dissociation curve. Reproduced from J.B. West, Respiratory Physiology, Williams and Wilkins, 1984.

Given these potential physiological alterations observable during impending respiratory failure, respiratory monitoring of the seriously ill child should systematically include a periodic assessment of respiratory effort, a continuous display of arterial oxygen saturation and an intermittent review of gas exchange and the adequacy of ventilation (Table 4.2).

The clinical observations recorded should include: skin colour, peripheral perfusion, respiratory rate and pattern, whether or not accessory muscles are being used, breath sounds and air entry and the level of consciousness and fatigue.

MONITORS

Pulse oximetry is a readily applicable clinical tool which non-invasively measures arterial oxyhaemoglobin (HbO_2) (Figure 4.2). This device functions by placing a pulsating arterial bed (e.g. finger or earlobe) between a two-wavelength light source and a light detector. The degree of change in transmitted light is proportional to the size of the arterial pulse change, the wavelengths of the light used and the HbO_2 saturations. Assuming that the pulsatile waveform is entirely due to the passage of arterial blood, the use of the appropriate light wavelengths

Table 4.2 Normal values

	Newborn	*Up to 3 years*	*3–6 years*	*Above 6 years*
Respiratory rate (breaths/minute)	40–60	20–30	20–30	15–20
Arterial blood				
pH	7.30–7.40	7.30–7.40	7.35–7.45	7.35–7.45
PCO_2 (mmHg, kPa)	30–35, 4.0.–4.7	30–35, 4.0–4.7	35–45, 4.7–6.0	35–45, 4.7–6.0
PO_2	60–90, 8.0–12	80–100, 10.7–13.3	80–100, 10.7–13.3	80–100, 10.7–13.3
Cardiovascular				
Heart rate (beats/minute)	100–200	100–180	70–150	70–150
Systolic blood pressure (mmHg)	60–90	75–130	90–140	90–140
Diastolic blood pressure (mmHg)	30–60	45–90	50–80	50–80

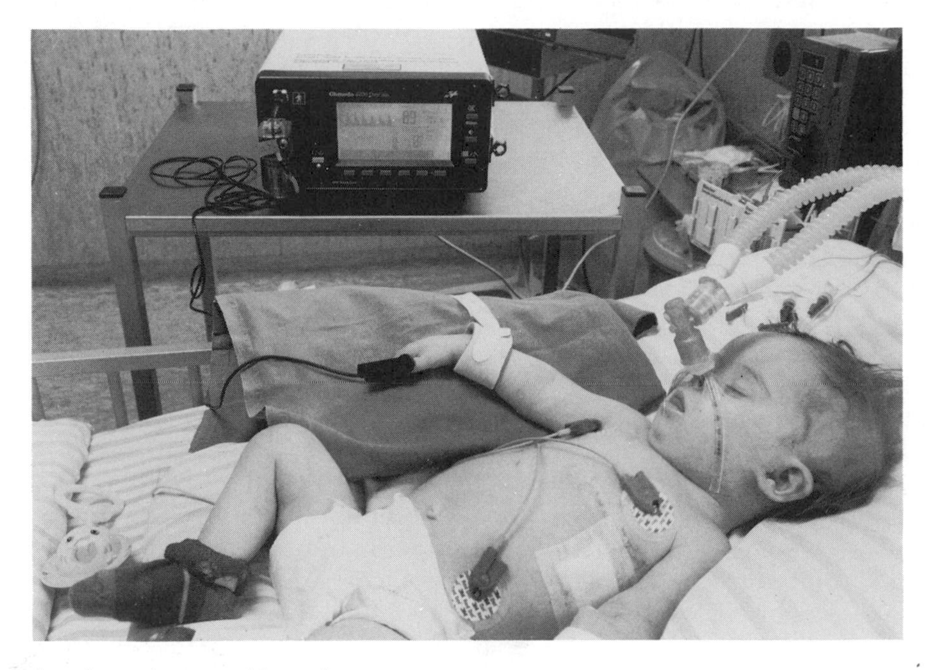

Figure 4.2 A pulse oximeter with probe.

allows the microprocessor inside the oximeter to calculate arterial oxygen saturation (SaO_2) continuously. However, although oximeters are generally reliable as trend monitors there are limitations of important clinical significance in paediatrics.

Walsh *et al.* (1987) examined the ability of pulse oximeters to predict the actual arterial oxygen tension (PaO_2) from the oxyhaemoglobin dissociation curve (see Figure 4.1) in two groups of infants – one with acute cardiopulmonary disease and the other with chronic lung disease. They found that the predicted and actual PaO_2 were within 10 mmHg (1.3 kPa) in 73% of instances in the group with chronic lung disease, but in only 50% of the instances in the group with acute cardiopulmonary disease. The explanation for this finding was that the infants with acute lung disease had fetal haemoglobin concentrations ranging from 26% to 83%, while those with chronic lung disease had less than 10% of fetal haemoglobin. When compared with adult haemoglobin, fetal haemoglobin has a greater oxygen affinity that shifts the oxyhaemoglobin dissociation curve to the left (Figure 4.1). Unfortunately these authors found that correction of the oxyhaemoglobin dissociation curve for the concentration of fetal haemoglobin in these infants failed to improve the value of pulse oximetry as a predictor of PaO_2. It was concluded that although pulse oximetry may be useful as a detector of clincal deterioration, in sick infants it is unreliable as a reflection of PaO_2. Nickerson *et al.* (1987) also demonstrated that pulse oximetry was an unreliable predictor of PaO_2 at saturations above 90% in infants in whom hyperoxia could be potentially harmful. Therefore, whilst pulse oximetry is a powerful tool which has revolutionized the monitoring of patients in respiratory failure, its use should be limited to following changes in arterial oxygenation and not as a quantitative substitute for arterial blood gas analysis.

Transcutaneous gas monitoring provides a reliable means of following trends in PaO_2 and $PaCO_2$ in patients with relatively normal cardiovascular function. In the early 1970s it was shown that transcutaneous measurements of oxygen ($tcPO_2$) through the skin heated to 44°C produced consistent, reliable reflections of PaO_2 in neonates (Huch *et al.*, 1973). However, in older patients such as haemodynamically stable adults, measured $tcPO_2$, although paralleling PaO_2, is only about 80% of its value (Tremper and Shoemaker, 1981). By the late 1970s the so-called 'Severinghaus transcutaneous oxygen electrode' was modified and used to measure carbon dioxide (Severinghaus *et al.*, 1978). Unlike $tcPO_2$, transcutaneous carbon dioxide ($tcPCO_2$) overestimates $PaCO_2$. Various correction factors based on temperature-induced changes in the CO_2 dissociation curve were applied to normalize the $tcPCO_2$ value and in both sick infants (Hansen and Tooley, 1979) and adults (Eletr *et al.*, 1978) correlations with $PaCO_2$ are very good.

In practice, transcutaneous monitoring offers two major advantages over conventional arterial or capillary blood gas monitoring: it is non-invasive and the information is continuous. However, there are potentially important disadvantages. The most important is skin burning, which can be minimized by limiting electrode temperatures to below 44°C, changing the electrode site every four hours and avoiding use in hypothermic patients. Under these circumstances cutaneous burns are unusual. Another disavantage is a 20–30 minute equilibration time whenever the site is changed and the need for regular electrode maintenance. Despite these problems, arterial hypoxaemia can be reliably tracked by $tcPO_2$ as long as cardiac output is maintained, with the $tcPO_2$ values being more sensitive to changes in blood flow than to blood pressure (Shapiro and Cane, 1989) and in both intubated and non-intubated patients $tcPCO_2$ monitoring is a reliable means of non-invasively assessing $PaCO_2$.

RESPIRATORY THERAPY

For practical purposes we can consider the treatment of respiratory dysfunction in terms of treating hypoxia and hypercarbia. Appropriate management is aimed firstly at prevention, secondly at early diagnosis and thirdly at a clear understanding of the pathophysiology and way in which the proposed treatment works to maintain or restore good lung function.

HYPOXIA

Hypoxia must be treated by the administration of supplementary oxygen. At the same time attempts should be made to correct the underlying problem (Table 4.3). Local processes such as atelectasis and bronchopneumonia can result in a portion of the pulmonary blood flow perfusing unventilated alveoli, so-called intrapulmonary shunt, which in some cases may be effectively treated by pulmonary toilet and postural change. With a large shunt fraction (i.e. greater than 25% of pulmonary blood flow 'seeing' non-ventilated lung), PaO_2 is not significantly improved by solely increasing the fractional inspired oxygen concentration (FiO_2). In these cases a diffuse pulmonary process is usually present and a form of assisted positive airways pressure is required. Such assistance may be required for severe impairment of chest wall mechanics from rib fractures, pain, weakness, etc., even in the absence of pulmonary parenchymal disease.

There are several methods of administering oxygen (Table 4.4). Nasal catheters and cannulae are not usually tolerated by younger patients. Oxygen delivered via the oxygen inlet of an incubator rarely exceeds an FiO_2 of 0.4. When oxygen is delivered into a tent the concentration varies depending on leaks. Regardless of the techniques, it is essential that the administered oxygen is heated and humidified. To avoid damage to the lungs, oxygen administration should be discontinued as soon as possible (as indicated by blood gas measurements). An FiO_2 below 0.6 is preferred so as to minimize the risk

Table 4.3 Causes of hypoxia

Decreased PaO_2 (hypoxaemia)
Impaired diffusion
Ventilation/perfusion mismatch
Alveolar hypoventilation
Increased pulmonary shunt
Decreased oxygen content in arterial blood
Decreased haemoglobin concentration
Decreased PaO_2
Carbon monoxide poisoning
Methaemoglobinaema
Shift to the right in the oxyhaemoglobin dissociation curve
Decreased cardiac output
Myocardial depression
Increased peripheral vascular resistance
Increased pulmonary vascular resistance
Decreased circulating blood volume

Table 4.4 Methods of oxygen administration

	Maximum achievable FiO_2 at 6–10 l/min of oxygen (%)
Nasopharyngeal catheter	50
Nasal prongs	50
Masks	
without reservoir bag	50
with reservoir bag (partial rebreathing)	70
with reservoir (non-rebreathing)	95
Venturi	24, 28, 35, 40
Incubator	40
Canopy tent	50
Head box	95

of oxygen toxicity. Reduction in the FiO_2 should be carried out cautiously in a stepwise manner. To facilitate this process both the concentration and duration of oxygen therapy must be recorded accurately. A well calibrated oxygen analyser must be used to check the inspired concentration at least every two hours. The necessity for monitoring PaO_2 in preterm newborn infants is related to both pulmonary oxygen toxicity and the danger of retinopathy of prematurity. In any patient, oxygen should be administered at the lowest concentration sufficient to maintain the PaO_2 between 50–100 mmHg (6.7–13.3 kPa). Continuous measurement or monitoring of $tcPO_2$ or SaO_2 has been used in addition to the direct measurement of arterial blood gases for following the adequacy of oxygenation (see above). Lastly, it should also be remembered that supplemental oxygen may cause further respiratory depression if there has been chronic respiratory failure and a loss of sensitivity to carbon dioxide – this is generally uncommon in paediatric practice, but has been encountered in children with cystic fibrosis.

Positive end expiratory pressure (PEEP) has also been used in the management of acute respiratory failure. PEEP or continuous positive airway pressure (CPAP) has been shown to increase lung compliance by recruiting additional areas of the lung for ventilation. PEEP or CPAP can therefore improve oxygenation by decreasing intrapulmonary shunt and can improve ventilatory mechanics by increasing compliance. The addition of some PEEP to all mechanical ventilation modes is a common practice in maintaining an adequate functional residual capacity. However, PEEP may adversely affect lung mechanics if hyperinflation occurs, which results in impaired pulmonary perfusion, further accentuating any ventilation/perfusion mismatch. Therefore PEEP is generally not indicated when there is already regional hyperinflation, such as occurs in bronchopulmonary dysplasia (Table 4.5). In this context a strategy for treating hypoxia is outlined in Table 4.6.

Table 4.5 Positive end expiratory pressure

Advantages
Increased functional residual capacity
Recruits additional lung units improving compliance
Reduces pulmonary shunt fraction
Allows for a decrease in FiO_2

Disadvantages
Increases mean airway pressure leading to reduced venous return
Can increase 'dead space' by impairing perfusion to hyperinflated regions
Can increase pulmonary vascular resistance and right heart dysfunction
Altered renal blood flow with increase in antidiuretic hormone release
Barotrauma caused by increased airway pressure

Table 4.6 Initial treatment of hypoxia

1. Increase FiO_2 to maintain $SaO_2 > 90\%$ (see Table 4.4)

2. Consider positive pressure and PEEP, if large shunt:
   Indications – hypoxaemia with $FiO_2 > 0.5$
   diffuse lung disease
   maintain lung volume

3. Initiate aggressive pulmonary toilet

4. Eliminate the underlying cause, e.g.:
   pain
   fluid overload
   atelectasis
   bronchopneumonia

5. Correct systemic abnormalities, e.g.:
   hypovolaemia
   sepsis
   carbon monoxide poisoning

HYPERCARBIA

Hypercarbia is treated by increasing alveolar minute ventilation, either by eliminating the cause of hypoventilation or by mechanical ventilation. The alveolar minute ventilation is that portion of the minute ventilation that is responsible for gas exchange. $PaCO_2$ is linearly related to alveolar ventilation, with the $PaCO_2$ value changing inversely with changes in alveolar ventilation. A decrease in the alveolar minute ventilation can be caused by mechanical or central nervous system impairment. Insufficient alveolar ventilation results in both hypoxia and hypercarbia, because neither gas will be exchanged. Administration of oxygen may maintain sufficient oxygen content in the alveolus, even during hypoventilation, which will provide reasonable oxygen exchange. Hence, a decrease in PaO_2 is a relatively late finding in those patients receiving supplemental oxygen. However, the alveolar CO_2 increases relatively rapidly and in direct proportion to the decrease in alveolar ventilation. The $PaCO_2$ increases in direct proportion to the alveolar CO_2, e.g. a halving of alveolar ventilation results in a doubling of $PaCO_2$.

When shallow (or ineffectual) breathing is present, the dead space (i.e. ventilated but non-perfused regions) becomes a larger fraction of each breath. This also results in a decrease in alveolar ventilation, even if the lung parenchyma is normal. The common causes of hypoventilation and increased dead space ventilation are listed in Table 4.7. When hypercarbia has been found and its cause considered, the most appropriate treatment can be effectively initiated. Increasing alveolar ventilation is relatively easy with mechanical ventilation, but an increase in mean airway pressure occurs, with its potential detrimental effects (see p. 44).

If the patient is already being treated with full mechanical ventilation the first step is to make sure that the patient is actually receiving an appropriate tidal volume and minute ventilation. Ventilatory system leaks and loss of a portion of the tidal volume through compression loss in the tubing, as well as abnormalities in endotracheal tube function, are common causes. Having excluded mechanical factors, the other causes of hypercarbia may be related to an increase in CO_2 production or an increase in dead space ventilation (Table 4.8). In the latter case, an increase in dead space due to excessive PEEP (particularly when there is already hyperinflation or hypovolaemia) can be corrected by intravenous volume loading.

Table 4.7 Causes of hypercarbia

Pulmonary
Airway obstruction
Impaired chest wall movement
Trauma
Pain
Neuromuscular disorders
Increased dead space ventilation
Shallow breathing (e.g. neuromuscular disease)
Low cardiac output (e.g. hypovolaemia and impaired perfusion)
Positive pressure ventilation
Increased airway pressure with impaired pulmonary perfusion
Extrapulmonary
Impaired ventilatory response to CO_2
Central nervous system depressant drugs (e.g. sedatives)
Central nervous system injury (e.g. head trauma)
Increased CO_2 production
Fever
Increased muscle activity (e.g. shivering, seizures)
Increased respiratory quotient from excess dietary carbohydrate
Sepsis

Table 4.8 Hypercarbia in patients receiving mechanical ventilation

Correct mechanical problems
- Endotracheal tube leak or plugging
- Airways plugging
- Airleak from lung or chest tubes
- Leak in ventilator

Correct increased dead space
- Treat hypovolaemia
- Decrease mean airway pressure

Correct increased CO_2 production
- Control fever
- Decrease activity
- Control sepsis
- Avoid excess carbohydrate leading to higher respiratory quotient

ENDOTRACHEAL INTUBATION

There are four absolute indications for controlling the airway by endotracheal intubation. Firstly, maintaining the patency of the airway where problems are present or anticipated, e.g. direct airway trauma, oedema or infection. Secondly, to protect the airway from aspiration in states of altered consciousness, where airway protective mechanisms may be lost or impaired. Thirdly, to facilitate pulmonary toilet and avoid airway obstruction when there is marked atelectasis and pulmonary infection – an inadequate cough might necessitate more direct access to the airways for suctioning. Fourthly, when positive pressure breathing is indicated because of inadequate spontaneous ventilation (see hypercarbia, p. 45).

In practice, establishing airway and respiratory support for the acutely ill child should be carried out by experienced staff, because such patients can deteriorate rapidly – particularly at the time of inducing anaesthesia. Following preoxygenation with 100% inspired oxygen, a variety of agents are used to facilitate endotracheal intubation, which include intravenous induction with drugs such as fentanyl, midazolam and suxamethonium and inhalational induction with gases such as halothane or isoflurane. Table 4.9 provides a guide to the appropriate endotracheal tube size, length and suction catheter used in the paediatric age range and Figure 4.3 illustrates two commonly used methods of fixation.

Table 4.9 Endotracheal tube size and suction catheters

Age	*Weight (kg)*	*Endotracheal tube (mm)*	*Length at lip (cm)*	*Length at nose (cm)*	*Suction catheter (French gauge)*
Newborn	<0.7	2.0	5.0	6.0	5.0
	<1	2.5	5.5	7.0	5.0
	1	3.0	6.0	7.5	6.0
	2	3.0	7.0	9.0	6.0
	3	3.0	8.5	10.5	6.0
	3.5	3.5	9.0	11	7.0
3 months	6.0	3.5	10	12	7.0
1 year	10	4.0	11	14	8.0
2 years	12	4.5	12	15	8.0
3 years	14	4.5	13	16	8.0
4 years	16	5.0	14	17	10
6 years	20	5.5	15	19	10
8 years	24	6.0	16	20	12
10 years	30	6.5	17	21	12
12 years	38	7.0	18	22	12–14
14 years	50	7.5	19	23	14

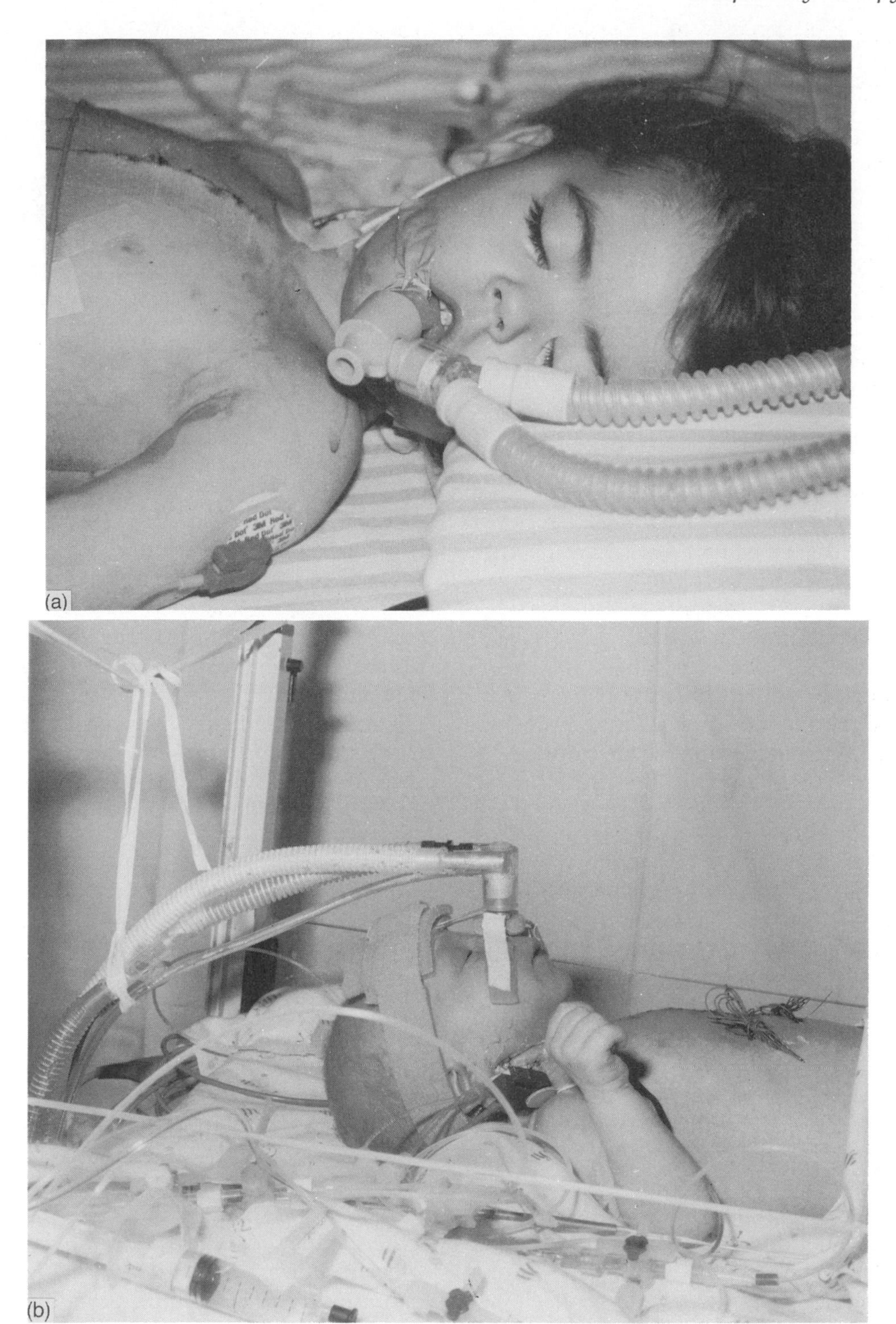

Figure 4.3 Endotracheal tube fixation for oral (a) and nasal (b) tubes.

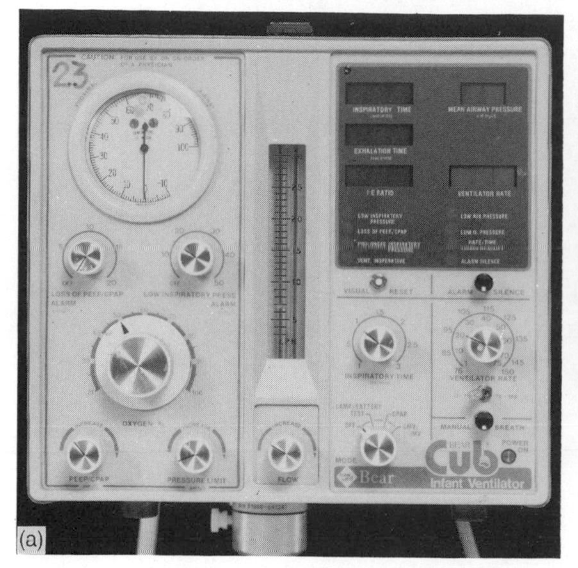

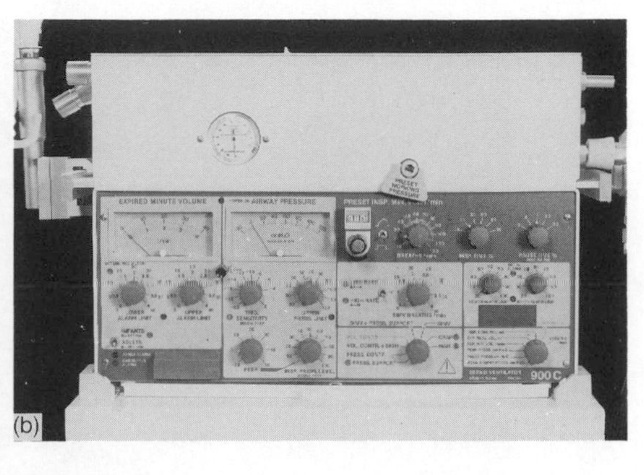

Figure 4.4 The infant Bear Cub (a) and Servo 900C (b) ventilators.

MECHANICAL VENTILATION

Mechanical ventilatory support using positive pressure ventilation is most commonly used. Positive pressure creates transairway pressure by increasing the intratracheal pressure relative to the pleural pressure. This action leads to lung expansion, which in turn leads to chest wall expansion. This approach provides the ability to ventilate adequately despite major impairments in the mechanics of the lung or chest wall. Lung volume can be maintained despite increased airways resistance and decreased lung compliance and a collapsed lung can be re-expanded, decreasing intrapulmonary shunting and increasing the PaO_2.

A variety of ventilators are used in paediatric mechanical ventilation (Figure 4.4). The effectiveness of a particular ventilator depends not least on the skill and experience of those administering this form of therapy – though of course, the functional characteristics of the machine itself are also an important factor! One type may best suit a particular age group under certain conditions (Tables 4.10 and 4.11). The volume cycled (pressure limited) machine (Figure 4.4b) is effective when airway resistance is markedly increased and lung compliance is decreased, because even under these circumstances the appropriate tidal volume will continue to be delivered to the patient. However, a sudden increase in lung compliance may lead to intrathoracic air leak or pneumothorax, which is difficult to detect unless inspiratory pressure is monitored. In contrast, use of the pressure cycled (flow rate limited) ventilator (Figure 4.4a) in the presence of leaks disturbs the attainment of the present pressure and thereby alters the cycling pattern. However, a decrease in lung compliance, such as that caused by accumulation of secretions, may be associated with a decrease in tidal volume. This situation may go unrecognized because the ventilator will continue to cycle at the preset pressure.

In conditions associated with low lung volumes, such as hyaline membrane disease, atelectasis and severe pneumonia (e.g. viral, *Pneumocystis carinii*), alveolar collapse may

Table 4.10 Advantages and disadvantages of pressure limited and volume limited ventilation

	Pressure limited	*Volume limited*
Advantages	Avoids excessive inflating pressures Decreased risk of barotrauma	Constant volume delivered High inflating pressures reflect changes in mechanics
Disadvantages	Variable volume delivered No signs of altered mechanics	Capable of generating very high inflating pressures Increased risk of barotrauma

Table 4.11 Comparison between ventilator types in common use for infants (Bear Cub) and children (Servo 900C)

	Bear Cub	*Servo 900C*
Inspiratory cycling	Time	Time or assist
Inspiratory limit	Time or pressure	Volume or pressure
Drive mechanism	Electric, pneumatic	Electric,pneumatic
Available inspiratory flow pattern	Constant	Constant or decelerating
Inspiratory pressure plateau	With pressure limit	Yes
IMV mode	Yes	Yes
Synchronized	No	Yes
Circuitry	Continuous flow	Demand valve
Continuous distending pressure range	0–20 cmH_20	0–30 cmH_20
Preset parameters	Flow, rate, inspiratory time	Volume, rate, flow
Inspiratory time	0.1–3.0 seconds	I:E of 4:1 and down
Alarms	Complete	High and low pressure High and low exhaled volume

be alleviated or prevented by the use of PEEP (see above). Alveolar pressure is not allowed to return to zero or atmospheric pressure but is held at 3–5 cmH_20 above atmospheric pressure during expiration.

Complications of ventilator therapy occur frequently and all intensive care staff should be continually aware of the potential hazards (Table 4.12). Aseptic technique is important for tracheal airway care because nosocomial infection constitutes a large and preventable problem. The application of PEEP, increased tidal volumes and increased airway pressure can also produce complications. Potential disruption of the normal ventilation/perfusion matching seen with spontaneous breathing can occur with lung overexpansion and leads to regional hypoperfusion. Cardiac output and oxygen delivery can be impaired by a decrease in venous return, an increase in pulmonary vascular resistance and a decrease in left ventricular output. The more compliant the lung or the less compliant the chest wall, the greater the transmission of positive airway pressure to the mediastinum and the greater the negative effect on cardiac function. The concomitant decrease in cardiac output, in large part, can be overcome by volume loading or inotropic support.

Table 4.12 Complications associated with mechanical ventilation

Respiratory
Tracheal lesions, i.e. erosions, oedema, stenosis, granuloma, obstruction
Accidental endotracheal tube displacement into bronchus, oesophagus or hypopharynx
Infection
Air leaks, i.e. pneumothorax, pneumomediastinum, interstitial emphysema
Air trapping causing hyperinflation
Excessive secretions resulting in atelectasis
Oxygen hazards, e.g depression of ventilation, bronchopulmonary dysplasia
Pulmonary haemorrhage

Circulatory
Impaired venous return resulting in decreased cardiac output and systemic hypotension
Oxygen hazards, e.g. retinopathy of prematurity, cerebral vasoconstriction
Septicaemia
Intracranial haemorrhage, i.e. intraventricular, subarachnoid
Hyperventilation leading to decreased cerebral blood flow

Metabolic
Increased work of breathing because of 'fighting' the ventilator
Alkalosis due to potassium depletion or excessive bicarbonate therapy

Renal and fluid balance
Antidiuresis
Excess water in the inspired gas

Equipment malfunction (mechanical)
Ventilator leaks or valve dysfunction
Overheating of inspired gases
Kinked or disconnected tubes

Barotrauma is the result of high airway inspiratory pressure causing alveolar disruption (Table 4.13). Airway pressure may be reduced by decreasing the tidal volume, PEEP, or peak inspiratory pressure or by paralysing the already sedated patient. Pulmonary interstitial emphysema, pneumomediastinum, pneumoperitoneum and subcutaneous emphysema do not require specific treatment unless there is significant haemodynamic impairment. Poor renal function, as exhibited by decreased glomerular filtration rate, urine production and sodium excretion, can be a consequence of hypoxia and hypercarbia. This may be further compounded by the effects of mechanical ventilation with PEEP on producing an antidiuretic hormone mediated salt and water retaining effect (probably secondary to decreased cardiac output), an increased renal vein pressure and a neural reflex from the pressure distorted atrial wall.

Table 4.13 Conditions associated with pulmonary barotrauma

Impaired expiratory phase
Obstructed endotracheal tube
Obstructive airways disease
Inadequate expiratory time

Excessive alveolar volume or pressure
High inflating pressure
Prolonged inspiration
Inspiratory pressure hold
High PEEP/CPAP

Various causes may result in an acute deterioration during mechanical ventilation. 'Trouble-shooting' should begin with disconnecting the patient from the ventilator and bagging with an FiO_2 of 1.0. Easy ventilation with the bag and patient stabilization suggests a ventilator problem, which should be systematically addressed (e.g. checking the circuit for leaks, checking ventilator function, checking gas flow). However, it should be remembered that 'hand-bagging' can result in an increased tidal volume, which can also be responsible for the patient's improvement. Patients with stiff lungs frequently are dyspnoeic, despite adequate gas exchange. Increasing the tidal volume will correct this subjective feeling and may also account for patient improvement. Difficult bagging at the time of disconnecting the ventilator strongly suggests a problem with the endotracheal tube or the lung to chest wall complex. A suction catheter (see Table 4.9) should be passed down the endotracheal tube to check for narrowing or blockage. Chest examination, blood gases and chest radiography should be ordered. A blocked endotracheal tube should be replaced. A pneumothorax requires chest tube placement. If neither of these are the cause of deterioration, then the possibilities may include new problems such as: an increased oxygen demand due to sepsis; impaired oxyen delivery due to heart failure; or acute pulmonary injury due to gastric aspiration. These and other causes need to be sought for and appropriately treated.

NEWER VENTILATORY SUPPORT TECHNIQUES

High frequency ventilation techniques including high frequency positive pressure ventilation, high frequency jet ventilation and high frequency oscillatory ventilation, achieve adequate ventilation by employing tidal volumes that are often less than actual dead space and respiratory rates of 60–3000 cycles/minute (Figure 4.5). The high velocity ventilations result in increased mixing by Brownian motion, which enhances gas diffusion and exchange. In theory, ventilation is more evenly distributed with the use of decreased airway pressures (Gertsmann *et al.*, 1991). Indications for this form of ventilation may include bronchopleural fistula and refractory hypoxaemia.

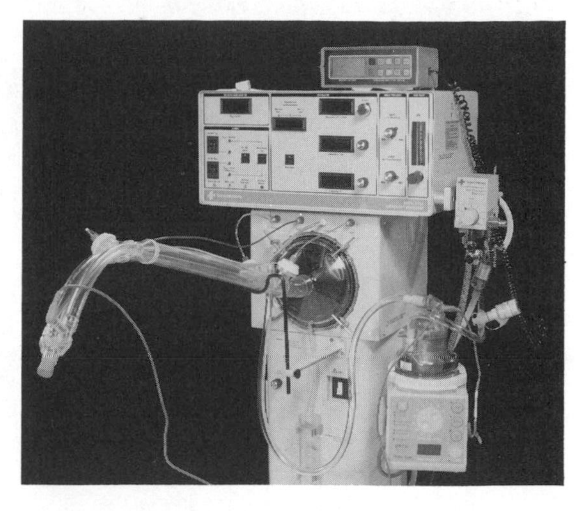

Figure 4.5 A ventilator used for high frequency oscillation.

Extracorporeal membrane oxygenation is designed to provide a variable degree of cardiopulmonary support for a predetermined period of time over which the underlying pulmonary disorder is expected to recover. Potentially, extracorporeal membrane oxygenation allows recovery without subjecting the lungs to the risks of barotrauma or oxygen toxicity. Venoarterial systems may be used to completely take over the child's own heart and lung function (Figure 4.6), although in practice extracorporeal flows may be limited by venous drainage (usually from the right internal jugular vein). Venovenous systems have

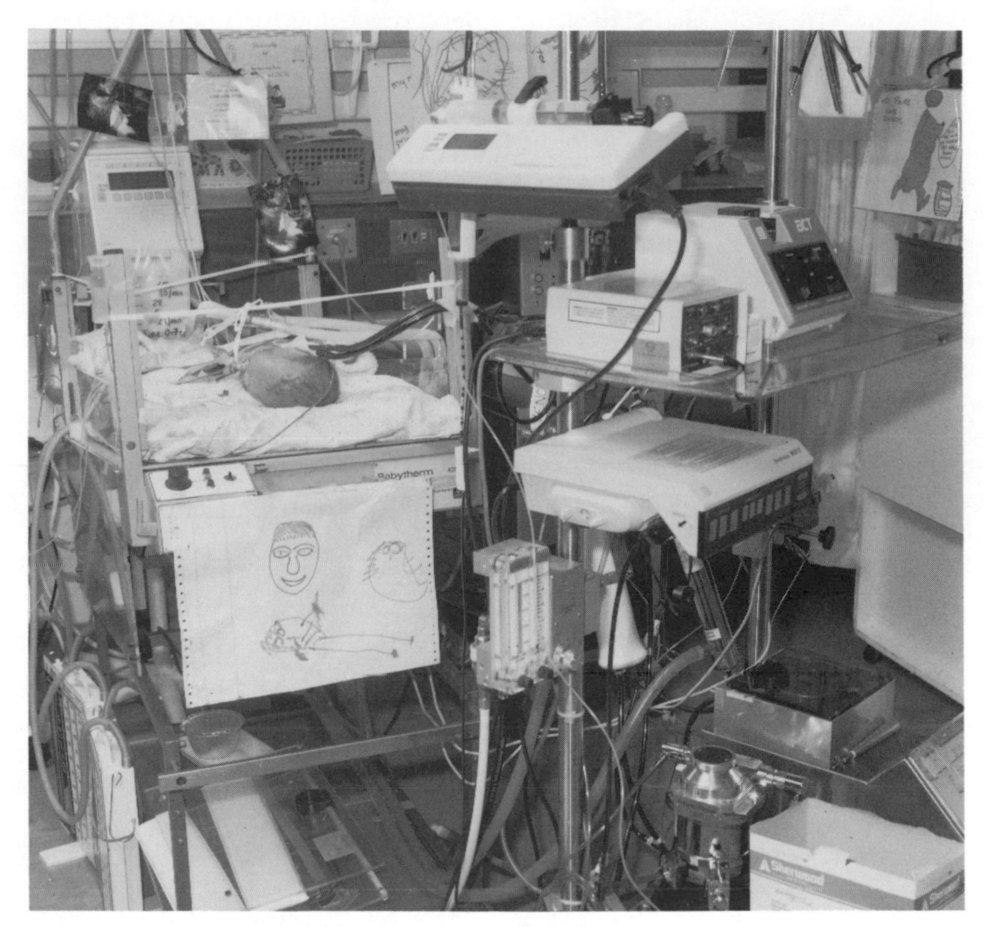

Figure 4.6 Extracorporeal membrane oxygenation.

been used for CO_2 removal and, in the complete absence of pulmonary function, will provide SaO_2 of 80%.

Using extracorporeal support, success has been achieved in neonates with persistent pulmonary hypertension who have failed to respond to conventional mechanical ventilation (Bartlett *et al.*, 1982) and some children with acute lung injury (Pearson *et al.*, 1993). However, appropriate patient selection is a critical and contentious issue. One method is that used by Bartlett (1990) who identifies neonates at high risk for failing to respond to conventional therapy by applying an index of oxygenation, which is related to the mean airway pressure and the FiO_2 used during mechanical ventilation and the achieved PaO_2:

$$\text{Oxygenation index (OI)} = \text{mean airway pressure} \times FiO_2 \times 100/PaO_2\ \text{(mmHg)}.$$

An OI greater than 25 predicts a 50% mortality rate and an OI greater than 40 predicts an 80% mortality rate. Prospective trials have documented an 83% survival rate with extracorporeal membrane oxygenation in neonates, but convincing data in older children and adults is lacking.

GENERAL MANAGEMENT

Finally, in any acutely ill child in respiratory failure the lungs are never treated in isolation. Optimal management includes addressing systemic and pathological factors which may influence the rate of recovery and outcome. In this section we will review some aspects of general treatment for cardiac impairment and sepsis.

CONGESTIVE HEART FAILURE

Congestive heart failure occurs when the heart is not able adequately to provide the tissues' circulatory needs. Since infants and children with this problem have frequent chest infections, it is worthwhile outlining some of its causes and the background to treatment. Clinically, congestive cardiac failure develops over time and can be described as being due to excessive preload, excessive afterload, decreased myocardial contractility or dysrhythmias or any combination of these derangements. An increased preload, or 'volume loaded' heart, is commonly seen in patients with a ventricular septal defect or patent ductus arteriosus, where blood is being 'shunted' from the left side of the heart to the right side. To ensure an adequate cardiac output the heart has to work harder. If there is inadequate myocardial reserve then failure will develop. This problem may also be encountered in patients with incompetent cardiac valves, arteriovenous fistulae, severe anaemia and renal failure with fluid overload. An increased afterload may be due to systemic hypertension or obstruction to the 'outflow' of a ventricle. Cardiac muscle dysfunction may be due to a variety of conditions, including: infectious myocarditis, cardiomyopathy, septicaemia, asphyxia, acidosis, hypocalcaemia and hypomagnesaemia.

To increase the cardiac output the heart has a limited number of compensatory mechanisms, which include dilation, hypertrophy and increasing sympathetic tone. Systemically, one important effect of congestive heart failure is an increased extracellular fluid volume resulting in weight gain, peripheral oedema, ascites and pleural effusions – which may further exacerbate cardiorespiratory function. Therefore, when treating such patients, the primary aim is to improve heart function and increase the tissue oxygen supply. This can be achieved by the use of specific measures when necessary (e.g. treatment of hypertension or with digoxin) as well as by correcting the electrolytes, pH, salt and water abnormalities.

MANAGEMENT OF SEPSIS AND SHOCK

The term sepsis describes a group of signs and symptoms associated with the presence of an infectious agent in the blood stream. Such infections may be transient or persistent and they may be clinically silent for hours to days. By the time of presentation, there may be a variety of signs and symptoms, including: an altered level of consciousness, seizures, tachypnoea, tachycardia, fever, shock, skin rashes and renal failure. Even in the child initially presenting with a pneumonia, one should remain vigilant about the possibility of more generalized sepsis, since worsening tachypnoea, hypoxia or hypercarbia may represent the development of systemic circulatory impairment which requires supportive therapy. In contrast to congestive heart failure, this state of 'shock' is a more acute state of circulatory dysfunction which has resulted in a failure to deliver sufficient amounts of oxygen and other nutrients to satisfy the body's requirements. Pathologically, we divide shock into three phases: compensated, uncompensated and irreversible. In the compensated state vital organ (heart, kidney, brain and liver) function is maintained by intrinsic compensatory mechanisms. As the underlying process progresses to an uncompensated state, the efficiency of the cardiovascular system deteriorates and tissue perfusion becomes compromised. Eventually, endogenous tissue and systemic mechanisms perpetuate and contribute to an irreversible state of vital organ damage or even death.

Unfortunately, it is only in the minority of cases that the specific aetiological agent causing the problem and its specific antimicrobial sensitivities is known at the time of treatment. Drug therapy is therefore based on the most likely pathogens for each age group and local patterns of antibiotic resistance (Table 4.14). However, even though the 'right' antibiotics may be being used, the place and importance of supportive therapy is to try and improve oxygen and nutrient delivery to the tissues, before an irreversible pathological process has had time to develop. In practice this entails optimizing cardiac output by manipulating 'preload' with adequate intravenous fluids, myocardial contractility, heart rate and 'afterload'. This often includes the use of drugs to augment myocardial function and change the pulmonary and systemic vascular resistances (Table 4.15).

Table 4.14 Common causative agents and sepsis

Organism	*Usual age*	*Other*
E. coli and other enterics	Neonate	Immunocompromised children, patients with central lines
Group B streptococcus	Neonate	Diabetics
Haemophilus influenzae	6 weeks–6 years	
Pneumococci		
Meningococci	6 weeks–adult	Immunodeficiency
Group A streptococcus		
Staphylococci	All ages	Patients with central lines

Table 4.15 Common cardiovascular drugs used in shock

Drug	*Effects*	
Dopamine	Increases	Myocardial contractility
		Systemic vascular resistance (at high doses)
		Renal, mesenteric, coronary, and cerebral blood flow
	Decreases	Systemic and pulmonary vascular resistance (at low dose) (pulmonary vascular resistance may be increased at high dose)
Dobutamine	Increases	Cardiac output
		Stroke volume
	Decreases	Systemic vascular resistance
Adrenaline	Increases	Myocardial contractility
		Heart rate
		Arteriolar resistance
		Pulmonary vascular resistance
	Decreases	Venous capacity
		Airway resistance
Nitroprusside	Decreases	Systemic and pulmonary vascular resistance

REFERENCES

Bartlett, R.H. (1990) Extracorporeal life support for cardiopulmonary failure. *Current Problems in Surgery*, **27**, 623.

Bartlett, R.H., Andrews, A.F. and Toomasian, J.M. (1982) Extracorporeal membrane oxygenation (ECMO) for newborn respiratory failure: 45 cases. *Surgery*, **92**, 425.

Eletr, S., Jimison, H., Ream, A.K. *et al.* (1978) Cutaneous monitoring of systemic PCO_2 on patients in the respiratory intensive care unit being weaned from the ventilator. *Acta Anaesthesiologica, Scandinavica*, **68**, 123.

Gertsmann, D.R., deLemos, R.A. and Clark, R.H. (1991) High frequency ventilation: issues of strategy. *Clinics in Perinatology*, **18**(3), 563.

Hansen, T.N. and Tooley, W.H. (1979) Skin surface carbon dioxide tension in sick infants. *Pediatrics*, **64**, 942.

Huch, R., Huch, A. and Lubbers, D.E. (1973) Transcutaneous measurement of blood PO_2 ($tcPO_2$): method and application in perinatal medicine. *Journal of Perinatal Medicine*, **1**, 183.

Nickerson, B.G., Sarkisan, C., Austin, P. *et al.* (1987) Performance of arterial and pulse oximeters over a wide range of saturations. *American Review of Respiratory Disease*, **135**, A69.

Pearson, G.A., Grant, J., Fields, D. *et al.* (1993) Extracorporeal life support in paediatrics. *Archives of Diseases of Childhood*, **68**, 94.

Rogers, M.C. (1987) The development of pediatric intensive care, in *Textbook of Pediatric Intensive Care*, (ed. M.C. Rogers), Williams and Wilkins, London, pp. 1–4.

Severinghaus, J.W., Stafford, M. and Bradley, A.F. (1978) $tcPCO_2$ electrode design, calibration and temperature gradient problems. *Acta Anaesthesiologica Scandinavica*, **68**, 118.

Shapiro, B.A. and Cane, R.D. (1989) Blood gas monitoring: yesterday, today, and tomorrow. *Critical Care Medicine*, **17**, 573.

Tremper, K.K. and Shoemaker, W.W. (1981) Transcutaneous oxygen monitoring of critically ill adults, with and without low flow shock. *Critical Care Medicine*, **9**, 706.

Walsh, M.C., Noble, L.M., Carlo, W.A. *et al.* (1987) Relationship of pulse oximetry to arterial oxygen tensions in infants. *Critical Care Medicine*, **15**, 1102.

ASSESSMENT OF THE CHILD WITH RESPIRATORY DISEASE

Juliette Hussey and S.Ammani Prasad

INDICATIONS FOR CHEST PHYSIOTHERAPY

Chest physiotherapy in the child with respiratory disease is indicated to prevent or to treat atelectasis and in the presence of retained bronchopulmonary secretions. It aims to remove such secretions, reduce airflow obstruction and reinflate areas of lung collapse, thereby improving oxygenation and reducing the work of breathing (Cochrane *et al.*, 1977). Changes in total lung and thoracic compliance reported following chest physiotherapy suggest an improvement in intrapulmonary shunting due to clearance of secretions from peripheral airways (Lyle *et al.*, 1979).

Atelectasis and retention of secretions cause ventilation/perfusion mismatch and if untreated may lead to infection and result in pneumonia (Bartlett *et al.*, 1973). Chest physiotherapy has been shown to be beneficial in the treatment of acute lobar atelectasis (Stiller *et al.*, 1990; Marini *et al.*, 1979; Johnson and Pierson, 1986; Mackenzie and Shin, 1985). Mackenzie *et al.* (1978) reported evidence of radiological improvement in 68% of patients when comparing chest radiographs taken prior to and 24 hours following chest physiotherapy. Treatment was most effective in unilobar densities and in atelectasis of acute onset. Loss of lung volume due to collapse as seen radiologically is a definite indication for chest physiotherapy and should be treated promptly. Positive bacteriological cultures from the airway are common in patients with artificial airways and the opening of obstructed airways by the removal of retained secretions may prevent the development of pneumonia. Other indications for chest physiotherapy include an impaired cough/gag reflex and respiratory muscle weakness which may occur in patients with neuromuscular disease.

ANAESTHESIA AND INTUBATION

Postoperative respiratory insufficiency may be a result of increased metabolic demands and impaired lung function (Fairshter and Williams, 1987). The characteristic postoperative pulmonary abnormality is of a restrictive nature, lung and chest wall compliance are reduced, resulting in a fall in both functional residual capacity (FRC) and vital capacity (VC) (Craig, 1981). The reduction in FRC has important consequences as small airways which lack cartilaginous support require transmitted positive transmural pressure to keep them open. With a low FRC these airways are narrowed or may close, resulting in low ventilation perfusion relationships and hypoxaemia. Failure of an airway to reopen leads to atelectasis of the lung unit it serves.

Inhaled anaesthetic agents may impair the compensatory mechanism of hypoxic pulmonary vasoconstriction (HPV) (Nunn, 1990). HPV is a component of a control system that matches ventilation and perfusion by increasing blood flow to areas of lung which are better aerated, thus preserving arterial oxygen tension (Voelkel, 1986). Under normal circumstances blood flow to atelectatic areas is reduced (Eisenkraft, 1990). Phagocytosis and ciliary activity normally provide adequate airway clearance, but these defence mechanisms may be impaired by anaesthetic drugs, hyperoxic mixtures of gas and intubation (Gamsu *et al.*, 1976; Voelkel, 1986; Fairshter and Williams, 1987). Hyperoxic mixtures with a fractional inspired oxygen concentration (FiO_2) of 0.4–1.0 decrease the rate of mucociliary clearance, diminish alveolar macrophage function and cause parenchymal damage to the lung (Stevens, 1977). Impairment of mucociliary clearance may be significant in the development of postoperative atelectasis (Gamsu *et al.*, 1976). The infant is particularly vulnerable to obstruction of the tracheobronchial tree due to the relatively small calibre of the conducting airways. The consequences of this may be more critical due to the lack of collateral ventilatory channels in the developing lungs (Johnson and Pierson, 1986). Intubation bypasses the defence mechanisms of filtration and humidification of inspired gas by the upper airway. Distortion and degeneration of cilia leading to impaired mucous transport for a period of two to seven days has been documented in animal studies following two hours of endotracheal intubation (Fairshter and Williams, 1987).

DETERIORATION IN RESPIRATORY STATUS

Changes in arterial blood gases, an increase in ventilatory requirement or respiratory support (unexplained by a change in metabolic status) are indicative of a deterioration in respiratory status. Such changes are often acute and are an indication for assessment of the patient by a physiotherapist and commencement of treatment if these changes are found to be a result of secretion retention or atelectasis.

CHEST RADIOLOGY

Radiological evidence of segmental, lobar or total lung collapse, as indicated by areas of opacity accompanied by loss of volume, indicate the need for assessment and possible chest physiotherapy intervention. It is important to note that clinical examination alone does not always indicate an area of lung pathology. The interpretation of chest radiology examinations is fully discussed in Chapter 3.

CHRONIC SPUTUM PRODUCTION

Chest physiotherapy is an integral part of the day-to-day management of patients with chronic lung disease and bronchial hypersecretion such as seen in cystic fibrosis (CF), bronchiectasis, chronic aspiration and cilial dyskinesia. Removal of mucopurulent secretions is aimed at preventing or delaying the progression of lung disease and complications such as atelectasis and hyperinflation.

NEUROLOGICAL DISORDERS

Respiratory muscle weakness, in neuromuscular disorders (e.g. Guillain–Barré syndrome, myasthenia gravis, muscular dystrophy) may lead to a fall in tidal volume and vital capacity leading to hypoventilation. In addition such patients often have a weak or ineffective cough (resulting from both respiratory and abdominal muscle weakness). Atelectasis and retention of secretions may result and such patients often require physiotherapy intervention. Reduced levels of consciousness (pathological or iatrogenic caused by sedatives and paralysing agents) may also impair the patient's respiratory function. Spinal cord injury interrupts the autonomic nervous system and results in loss of motor function below the level of injury. Chest physiotherapy on a prophylactic basis may be required for tetraplegic patients where chest complications are common.

CONTRAINDICATIONS TO CHEST PHYSIOTHERAPY INTERVENTION

In certain situations chest physiotherapy may be of no value or indeed detrimental. It is vital that those involved in the care of the child with respiratory disease are aware that physiotherapy is neither necessary or appropriate in several situations, thereby avoiding distress to both the child and family and the potential serious consequences of inappropriate intervention.

INHALED FOREIGN BODY

Inhalation of a foreign body usually results in the impaction of the object in a main or stem bronchus. Chest physiotherapy aiming to remove the foreign body is absolutely contraindicated and its application may have potentially dangerous consequences. If applied the object may be mobilized either into a central airway, where it may completely occlude any airflow, or into the laryngeal region, where a vagal response may lead to devastating airway spasm and the need for emergency tracheostomy. Removal of the foreign body should only be performed under controlled conditions using bronchoscopic techniques (Phelan *et al.*, 1990). Following bronchoscopic removal, chest physiotherapy may be indicated due to the associated bacterial colonization of the lower respiratory tract and the inflammatory pneumonic process which commonly occurs distal to the site of obstruction (Dinwiddie, 1990).

SEVERE BRONCHOSPASM

In infants and children with severe respiratory embarrassment due to bronchospasm, chest physiotherapy manoeuvres such as percussion, vibrations and forced expirations are likely to further exacerbate airflow obstruction. Treatment should only be performed if indicated (e.g. in the presence of mucous plugging) and with extreme care, after bronchodilators have been administered and the patient is responding well. In ventilated patients particular care should be taken with manual hyperinflation as high peak pressures may lead to air leak (e.g. pnuemothorax).

ACUTE BRONCHIOLITIS

Acute bronchiolitis is a disease of infancy, characterized by a harsh cough, hyperinflation of the chest and respiratory distress. It is not usually associated with an increase in lower respiratory tract secretions. These infants respond very poorly to handling and should be nursed with a minimal handling policy, appropriate respiratory support with well humidified inspired gas and careful nasopharyngeal suction as necessary. In the acute stages of the disease physiotherapy procedures may result in an acute exacerbation of respiratory difficulty and are usually contraindicated. Webb *et al.* (1985) and Dick *et al.* (1992) reported no positive benefit from chest physiotherapy in the natural course of acute viral bronchiolitis and therefore, unless complicated by other acute lung pathology, physiotherapy is usually inappropriate for this condition.

LOBAR PNEUMONIA

Chest physiotherapy has been demonstrated to be of little value in the acute or consolidatory phase of lobar pneumonia, unless complicated by additional pulmonary pathology (Graham and Bradley, 1978). However, in the productive phase of the disease chest physiotherapy may be helpful.

INVESTIGATIONS OF RESPIRATORY FUNCTION

BLOOD GAS ANALYSIS

Measurement of arterial blood gas parameters such as arterial oxygen tension (PaO_2), arterial carbon dioxide tension ($PaCO_2$), hydrogen ion concentration (pH), standard bicarbonate and base excess is an essential tool in the assessment of the severity of lung disease and response to treatment in the acutely ill infant or child. An alteration of blood gas indices from normal indicates the nature of the problem, including whether it is respiratory or metabolic in origin. If associated with respiratory insufficiency appropriate adjustments to respiratory support can be made. In infancy and childhood the normal arterial oxygen tension is lower than that of the adult. This may be due to the higher closing volume, exceeding the FRC and resulting in airway closure during normal ventilation (Mansell *et al.* 1972). From birth to approximately one year of age normal PaO_2 levels range from 8.0–12.0 kPa and gradually rise to between 10.7–13.3 kPa by six years of age. Normal adult values (12–14 kPa) are usually reached during the teenage years. The normal $PaCO_2$ is 4.0–4.7 kPa between birth and three years of age, increasing slightly to 4.7–6.0 kPa in subsequent years (see also Table 4.2).

A low arterial PaO_2 may be due to hypoventilation, diffusion impairment, ventilation/perfusion inequality or intrapulmonary shunting. A raised $PaCO_2$ is always observed in the presence of hypoventilation and may occur in conjunction with ventilation/perfusion inequality. The acid-base status of the blood is closely linked to $PaCO_2$. Carbon dioxide retention is associated with a respiratory acidosis. If acute falls in pH are not corrected, a compensatory acidosis results with the excretion of hydrogen ions by the renal system, thereby tending to return the pH towards normal. A high $PaCO_2$ with a normal pH indicates chronic respiratory acidosis. In contrast respiratory alkalosis is characterized by a low $PaCO_2$ and a high pH. Capillary blood gas analysis, which gives accurate measurements of PCO_2 and pH, may be used if arterial samples are not readily obtainable.

Transcutaneous oxygen measurements are frequently used in neonatal units and allow continuous monitoring of oxygen tension. Such devices need to be regularly calibrated and the probe site changed frequently in order to prevent skin damage (Southall *et al.*, 1987; Fanconi *et al.*, 1985). Pulse oximetry is also very valuable as a continual non-invasive measurement of oxygen saturation (SaO_2). It allows safe monitoring of patients at risk of developing acute hypoxic episodes (Taylor and Whitwam, 1988). Although good correlations with arterial blood gas values at saturation levels greater than 80% are documented (Fanconi, 1988, 1989; Sidi *et al.*, 1987), these devices have significant limitations and should be used only to follow trends in arterial oxygenation as discussed in Chapter 4. Malposition of the probe leading to an inadequate trace and therefore unreliable values can be problematic, particularly in the more active child. In low perfusion states readings may be inaccurate and therefore may not be so useful in patients with low cardiac output. However, when care is taken to use high quality arterial wave forms, pulse oximetry in children is particularly useful as a means of continual monitoring of patient well-being during procedures such as chest physiotherapy.

PULMONARY FUNCTION TESTS

The simplest device for the measurement of

Table 5.1 Normal values

Respiratory rate

Age/years	*Breaths/minute*
0	40–60
1–3	20–30
3–6	20–30
>6	15–20
Adult	15

Heart rate

Age/years	*Average rate/minute*	*Minimum/maximum*
0	125	100–200
1–3	130	100–180
3–8	105	70–150
8–12	85	55–25

Respiratory function

	Neonate (per kg)	*Age 7 (per kg)*	*Adult (per kg)*
VC (ml)	35	65	54
FEV1 (ml)	–	60	51
PEFR (l/min)	2.5	8	7
TV (ml/breath)	7	7	7
RV (ml)	23	18	16
FRC (ml)	28	30	30

pulmonary function is the peak flow meter. This is an inexpensive tool providing readily repeatable results. It may be used for the evaluation of progress and home monitoring of bronchial reactivity. Peak expiratory flow rate is usually measured using a Wright peak flow meter or a mini peak flow meter. It requires the patient to be able to perform a fast expiration and is effort dependent. Measurements are in litres per minute or as a percentage of predicted normal (Table 5.1). Spirometry is usually performed in a pulmonary function laboratory or using a portable spirometer to assess VC, forced vital capacity (FVC), forced expiratory volume in one second (FEV1) and forced expiratory flow rates (FEF 25–75%). VC and FVC are expressed as volume in ml or litres and also as a percentage of predicted normal. The FEV1 is often expressed as a ratio of FVC. An FEV1:FVC ratio of less than 70% is diagnostic of airway obstruction. Static lung volume measurements are performed using plethysmography or gas dilution techniques in a respiratory laboratory. The FRC is usually measured using spirometry with a helium dilution technique; total gas volume (TGV) requires the use of whole body plethysmography and measures the total gas within the chest including FRC and trapped gas. It is likely to be abnormal in chronic airway obstruction, e.g. cystic fibrosis. Measurement of the residual volume (RV) and total lung capacity (TLC) ratio also assesses the degree of gas trapping and is usually below 30% in normal, healthy children. FEF at 25%–75% of VC is a more sensitive indicator of small airways obstruction than FEV1. These basic tests of lung function can usually only be performed in children over the age of 4–5 years who are co-operative and understand the requirements of the tests. Measurements of compliance, resistance and FRC can be performed in infants using whole body plethysmography with face mask and airway occlusion techniques and gas dilution (England, 1988; Stocks, 1993). Between the ages of 2–5 years it is not possible to perform accurate pulmonary function testing.

BRONCHOSCOPY

Bronchoscopy allows direct visualization of the tracheobronchial tree and may be performed using a rigid bronchoscope or a flexible fibreoptic device. It enables the detection of a variety of both upper and lower respiratory tract disorders. Transbronchial biopsy and bronchial washings may be taken for diagnostic purposes and bronchoalveolar lavage can be performed under direct vision.

RADIOLOGICAL IMAGING

Chest radiographs are the simplest ways of radiologically diagnosing respiratory tract problems and are invaluable in the physiotherapy assessment of respiratory status. The concept and interpretation of these studies and of more sophisticated imaging modalities such as computerized tomography (CT) and magnetic resonance imaging (MRI) have been discussed fully in Chapter 3, p. 26.

EXERCISE TESTING

A progressive workload on a bicycle ergometer or treadmill may be used to measure the response of heart rate, ventilation, oxygen uptake and carbon dioxide production to exercise. These tests indicate whether a decrease in exercise tolerance is due to abnormalities of ventilation, gas exchange or cardiac status. In its simplest form exercise testing involves a six minute walk or running test. Pulse rate, oxygen saturation and peak flow can be recorded throughout the study. This is a useful way of assessing airway lability and levels of exercise tolerance in the asymptomatic child.

ASSESSMENT OF RESPIRATORY STATUS

Accurate assessment of respiratory status is essential prior to chest physiotherapy. This involves collating information from the case notes and relevant investigations (e.g. chest X-ray), discussion with the medical and nursing team, obtaining a history from the patient or parents as appropriate and observation and examination of the child. This allows the identification of problems and the formulation of a safe and effective treatment plan with both long and short term goals. The relative risks and benefits of each intervention need to be considered carefully and treatment should only be given in the belief that it is indicated and will be effective.

HISTORY

The details of the patient's previous medical history (including birth history), history of the present condition (including relevant investigations), family history, psychological and social situation should be taken from the case notes. If appropriate, the parents and child are questioned in order to obtain a summary of the child's present status. This should include the onset and type of symptoms, details of cough, exercise tolerance, wheeze, dyspnoea, pain and any relevant environmental factors such as passive smoking and household pets. It is also important to assess both the physical and mental development of the child (particularly those with chronic disorders), recording the achievement of relevant milestones. Chronic respiratory or congenital heart disease may result in frequent hospitalization and a degree of parental overprotection, leading to developmental delay. Such detailed assessment may also reveal previously unrecognized mild neurological or developmental disorders. In such instances appropriate referral can then be made and advice should be sought from other specialist disciplines. Valuable

Table 5.2 Physical examination

1. Inspection	*2. Palpation*	*3. Auscultation*
State of consciousness	Pain/tenderness	Breath sounds
Breathing pattern and rate	Expansion and crepitus	Stridor
Respiratory effort	Swelling	Wheeze
Clubbing	Tracheal position/tug	Crackles/crepitations
Cyanosis	Subcutaneous emphysema	Pleural sounds
Structural abnormalities	Percussion	Heart rate

information can also be obtained from the nursing and medical staff caring for the child with regard to the patient's general status, ability to tolerate handling or previous physiotherapy treatments, the amount of secretions and response to suction.

PHYSICAL EXAMINATION

Prior to the commencement of physical examination, the type and degree of respiratory support the patient requires, baseline values of vital signs such as temperature, heart rate, respiratory rate and blood pressure (normal values are listed in Table 5.1) and any analgesia required should be noted. In the intensive care setting note should also be made of any additional monitoring (e.g. central venous pressure, intracranial pressure) or drug support (e.g. inotropes, paralysis and sedative agents) which may influence the application of treatment. The examination of the infant or child should include inspection, palpation and auscultation (Table 5.2). In toddlers physical examination may be quite a challenge as the patient is often unable to or not in the mood to co-operate. The use of play may facilitate the assessment process. Often much of the assessment can be performed in sleeping infants and children. The clinical signs of respiratory failure are listed in Table 5.3.

Inspection

The state of consciousness of the patient should be noted. This may be depressed in patients with neurological deficit, but decreased levels of activity are also seen in other situations, for example, following the use of opiate analgesia and particularly in infants with respiratory distress. Breathing patterns show great variability in newborn and young infants (Pasterkamp, 1990). Significant changes in respiratory rhythm are seen during the first few months of life and respiratory pauses of up to ten seconds are common up to three months of age. Apnoea of more than 15 seconds' duration is abnormal and may be accompanied by bradycardia and cyanosis. Respiratory rate should be noted, bearing in mind that this is variable according to sleep state and wakefulness. Tachypnoea is seen in states of decreased respiratory compliance and in the presence of a metabolic acidosis. Bradypnoea is observed in metabolic alkalosis. Normal values of respiratory rate are listed in Table 5.1.

Table 5.3 Clinical signs of respiratory failure

Tachypnoea	Sweating
(>60–70 in infants)	Pallor
(>40 in older children	Tachycardia
Expiratory grunting	Cool peripheries
Rib cage distortion	Restlessness
Nasal flaring	Reduced activity
Tracheal tug	Inability to feed or cry
Cyanosis	

The child's respiratory effort should be observed with care to note any retraction of the chest wall during inspiration, whether subcostal, intercostal or sternal. In disease states where the lungs are stiff, the negative pleural pressure required to inflate the lungs may lead to distortion of the rib cage (due to the action of the diaphragm). If severe, this will result in paradoxical movement of the chest where the lower rib cage is sucked in as the abdomen moves outward during inspiration (see-sawing). Symmetry of chest excursion should also be noted as unilateral lung disease may result in asymmetric breathing movements. Note should be made of any respiratory noise, such as inspiratory or expiratory stridor or grunting. The latter is an expiratory sound caused by partial closure of the glottis, which helps to slow expiration, maintaining a high expiratory pressure and lung volume in an attempt to keep small airways and alveoli open (i.e. a form of self-applied PEEP). The presence of flaring of the alae nasi is a sensitive sign of respiratory distress. Nasal flaring enlarges the anterior nasal passages and reduces the upper and total airway resistance.

Clubbing of the digits is an enlargement of the connective tissue in the terminal phalanges, the pathogenesis of which is unclear. Clubbing may be idiopathic, acquired or hereditary and is an indicator of chest disease. Acquired clubbing is frequently seen in chronic lung disease such as CF. The colour of the peripheries and mucous membranes should be observed for evidence of cyanosis which indicates poor oxygenation. Areas with a high blood flow and small arteriovenous oxygen difference (e.g. the tongue and mucous membranes) will not become cyanotic as readily as those areas with low blood flow and a large arteriovenous oxygen difference. Peripheral cyanosis refers therefore to bluish colouring of the skin in the extremities and central cyanosis includes the tongue and mucous membranes. The clinical impression of cyanosis may be confirmed by blood gas analysis or pulse oximetry.

Palpation

Palpation should follow inspection and allows the observed abnormalities to be confirmed or further investigated (Table 5.2). Any areas of pain, tenderness or swelling should be noted, particularly with regard to application of manual techniques during future treatment. Deviation of the trachea from its normal position (midline or very slightly to the right) may indicate significant abnormality, either extrathoracic (e.g. external compression by a space occupying lesion) or intrathoracic (e.g. atelectasis pulling or pleural effusion pushing the trachea to the contralateral side). The trachea can be palpated by sliding the index finger inward over the suprasternal notch. In patients with respiratory distress retraction of the suprasternal fossa may be seen and a tracheal tug palpated. Placing the hands on the chest allows the assessment of expansion and symmetry of movement. During this time crepitations (either pulmonary in origin or due to subcutaneous emphysema) may be noted. Palpation may include percussion of the chest wall in order to assess resonance. This may be increased (indicating air) or decreased (indicating solid or fluid). It is performed by tapping on a finger placed over an intercostal space, whilst listening for the different qualities of resonance.

Auscultation

Auscultation of the chest is performed using a stethoscope to determine the presence and character of breath sounds, adventitious sounds and sometimes vocal resonance (Forgaes, 1978). Breath sounds are caused by the turbulent flow of air during inspiration and expiration and are altered in intensity and frequency as they pass through the lungs. Vesicular breathing is normally heard over peripheral lung fields and its intensity increases during inspiration and fades quickly during expiration, without a pause between the two. Bronchial, pulmonary and pleural disease may alter these breath sounds (Macleod and Munro, 1986).

A reduction in air entry to the underlying lung secondary to a disease process such as a pleural effusion, pneumothorax or major lobar collapse leads to diminished or absent breath sounds over the affected area. If present the breath sounds will remain vesicular. If the lung tissue through which the breath sounds are transmitted has lost its normal consistency and there is loss of the normal air/alveolus interface (e.g. consolidation, fibrosis or collapse), the sounds are harsh and abnormal (similar to those heard normally at the larynx or directly over the trachea). This is termed bronchial breathing which is heard over the affected area and may be recognized by being clearer than vesicular breathing. The expiratory sound is as loud and as long as the inspiratory sound and there is a pause between the two.

The presence of adventitious sounds should be noted; these are described in many ways, but for the purpose of this description will be divided into crackles (or crepitations) and wheeze. Crackles are usually attributed to secretions within the airways, although they may be present in disease states where there is no sputum, such as interstitial fibrosis. They are coarse or fine discontinuous, non-musical sounds. Crackles heard in late inspiration are usually due to the explosive reopening of small peripheral airways which have been occluded during expiration. These are usually fine high-pitched sounds and are associated with pulmonary oedema and interstitial fibrosis. Coarser sounding crackles are associated with secretions in both chronic and acute disease. Early inspiratory crackling may be heard in chronic obstructive pulmonary disease and may be audible at the mouth as well as over the lower lobes. Wheezes are musical sounds produced by the passage of air through narrowed bronchi, as a result of mucosal oedema or bronchospasm. They are usually superimposed over expiration which is generally prolonged. Localized wheezing may be heard over a partially obstructed bronchus (e.g. in the presence of a foreign body). A pleural rub is a creaking sound produced by friction between the pleural layers if the surfaces are roughened (e.g. in the presence of fibrinous exudate) and is usually heard toward the end of inspiration or very early in expiration.

EVALUATION FOLLOWING TREATMENT

It is essential to note the efficacy and any detrimental effects of intervention. This may be performed immediately following treatment or some time after treatment but prior to the next intervention. Appropriate measurements should be made with regard to the expected outcome. These may include changes in ventilatory requirement or in oxygen saturation and arterial blood gas analysis. A verbal report from nursing staff caring for the child, any radiological evidence of improvement if this is available and auscultation to assess any changes in breath sounds should also be noted. Goals initially set may need to be refined on the basis of the outcome of the initial or subsequent interventions and the treatment plan modified accordingly. Chest physiotherapy in the child with respiratory disease, whether acute or chronic, is only part of the overall management plan. Close liaison and communication with other members of the multidisciplinary team is essential to ensure optimal treatment and maximum therapeutic value.

REFERENCES

Bartlett, R.H., Gazzangia, A.B. and Geraghty, T.R. (1973) Respiratory manoeuvres to prevent postoperative complications. *Journal of the American Medical Association*, **224**, 1017–21.

Cochrane, G.M., Webber, B.A. and Clarke, S.W. (1977) Effects of sputum on pulmonary function. *British Medical Journal*, **2**, 1181–3.

Craig, D.B. (1981) Postoperative recovery of pulmonary function. *Anaesthesia & Analgesia*, **60**, 46–52.

Dick, K.J., Dhoueib, E., Edmunds, A.T. *et al.* (1992) Investigation and evaluation of physiotherapy evaluation in acute bronchiolitis. (Abstract) Course proceedings, Paediatric Respiratory Care for Physiotherapists, London.

Dinwiddie, R. (1990) Aspiration syndromes, in *The Diagnosis and Management of Paediatric Respiratory Disease*, (ed. R. Dinwiddie), Churchill Livingstone, London, pp. 223–35.

Eisenkraft, J.B. (1990) Effects of anaesthesia on the pulmonary circulation. *British Medical Journal*, **65**, 63–78.

England, S. (1988) Current techniques for assessing pulmonary function in the newborn infant: advantages and limitations. *Pediatric Pulmonology*, **4**, 48–53.

Fairshter, R.D. and Williams, J.H. (1987) Pulmonary physiology in the postoperative period. *Critical Care Clinics*, **3**, 287–305.

Fanconi, S. (1988) Reliability of pulse oximetry in hypoxic infants. *Journal of Pediatrics*, **112**, 424–7.

Fanconi, S. (1989) Pulse oximetry for hypoxemia: a warning to users and manufacturers. *Intensive Care Medicine*, **15**, 540–2.

Fanconi, S., Doherty, P., Edmunds, J.F. *et al.* (1985) Pulse oximetry in pediatric intensive care: comparison with measured saturations and transcutaneous oxygen tension. *Journal of Pediatrics*, **107**, 362–6.

Forgaes, P. (1978) The functional basis of pulmonary sounds. *Chest*, **73**, 399–405.

Gamsu, G., Singer, M.M., Vincent, H.H. *et al.* (1976) Postoperative impairment of mucous transport in the lung. *American Review of Respiratory Diseases*, **114**, 673–9.

Graham, W.G. and Bradley, D.A. (1978) Efficacy of chest physiotherapy and IPPB in the resolution of pneumonia. *New England Journal of Medicine*, **12**, 624–7.

Johnson, N.J. and Pierson, D.J. (1986) The spectrum of pulmonary atelectasis: pathophysiology, diagnosis and therapy. *Respiratory Care*, **331**, 1107–20.

Lyle, C.D., Blanch, R.F. and Harris, J.H. (1979) Evaluation of respiratory physical therapy. *New England Journal of Medicine*, **30**, 665–6.

Mackenzie, C. and Shin, B. (1985) Cardiorespiratory function before and after physiotherapy in mechanically ventilated patients with post-traumatic respiratory failure. *Critical Care Medicine*, **13**, 483–6.

Mackenzie, C., Shin, B. and McAslan, T.C. (1978) Chest physiotherapy: the effect on arterial oxygenation. *Anaesthesia & Analgesia*, **57**, 28–30.

Macleod, J. and Munro, J. (1986) The respiratory system, in *Clinical Examination*, 7th edn, (eds J. MacLeod and J. Munro), Churchill Livingstone, London, pp. 153–91.

Mansell, A., Bryan, C. and Levinson, H. (1972) Airway closure in children. *Journal of Applied Physiology*, **33**, 711.

Marini, J., Pierson, D. and Hudson, L. (1979) Acute lobar atelectasis: a prospective comparison of fibreoptic bronchoscopy and respiratory therapy. *American Review of Respiratory Disease*, **119**, 971–8.

Nunn, J.F. (1990) Effects of anaesthesia on respiration. *British Medical Journal*, **65**, 54–62.

Pasterkamp, H. (1990) The history and physical examination, in *Kendigs Disorders of the Respiratory Tract in Children*, 2nd edn, (ed. V. Chernick), W.B. Saunders, Philadelphia, pp. 56–77.

Phelan, P.D., Landau, L.I. and Olinsky, A. (1990) Pulmonary complications of inhalation, in *Respiratory Illness in Children*, 3rd edn, (eds P.D. Phelan, L.I. Landau and A. Olinsky), Blackwell Scientific Publications, Oxford, pp. 357–88.

Sidi, A., Rush, W., Gravenstein, N. *et al.* (1987) Pulse oximetry fails to accurately detect low levels of arterial haemoglobin oxygen saturation in dogs. *Journal of Clinical Monitoring*, **3**, 257–62.

Southall, D.P., Bignall, S., Stebbens, V.A. *et al.* (1987) Pulse oximeter and transcutaneous oxygen measurements in neonatal and paediatric intensive care. *Archives of Disease in Childhood*, **62**, 882–8.

Stevens, P.M. (1977) Positive end expiratory pressure breathing. *Journal of the American Thoracic Society*, **5**, 1–6.

Stiller, K., Geake, T., Taylor, J. *et al.* (1990) Acute lobar atelectasis. A comparison of two chest physiotherapy regimens. *Chest*, **98**, 1336–40.

Stocks, J. (1993) Assessment of lung function in infants. *Perfusion*, **8**, 71–80.

Taylor, M.B. and Whitwam, J.C. (1988) The accuracy of pulse oximeters: a comparative clinical evaluation of five pulse oximeters. *Anaesthesia*, **43**, 229–32.

Voelkel, N.F. (1986) Mechanisms of hypoxic pulmonary vasoconstriction. *American Review of Respiratory Disease*, **113**, 1186–91.

Webb, M., Martin, J.A., Cartlidge, P.H.T. *et al.* (1985) Chest physiotherapy in acute bronchiolitis. *Archives of Disease in Childhood*, **60**, 1078–9.

CHEST PHYSIOTHERAPY TECHNIQUES AND ADJUNCTS TO CHEST PHYSIOTHERAPY 6

S. Ammani Prasad and Juliette Hussey

INTRODUCTION

In normal health mucus produced by the tracheobronchial tree is continually propelled upstream by cilial action toward the upper respiratory tract, from where it can be expectorated or swallowed, thus maintaining a clear and patent airway. Respiratory pathology may alter this process in different ways. Tracheobronchial secretions may increase in quantity, change in consistency or there may be a disruption of the normal mucociliary clearance process due to direct cilial damage. Under these circumstances a variety of chest physiotherapy techniques may be employed to enhance tracheobronchial clearance. In addition respiratory physiotherapy can reduce the work of breathing, improve oxygenation, may help to maintain lung volume and improve exercise tolerance. Functional and postural re-education are also important elements of chest physiotherapy.

The safe and effective physiotherapy management of infants and children with respiratory disorders necessitates an understanding of treatment aims, careful and accurate individual assessment and the judicious use of appropriate physiotherapy techniques. Optimal care of respiratory disease relies on a multidisciplinary approach to patient care, dependent on close co-operation and communication between all members of the care team, support services, the child and family. Perhaps the most important difference in the treatment of adults and children is the need and ability to communicate effectively not only with the child but also with the parents/guardians, particularly those with acutely ill children requiring intensive care who may feel they can no longer contribute to their child's recovery. The hospital environment generally and particularly the intensive care setting will be unfamiliar and is likely to be frightening for most parents and relatives. Physiotherapy treatments themselves may cause distress to the parents. A careful explanation of the indication for intervention and treatment techniques provides both reassurance and psychological support. Following treatment the benefits and the timing of further intervention should be discussed. Parents should be encouraged to participate in the treatment if they wish and if the clinical condition of the patient allows. Even a small contribution such as holding a hand may provide comfort to both the parent and child.

In this chapter the various physiotherapy techniques and adjuncts listed in Table 6.1 will be described and discussed.

POSITIONING AND POSTURAL DRAINAGE

Positioning is used to optimize lung function, including ventilation and perfusion, and as a technique, postural drainage, to enhance tracheobronchial clearance.

Table 6.1 Chest physiotherapy techniques and adjuncts to chest physiotherapy

Techniques	*Adjuncts*
Positioning	Continuous positive airway pressure (CPAP)
Postural drainage	Intermittent positive pressure breathing (IPPB)
Chest percussion	Incentive spirometry (IS)
Chest vibrations	Positive expiratory pressure (PEP)
Manual hyperinflation	Inhalation therapies
Breathing exercises/forced expirations	
Irrigant instillation/airway suction	

SUPINE

The supine position is often considered the most convenient position in which to nurse acutely ill infants and children (Figure 6.1a). Although monitoring and management may be easier, this position compromises pulmonary function and arterial blood gas composition. Even in healthy neonates Schwartz *et al.*, (1975) showed reduced arterial oxygenation (PaO_2) levels during supine lying. Three mechanisms have been

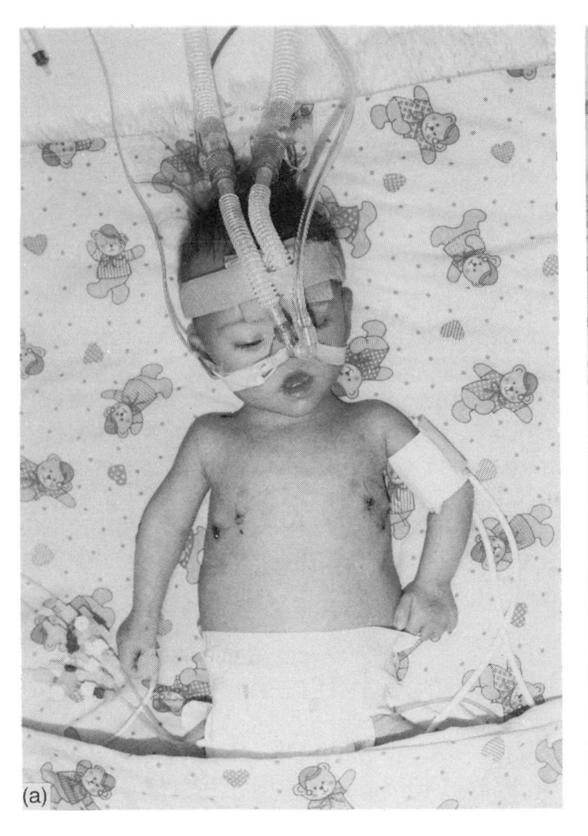

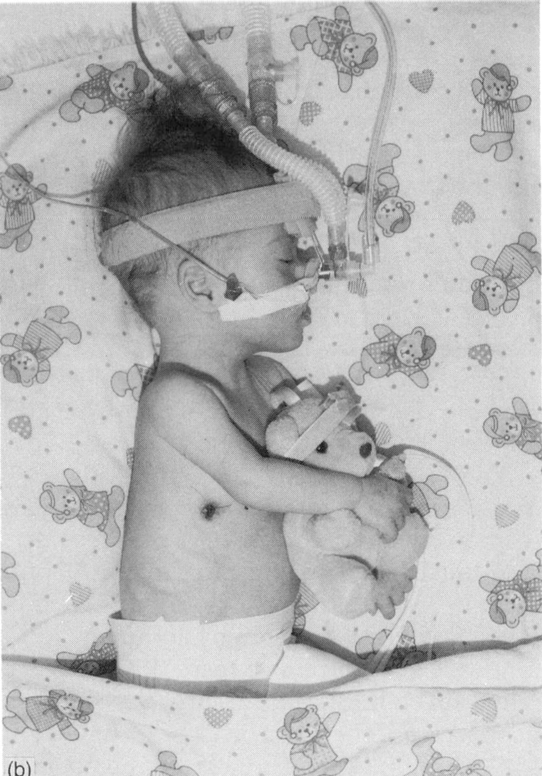

Figure 6.1 Patient rolled from supine (a) to side lying (b).

postulated to account for these positional changes in lung function. Firstly, in the upright posture the abdominal contents hang as a weight suspended from the undersurface of the diaphragm, applying a uniform negative pressure to it. In contrast, in the supine position the abdominal contents apply a non-uniform positive pressure to the undersurface of the diaphragm, compressing the bases of the lungs. Thus lung volume is at its lowest in the supine posture (Muller and Bryan, 1979).

Secondly, secretions will tend to pool in dependent lung regions and in the supine position the posterior regions of both the upper and lower lobes will be principally affected. Thirdly, mechanical coupling between the rib cage and abdomen is lost and diaphragmatic contraction tends to pull the anterior rib cage posteriorly rather than upward (Muller and Bryan, 1979). Appropriate positioning is also important in the ventilated patient, as during intermittent positive pressure ventilation (IPPV) the diaphragm moves passively and there is less excursion posteriorly where opposing pressure from the viscera is greatest (Agostini and Hyatt, 1986), thus contributing to the development of basal atelectasis.

SIDE LYING

The lateral decubitus position with the patient rolled well forward into side lying (Figure 6.1b) releases the diaphragm from the pressure of the abdominal viscera and allows for more effective basal expansion. In addition this position facilitates drainage of secretions from the uppermost lung. Even in the most unstable patient, with particular attention to monitoring and access lines, it is usually possible to roll the patient from supine into the side lying position. Though the change in position itself may lead to an immediate fall in oxygen saturation, if the position achieved is comfortable a return to baseline values should readily occur.

Gravity has been shown to have an important effect on pulmonary gas exchange in adults, with dependent lung regions being preferentially ventilated and perfused. However, ventilation in infants has been shown to be preferentially distributed to the uppermost lung regions (Heaf *et al.*, 1983; Davies *et al.*, 1985). The differences between distribution of ventilation in the adult and infant are fully discussed in Chapter 2. It is well established that adults with unilateral lung disease should be nursed in the lateral decubitus position with the unaffected lung down in order to achieve optimal arterial oxygenation (Zack *et al.*, 1974; Ibanez *et al.*, 1981). This position also facilitates the application of chest physiotherapy to the affected side. However, in infants with unilateral lung disease, altered rib cage and lung mechanics mean that the affected lung should be placed down to achieve maximal oxygenation. This may dictate the ability to apply chest physiotherapy directly to the affected area and highlights the need for individual patient assessment. Close monitoring of vital signs allows one to determine whether and for how long a side lying position can be tolerated in infants and small children with unilateral lung disease, bearing in mind that physiotherapy procedures themselves may lead to a further fall in oxygen saturation (Hussey *et al.*, 1992). It may be necessary to increase the level of inspired oxygen during treatment in order to maintain adequate patient oxygenation and yet achieve maximal therapeutic effect. Occasionally if a position is not tolerated treatment techniques may have to be performed in a modified position, e.g. a quarter turn only into the side lying position. A practical benefit of side lying is the convenience of administration and delivery of aerosol/inhalation therapy in acutely

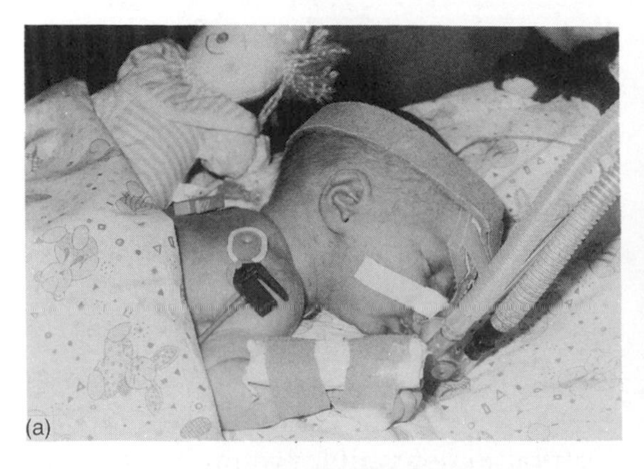

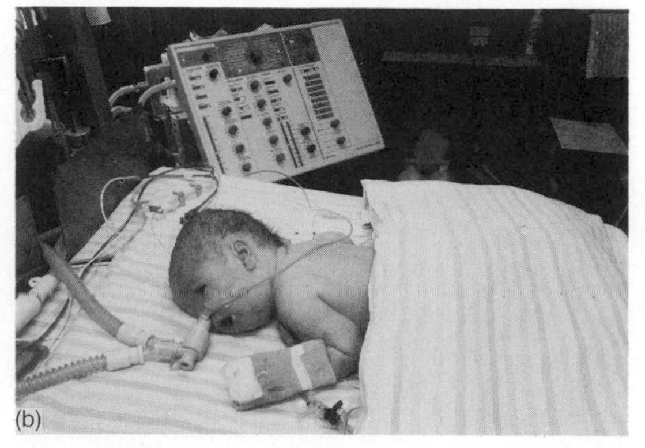

Figure 6.2 (a and b) Prone positioning.

ill patients unable to adopt a more upright posture.

PRONE

The prone position (Figure 6.2) improves anterior chest wall stability as the pressure from the abdominal contents transmitted to the chest helps to prevent inward collapse of the rib cage. This leads to improved co-ordination between the rib cage, diaphragm and abdomen. The release of visceral pressure on the posterior arc of the diaphragm allows it to descend more efficiently, thus improving tidal volume. Piehl and Brown (1976) compared PaO_2 in adults with acute respiratory failure in the prone and supine positions and found oxygenation to be improved in prone. Supporting evidence for advocating the prone position has been provided by studies in neonates. Wagaman *et al.* (1979) showed improved oxygenation, tidal volume and lung compliance in neonates with prone positioning and similarly Martin *et al.* (1979) showed an improvement in gas exchange of 15% in normal neonates and 25% in those with respiratory disease when turned from supine to prone.

A further advantage of the prone position is that it reduces the incidence of gastro-oesophageal reflux (Blumenthal and Lealman, 1982). Brackbill *et al.* (1973) demonstrated a fall in energy expenditure in infants nursed in the prone position, with more time spent sleeping and less time crying. However, the position is less likely to be tolerated in patients with abdominal distension or who have undergone recent major abdominal surgery.

Recent evidence has shown a strong association between the prone position and sudden infant death syndrome (SIDS) (Southall and Samuels, 1992). It is important to note that a child in intensive care or on a respiratory medical ward is constantly monitored and observed and therefore the risk is negligible. However this position should not be advocated in infants for long periods at home, when the child may be unattended, and this should be explained to the parents. At the same time it is important to note that prone positioning is important in terms of normal development and therefore should be encouraged during play.

SITTING

The sitting position increases lung volume

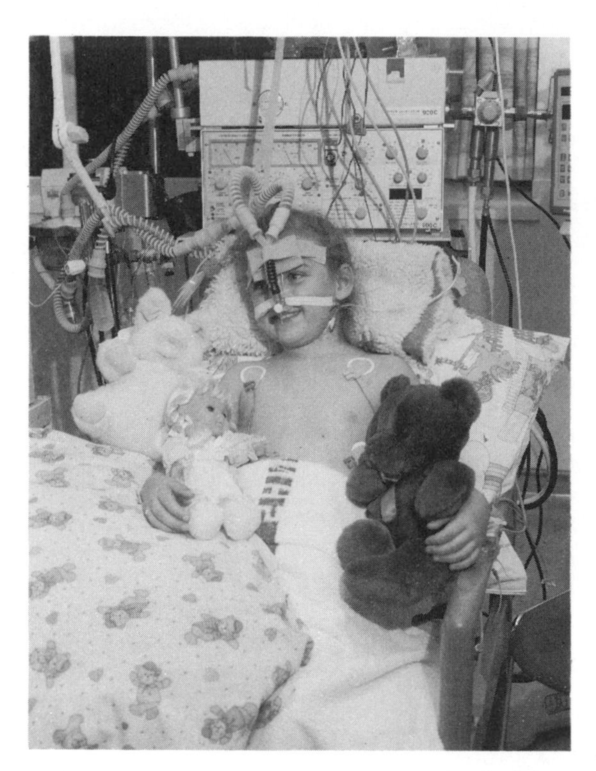

Figure 6.3 Sitting position with nasotracheal intubation.

and functional residual capacity (FRC) as compared to supine. To attain maximal benefit it is important to ensure that the patient is kept upright (Figure 6.3) and not allowed to slump forward, therefore negating any advantageous effects. Hospitalization can adversely affect normal motor and cognitive development and an additional benefit of sitting is that it allows the patient to observe their environment from a more normal perspective and encourages activities of play. A sitting posture can be easily achieved in stable patients undergoing mechanical ventilation via nasotracheal intubation or tracheostomy.

The development of rib cage configuration to the oblique rather than horizontal lie is associated with the adoption of an upright posture (Oppenshaw *et al.*, 1984). It may be postulated that in infants who are chronically sick the sitting position may encourage maturation of rib cage configuration. This in turn may facilitate intercostal function and therefore the ability to increase the anteroposterior and transverse diameters of the chest.

POSTURAL DRAINAGE

Postural drainage (PD) or gravity assisted positioning enhances the drainage of pulmonary secretions by positioning lung segments above their respective bronchi and allowing gravity to assist the drainage of secretions into the more central airways. It has also been suggested that gravity could assist cilial action and therefore the mobilization of mucus toward major bronchi (Zausmer, 1968). The benefits of postural drainage have been demonstrated using radioaerosol clearance studies. In ten patients with copious secretions, sputum clearance increased in those patients in whom a regime of treatment included postural drainage. (Sutton *et al.*, 1983; Maloney *et al.*, 1981). Postural drainage may also increase the rate of tracheal transport of sputum (Wong *et al.*, 1977).

There are few studies evaluating the benefit of postural drainage as a single treatment modality. Most studies have evaluated the use of postural drainage in combination with other techniques and most of these studies were undertaken in patients with chronic lung disease. Newhouse and Rossman (1984) suggested that postural drainage is most likely to be effective in the presence of copious amounts of thin secretions, but that PD was not as effective as physiotherapy including cough or even cough alone. This finding is in agreement with an earlier study by Oldenberg *et al.* (1979) who stated that intermittent postural

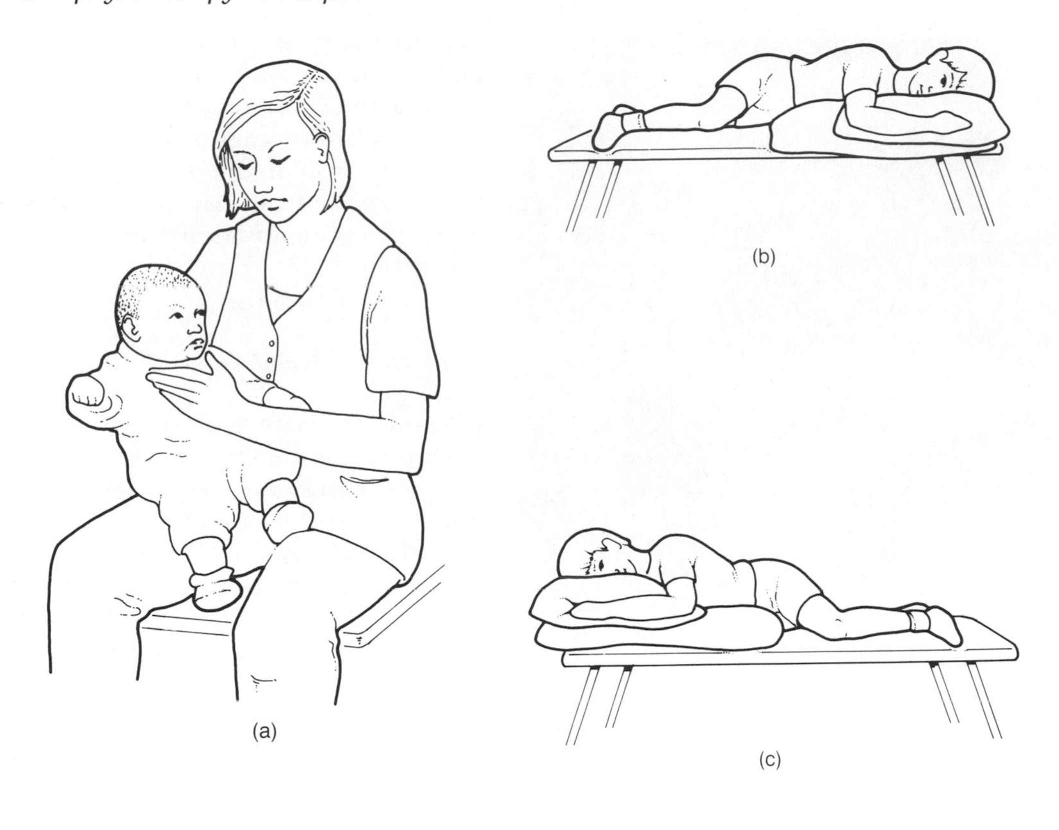

(a) (b) (c)

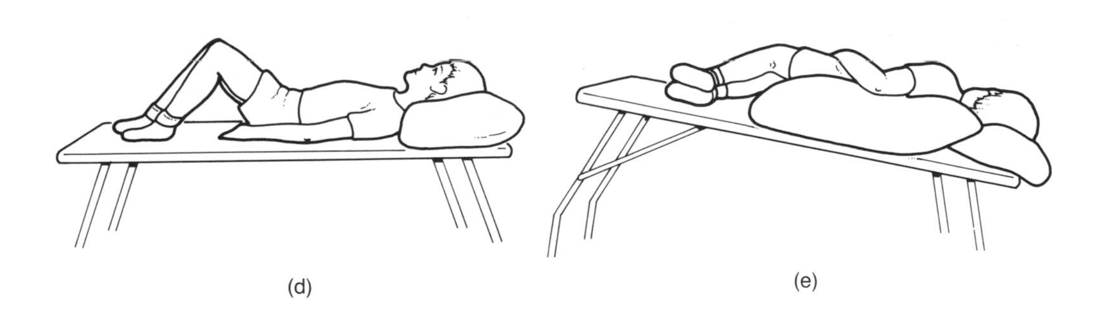

(d) (e)

aerosols into diseased peripheral airways is likely to be impeded by bronchial thickening and retained secretions, probably resulting in greater deposition to the larger airways.

In animal studies Rowe *et al.* (1973) showed improved radiological clearance of dye that had been injected into the tracheobronchial tree of piglets when using vibrations. In humans bronchoscopy has shown that vibrations performed during expiration can mobilize secretions toward the larger segmental bronchi (Kigin, 1981, 1984). However this information can only be used to confirm large airway clearance as bronchoscopy is reported to reach only the fourth generation of bronchi (Kovnat *et al.*, 1974). In adults with acute lobar atelectasis chest physiotherapy, including postural drainage, percussion and deep breathing exercises, has been reported to be as effective as therapeutic fibreoptic bronchoscopy in reversing atelectasis (Marini *et al.*, 1979). Stiller *et al.* (1990) also reported that positioning and vibrations added to a treatment of hyperinflation and suctioning led to an improvement in the resolution of acute lobar atelectasis. In the paediatric population, Finer *et al.* (1979) investigated the role of postural drainage, vibration and suctioning in preventing and reversing postextubation atelectasis in 85 neonates. The right upper lobe was the most common site of collapse. A significant decrease in atelectasis was reported in the group receiving chest physiotherapy despite the control group also being frequently placed in the appropriate postural drainage position for the right upper lobe. Chest percussion and vibrations have been reported to help reinflate areas of acute lung collapse (unresponsive to other treatment) and may enhance the removal of secretions as compared to suction alone (Mellins, 1974; Etches and Scott, 1978). Crane *et al.* (1978) studied the effects of manual techniques in infants with hyaline membrane disease (HMD), with percussion followed by vibrations in both the head down and flat positions. Significant increases in respiratory rate, heart rate and systolic blood pressure were found in all four treatment regimes including suctioning, but it was unclear as to whether these increases were due to suction alone or a combination of one or more of the procedures.

Following a study investigating the effects of postural drainage with and without percussion in neonates recovering from respiratory distress PaO_2 was improved in those receiving percussion. Finer and Boyd (1978) suggested that premature infants may be unable to effectively clear secretions without mechanical assistance in the form of percussion or vibrations due to their narrower airways. In a comparison of the effects of contact heel percussion, manual percussion (with a face mask) and chest vibration (using an electric toothbrush) used in combination with postural drainage and followed by airway suctioning in preterm neonates, a rise in PaO_2 which was maintained for up to one hour post-treatment was reported with both groups receiving percussion (Tudehope and Bagley, 1980). It was postulated that the loosened terminal airway secretions were responsible for the improvement of PaO_2 in those treated with percussion.

However, percussion has received much criticism (Kiriloff *et al.*, 1985; Sutton *et al*, 1985; Selsby, 1989) though much of this may result from a miscomprehension of the use of the technique (Gallon, 1992). In some studies efficacy of percussion was evaluated in patients who did not have excessive or retained airway secretions and in such instances one must question why percussion was being used (Connors *et al.*, 1980; Campbell *et al.*, 1975). Clinically percussion and vibrations are rarely used in isolation but in combination with positioning, postural drainage, breathing exercises, coughing or airway suction. It is therefore difficult to assess the efficacy of each treatment component separately.

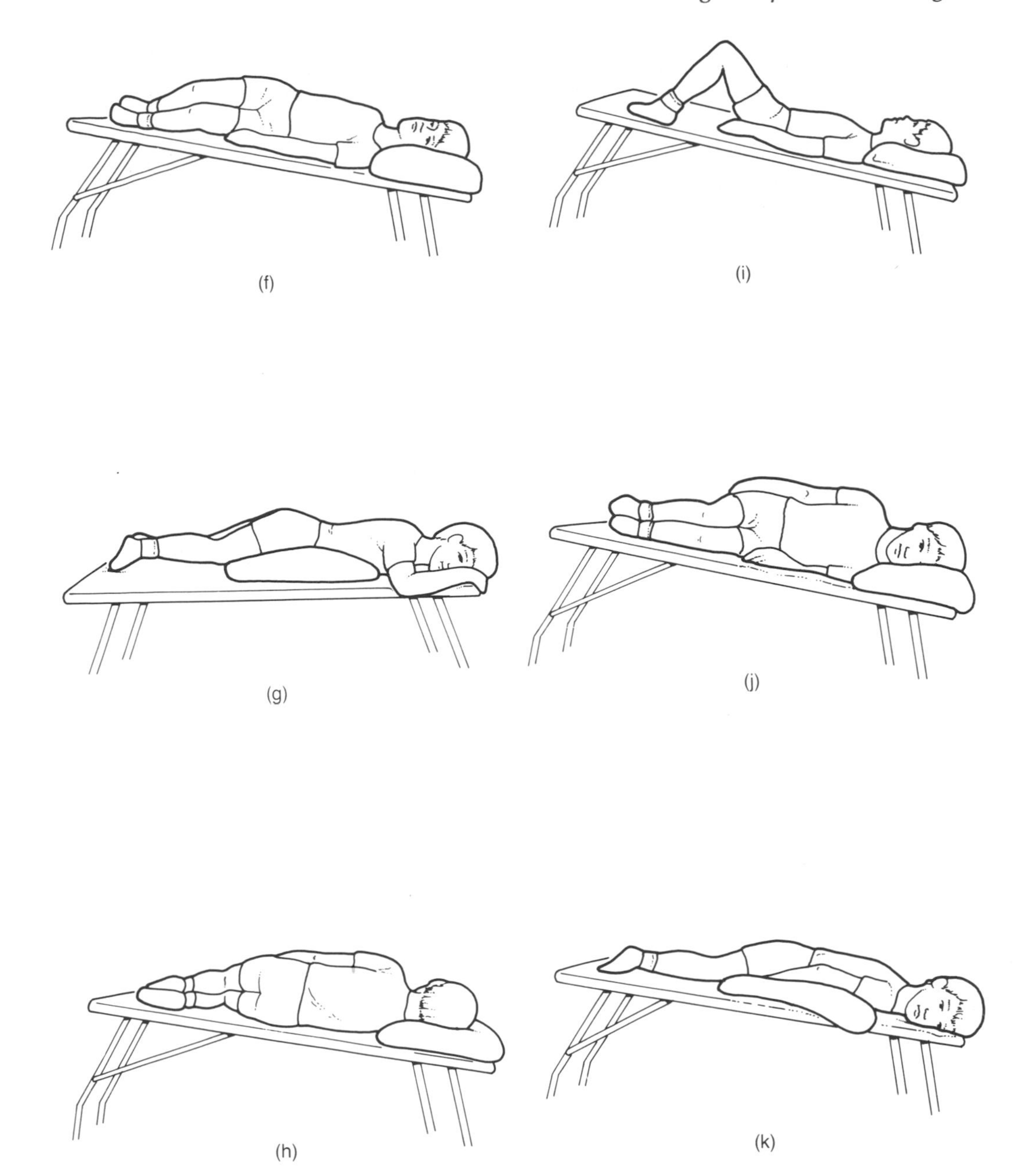

Figure 6.4 Positions for postural drainage of the various lung segments. (a) Apical segments upper lobes (b) Posterior segment right upper lobe (c) Posterior segment left upper lobe (d) Anterior segments upper lobes (e) Lingular (f) Right middle lobe (g) Apical segments lower lobes (h) Right medial basal and left lateral basal segments lower lobes (i) Anterior basal segments (j) Lateral basal segment right lower lobe (k) Posterior basal segments lower lobes.

drainage alone is less effective unless accompanied by cough or exercise. Similarly, Bateman *et al.* (1981) concluded that peripheral lung clearance was enhanced when postural drainage was performed in addition to coughing alone in patients with chronic obstructive airways disease. In contrast, Zinman (1984), in a study of nine patients with cystic fibrosis, compared a regime of cough versus chest physiotherapy (including postural drainage) and demonstrated cough alone to be as effective. Despite these apparently contrasting studies it is widely accepted that a regime of postural drainage, accompanied by other chest physiotherapy techniques, assists in the mobilization of peripheral secretions to central airways from where they can be cleared by forced expiration manoeuvres such as coughing.

The positions of postural drainage are shown in Figure 6.4. Particular care is required when considering the use of the technique in the preterm neonate or acutely ill infant and these are illustrated in Table 6.2. Neonates, and particularly preterm infants, rely to a much greater extent on diaphragmatic function during respiration and may not tolerate the head down position which puts the diaphragm at a mechanical disadvantage. In the presence of raised intracranial pressure (ICP) the optimal position to nurse infants has been shown to be midline with a 30° head up tilt (Feldman *et al.*, 1992). The use of postural drainage may lead to a further increase in ICP and therefore a possible fall in cerebral perfusion pressure (CPP) (Chapter 9, p. 145). Abdominal distension (as may occur postsurgery or during peritoneal dialysis) may increase intra-abdominal pressure on the undersurface of the diaphragm. This is exacerbated by the head down position, increasing respiratory embarrassment, and this position should therefore be avoided.

Table 6.2 Special precautions for the use of postural drainage

1. Preterm infants/neonates
2. Abdominal distension
3. Phrenic nerve palsy
4. Raised intracranial pressure
5. Postsurgery
   abdominal surgery
   neurosurgery
   cardiac surgery
6. Gastro-oesophageal reflux

PERCUSSION AND VIBRATIONS

Percussion is the rhythmic clapping of the chest wall with a cupped hand over an involved lung segment/lobe and is used to assist the mobilization of bronchopulmonary secretions. It is thought to produce an energy wave which is transmitted through the chest wall to the airways, loosening secretions from the bronchial walls (Sutton *et al.*, 1985). Percussion is performed throughout the respiratory cycle. Vibrations are intermittent chest wall compressions performed during expiration in the direction in which the ribs and soft tissues move during exhalation (Imle, 1989). Vibrations may dislodge both peripheral and central secretions.

Percussion should produce a hollow sound by the creation of an 'air cushion' on impact. The rate at which percussion is performed is usually determined by the therapists' bias and in children is often performed using a single handed technique (Figure 6.5a) rather than double handed. Slower rates of percussion may be better tolerated by critically ill infants and those with a tendency to develop bronchospasm. Therapist preference dictates whether percussion is performed over bare skin, allowing the visualization of anatomical landmarks, or over a thin layer of clothing or towelling. The use of bulky towels requires a greater force to achieve the same effect as much of the air cushion is lost.

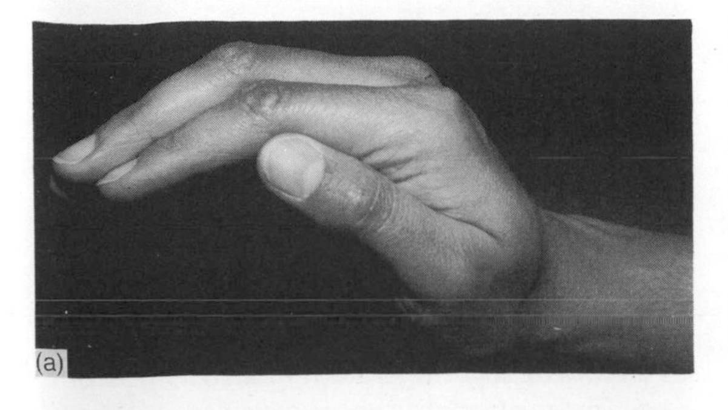
(a)

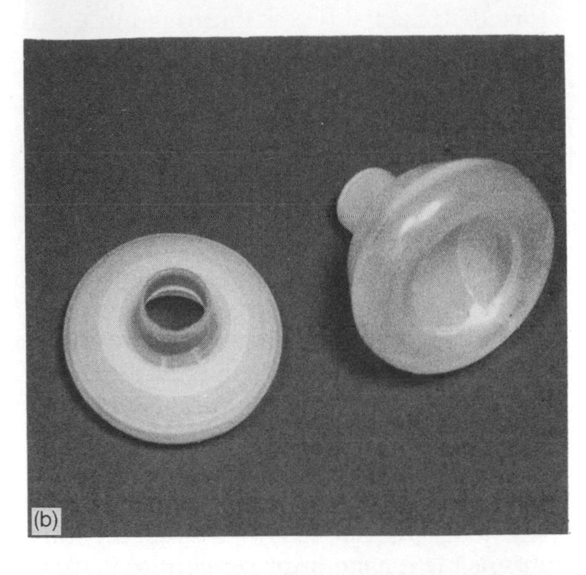
(b)

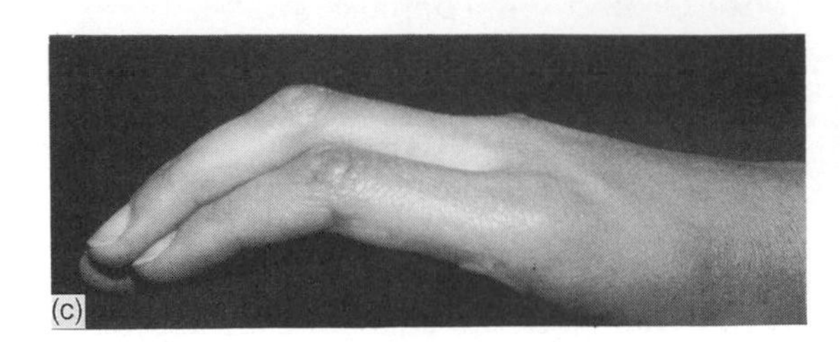
(c)

Figure 6.5 Methods of chest percussion: (a) single handed technique, (b) using infant face mask, (c) 'tenting' using three fingers.

The technique should not cause pain or discomfort and therefore should not be performed over or too close to incision or chest drain sites. In the paediatric population infant sized anaesthetic masks or similar padded cup shaped objects may be preferred (Figure 6.5b); others may prefer to use the three-fingered 'tenting' technique with the middle finger raised to overlap the first and third (Figure 6.5c). Contact heel percussion uses the thenar and hypothenar eminence to apply percussion (usually at a rate of approximately 40/minute). No conclusive evidence shows one technique to be superior to another though in a study by Tudehope and Bagley (1980) vibrations applied with an electric toothbrush were shown to be less effective than either percussion using an anaesthetic mask or the contact heel method. Vibrations refer to an oscillatory movement performed with the hands placed over the chest wall. The amount of pressure applied to the thorax is modified according to the size and condition of the patient and is also dependent on the therapist's own bias. The technique is usually commenced just prior to the start of expiration and may be continued to just before the start of the following inspiration.

These manual techniques aim to facilitate both large and small airway clearance by advancing secretions centrally from where they can be expectorated by coughing or removed by airway suction. Radiological clearance of segmental, lobar and multilobar atelectasis following chest physiotherapy regimes which include percussion are well documented (Mackenzie *et al.*, 1978; Imle, 1989; Finer and Boyd, 1978), as is peripheral lung clearance (Bateman *et al.*, 1979). Bateman *et al.* (1981), using radioisotope aerosol imaging, found peripheral lung clearance was enhanced by physiotherapy regimes which included postural drainage, percussion, vibration and cough compared to cough alone. However, it is difficult to objectively measure peripheral lung clearance and DeCesare *et al.* (1982) questioned methods using inhalation of radioactive aerosols to measure mucus clearance. It was suggested that the particle sizes are relatively large and uniform penetration of these

Percussion and vibrations can be used in both spontaneously breathing and artificially ventilated patients. Vibrations are often used in conjunction with manual hyperinflation. This combination may be used following a period of percussion in ventilated infants and children with areas of atelectasis and/or retained secretions. Mechanical percussors and vibrators have been introduced both in chronic lung disease and in acute states but few studies have investigated their efficacy in the acute setting. Though Curran and Kachoyeanos (1979) reported some benefit from vibrations using an electric toothbrush in neonates, mechanical devices have generally been found to be inferior to manual techniques (Tudehope and Bagley, 1980; Parker, 1985). In the acutely ill child manual techniques may be preferred because they allow palpation or 'feel' and visual inspection of the chest during treatment. Thus they may be more easily adapted to the patient's need and tolerance. However, certain precautions should be considered before application of these techniques (Table 6.3) and neither should be performed as a routine part of chest physiotherapy in the younger age group.

Table 6.3 Special precautions for the use of percussion and vibrations

Percussion	*Vibrations*
Low platelet count/ coagulopathy	Low platelet count/ coagulopathy
Active pulmonary haemorrhage	Osteoporosis/mineral deficiency
Severe bronchospasm	Active pulmonary haemorrhage
Osteoporosis/mineral deficiency	Pain
Pain	

It must be acknowledged that infants and small children, unlike adults, cannot or may not co-operate with other mucus clearance techniques such as the active cycle of breathing techniques (ACBT) and treatment has to be based on techniques that can be performed effectively depending on each individual situation. This is supported by Gallon (1992) who recommends the use of percussion in those patients, e.g. unconscious patients or those with neuromuscular disease, who have retained secretions but are unable to participate in breathing exercises.

Based on limited research and on our own clinical experience it appears that percussion and vibrations are effective in children in enhancing the clearance of bronchopulmonary secretions. This conclusion has been reached by frequent observations of improved clinical status and radiological evidence particularly in infants and children with acute lung pathology.

In patients with low platelet counts or coagulopathies percussion may cause petechiae or localized bruising and patients with mineral deficiency may be more susceptible to rib fracture. In these instances percussion should be avoided or performed only with extreme care. The technique itself should not cause pain and should be avoided in patients complaining of chest pain. Active pulmonary haemorrhage is a contraindication to treatment with percussion and vibrations as it may potentially exacerbate bleeding. Percussion has been reported to cause bronchospasm in patients with chronic lung disease (Campbell *et al.*, 1975; Wollmer *et al.*, 1985) and we have occasionally noted this in acutely ill infants and small children. Percussion should therefore only be used cautiously in children who are susceptible to bronchospasm or who are wheezy prior to commencement of treatment. In such cases the adverse effects can often be obviated by premedication with bronchodilator therapy and modification of treatment techniques.

MANUAL HYPERINFLATION

Manual hyperinflation is a means of delivering breaths by the use of a gas supply and a manual reservoir bag. In the intubated patient the bag is connected to the artificial airway (endotracheal or tracheostomy tube) and squeezed at a rate similar to the required respiratory rate of the child, in order to deliver a volume of gas to the patient. The technique was first described as part of a physiotherapeutic regimen by Clement and Hubsch (1968) used to clear bronchial secretions and reinflate areas of lung collapse. Its role has since been extended and the technique may be used as a means of evacuating secretions from the bronchioles and alveoli in patients in whom the natural process of clearance of pulmonary secretions is inadequate (Windsor *et al.*, 1972). The principal use of the technique is to assist in the removal of obstructive secretions causing atelectatic areas, thereby opening up previously unventilated areas. When applied as part of a physiotherapy treatment manual hyperinflation may be performed by applying a slow inspiration with a short inspiratory hold, followed by quick release of the bag in order to generate a fast expiratory flow rate which may be enhanced by chest wall vibrations. The purpose of a slow inspiration with end inspiratory hold is to increase lung volume and promote collateral ventilatory flow, allowing a pressure gradient to build up behind bronchial secretions. The quick release is believed to move secretions toward the larger airways and simulates the effect of a cough. The application of three or four tidal volume breaths followed by a larger volume breath, accompanied by chest vibrations if appropriate, is particularly useful in patients who are haemodynamically unstable or at risk from spikes in intracranial pressure.

A 500 ml bag is recommended for infants and small children and a 1 litre bag for the older child. They may be open ended, allowing the therapist to control the volume of gas filling the bag, or they may incorporate a valve which restricts the amount of gas expelled (Figure 6.6). The gas flow to the bag is dependent on the size of the patient; approximately 4 l/min for an infant and up to 8–10 l/min for an older child. When using smaller sized bags in paediatric practice it is often possible to control and compress the bag using one hand whilst applying vibrations to the chest wall with the other. This allows for effective co-ordination of the two manoeuvres whilst simultaneously allowing accurate palpation of the chest wall. Ideally a manometer should be incorporated into the bagging circuit to monitor the peak inflation pressures (Figure 6.6).

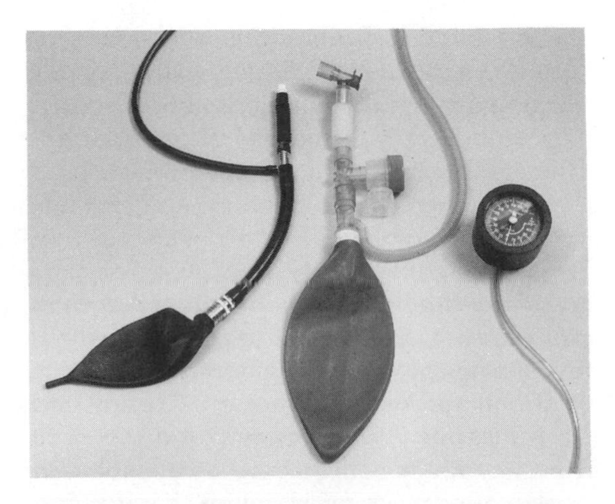

Figure 6.6 Circuit for manual hyperinflation (left to right): open ended; valved; gauge for monitoring peak inflation pressures.

Manual hyperinflation has been used to expand areas of lung which are not inflated during the inspiratory cycle of the ventilator; however, this remains contentious as it could be argued that air follows the pathway of least resistance and this may result in hyperinflation of the area already ventilated with no effect on the area of collapse. Another debatable benefit attributed to manual hyperinflation is that it may improve lung compliance (Rhodes, 1987). This is disputed by Mackenzie and Shin (1985) who reported that secretion removal by chest physiotherapy techniques which did not include manual hyperinflation improved total lung/thoracic compliance and did not cause changes in cardiac function. The improvement in compliance was thought to be due to effective mobilization of secretions from peripheral to central airways with subsequent recruitment of more functional alveolar units. In patients without lung pathology significant increases in total static compliance have been reported after bagging; however, the relevance of this to disease states is questionable (Jones *et al.*, 1992).

Table 6.4 Special precautions for manual hyperinflation

1. Preterm neonates
2. Hypovolaemia, low cardiac output
3. Raised intracranial pressure
4. Emphysematous bullae, multiple cysts
5. Undrained pneumothorax

In certain situations manual hyperinflation should only be used with extreme caution (Table 6.4). In preterm neonates manual hyperinflation should only be carried out if absolutely necessary and with extreme care due to the risk of barotrauma and pneumothorax (see Chapter 7, p. 118). In patients with low blood pressure increases in intrathoracic pressure may lead to a further fall in cardiac output, thereby exacerbating pre-existing hypotension. Patients with high pulmonary artery pressures may show an adverse reaction to bag squeezing unless the cause is related to insufficient oxygenation. In patients with a low cardiac output, the rise in intrathoracic pressure associated with manual hyperinflation may also lead to a reduction in arterial oxygenation despite delivery of 100% oxygen therapy. It could be postulated that this is due to the resulting reduction in venous return and therefore a further fall in cardiac output. In addition pressure changes in the thorax can also effect cardiac performance through the thoracic pump mechanism and may interfere with pulmonary blood flow (Paratz, 1992; Scharf *et al.*, 1980). Gormezano and Branthwaite (1972a) reported increases in intrathoracic pressure leading to a fall in arterial oxygen tension in adults with unstable cardiovascular status.

Manual hyperinflation with vibrations in supine and side lying positions in unconscious patients or in those unable to resist the operator's efforts has been associated with a 50% reduction in cardiac output. In contrast, in patients who actively resisted the manoeuvres cardiac output increased up to 50% (Laws and McIntyre, 1969). Patients with evidence of pulmonary air leak should not receive manual hyperinflation until a drain is inserted. The technique is also associated with rapid rises in intracranial pressure (Garrad and Bullock, 1986) and extreme care should be taken if using this technique in such patients (Chapter 9, p. 146).

The majority of research into manual hyperinflation has been conducted in the adult population and the findings applied to the paediatric population. Patients unable to tolerate a reduction in preload or coronary blood flow may experience haemodynamic instability during such procedures (Paratz, 1992). This necessitates constant observation of haemodynamic parameters during treatment in order to avoid excessive and potentially dangerous changes in cardiovascular status. Due to these potential changes it is recommended that in infants and young children the technique is performed using one hyperinflation (larger than tidal volume and at approximately 20% above the ventilator inspiratory pressure) with three to four tidal volume breaths. Using this method, accompanied by vibrations and airway suction, Hussey (1991) found that chest physiotherapy in children post cardiac surgery caused only a minimal fall in oxygen saturation (SaO_2). Holloway *et al.* (1969) demonstrated a significantly higher oxygen saturation after bagging neonates with lung pathology, with a period of manual hyperinflation post-treatment initiating a more rapid return of arterial oxygen tension to pretreatment values. This is supported by Hussey (1991) who found an immediate return to baseline oxygen saturation levels in chest physiotherapy treatments which included manual hyperinflation. Manual hyperinflation can be an invaluable tool in the management of patients with acute lung pathology, if after appropriate assessment its use is indicated.

BREATHING EXERCISES

Breathing exercises may be used to assist airway clearance, improve respiratory muscle strength and endurance, increase and maintain thoracic gas volume and rib cage mobility. Techniques of breathing control may also be taught to promote relaxation either in isolation for the relief of shortness of breath or respiratory distress or as part of a more active technique to clear secretions, e.g. the active cycle of breathing techniques.

Thoracic expansion exercises are deep breaths which emphasize inspiration and incorporate the concept of interdependence (Chapter 2, p. 16) and the promotion of collateral ventilatory flow (Chapter 1, p. 5). They cause an increase in lung volume which may assist the reinflation of atelectatic areas and the mobilization of obstructive secretions. Breathing exercises may be used in both acute and chronic lung disease as part of the ACBT for clearance of secretions. They have also been advocated postoperatively to assist the return to preoperative lung volumes by encouraging expansion which may be limited by incisional pain, splinting of the chest and consequent hypoventilation. In small children breathing exercises can often be executed in the form of play until the child is old enough to co-operate with more formal exercises as part of a physiotherapy treatment.

Breathing control consists of periods of quiet relaxed breathing at the patient's own rate and rhythm and may be taught to those suffering from asthma or chronic lung disease for use during episodes of respiratory distress. It is also an integral part of the forced expiration technique (FET) and is used to avoid a potential increase in airflow obstruction caused by forced expiratory manoeuvres. The forced expiration technique (Partridge *et al.*, 1989), based on the concept of the equal pressure point, consists of a forced expiratory manoeuvre from mid to low lung volume and is used to mobilize peripheral secretions (see Chapter 11, p. 166).

The previously described techniques of thoracic expansion exercises, breathing control and the FET are the components of the ACBT and may be accompanied by gravity assisted positioning. The ACBT is a modality of airway clearance which allows patients to perform treatment independently and is discussed fully in Chapter 11, p. 166.

AIRWAY SUCTION

In patients who are unable to effectively clear tracheobronchial secretions, airway suction using negative pressure may be used to remove excessive or retained secretions from the respiratory tract. It is a common procedure in the nursing and physiotherapy management of children with respiratory pathology. Secretions may be retained due to:

1. respiratory pathology with an inability to clear secretions normally;

2. neurological disorders which inhibit/ depress the normal cough reflex;
3. the presence of an artificial airway. This may impair the natural ability to mobilize and expectorate secretions due to an open intubated glottis and a reduction in the effectiveness of normal mucociliary clearance. In addition, the presence of an endotracheal tube may itself irritate the airway and cause an increase in the production of secretions (Sumner, 1990).

Airway suction may be performed as a single procedure by nursing and medical staff (and occasionally parents) or it may be incorporated into a chest physiotherapy regime. The aim of the procedure is to clear secretions thereby maintaining a patent airway and improving ventilation and oxygenation. Removal of such secretions will also help to minimize the risk of atelectasis. However, deleterious physiological effects directly attributed to this procedure are well documented (Table 6.5).

Table 6.5 Deleterious effects of airway suction

Tracheobronchial trauma
Hypoxia
Cardiovascular changes
Atelectasis
Changes in intracranial pressure
Pneumothorax
Bacterial infection

COMPLICATIONS

Tracheobronchial trauma

The mucosa of the tracheobronchial tree may be damaged merely by the passage of a catheter, even without the application of negative pressure (Kleiber *et al.*, 1988; Kuzenski, 1978; Link *et al.*, 1976). Once negative pressure is applied invagination of mucosal tissue into the catheter further

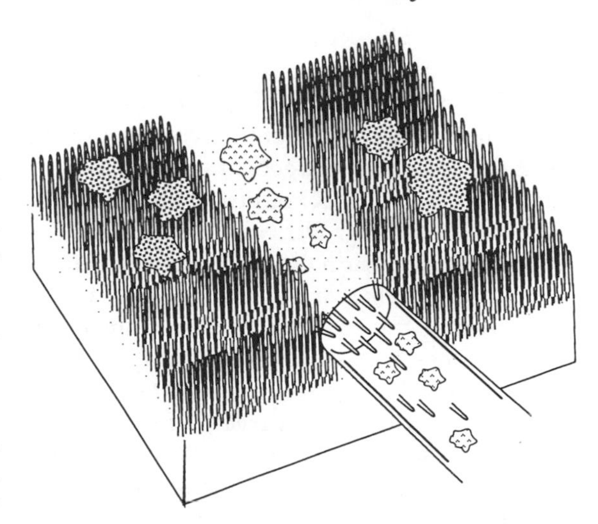

Figure 6.7 Diagrammatic representation of tracheobronchial trauma caused by application of negative pressure. Reproduced with permission from UnoPlast (UK) Ltd.

exacerbates trauma (Figure 6.7) (Sackner *et al.*, 1973; Landa *et al.*, 1973). Mucosal trauma may lead to the replacement of normal ciliated epithelium by squamous cells which are less efficient in achieving mucocilary clearance (Summer, 1990).

A post mortem study of intubated low birthweight infants documented significant tracheal damage and found a correlation between tracheal pathology and suction (Brodsky *et al.*, 1987). Although this study suggested that tracheal damage may be reduced if suction is limited to the end of the artificial airway, such practice may not always lead to effective clearance of secretions.

Further histological evidence for the damage caused by repeated airway suction is the finding of granulation tissue in repeatedly suctioned airways. This may result in bronchial stenosis and compromise of respiratory function (Kleiber *et al.*, 1988). Mechanical ventilation for more than 20 days has been observed to cause bronchial obstruction leading to atelectasis in infants

(Nagaraj *et al.*, 1980). However, Fisk and Baker (1975), at post mortem of two infants ventilated for 50 days, found regeneration of normal ciliated epithelium which suggests that the long term effects of suction and its effect on the tracheobronchial mucosa remain uncertain. However, it is essential that the association of suction and tracheobronchial trauma are borne in mind when performing the procedure. The number of suction passes is highly significant (Sackner *et al.*, 1973; Link *et al.*, 1976). Despite the existing evidence, a survey of paediatric suction practice by Young (1988) reported that suction practice was frequently undertaken using a rigid protocol with frequent catheter passes being commonplace (more than five reported by some respondents). Suction should only be undertaken when indicated and not at routine or predetermined intervals.

The type and size of catheter may also influence the degree of trauma. The larger the size of catheter, the greater the contact between mucosa and catheter and subsequent trauma. Several designs of catheter are now available, although frequently choice is limited by cost. Catheter tip design has become an important feature (Figure 6.8). Whistle tip catheters may lead to increased trauma as they easily become adherent to the tracheal wall (Link *et al.*, 1976). It is recommended therefore that catheters should have more than one lateral eye, smaller in size than the end hole. Although catheters with a beaded tip are designed to cushion the mucosal wall from the lateral eyes of the suction catheter, further reducing the degree of trauma caused, studies have not conclusively shown that they are effective in achieving this aim (Jung and Gotleib, 1976; Link *et al.*, 1976). In paediatric practice the use of such catheters may be limited due to the need to use a smaller than desired size of catheter in order to allow the beaded tip to pass through the airway, thereby reducing the efficiency of suction of thick secretions.

The vigour of insertion of the catheter into the airway may be another contributory factor causing tracheobronchial trauma (Jung and Gotleib, 1976) and it is recommended that the catheter be introduced into the airway gently and withdrawn without rotation of the catheter around the tracheal wall. Some authors recommend vacuum interrupted suction techniques (Young, 1984), but Czarnik *et al.* (1991) reported no difference in the amount of trauma caused by continuous and intermittent negative pressure application. However, the greater the negative pressure, the greater the risk of trauma. Vacuum control valves or Y-connectors should be used to minimize the risk of trauma from the application of negative pressure during the introduction of the catheter into the airway. Kinking of catheters to prevent suction during introduction is undesirable, because this may result in an increased vacuum suddenly being relayed to the airway when the kink is released.

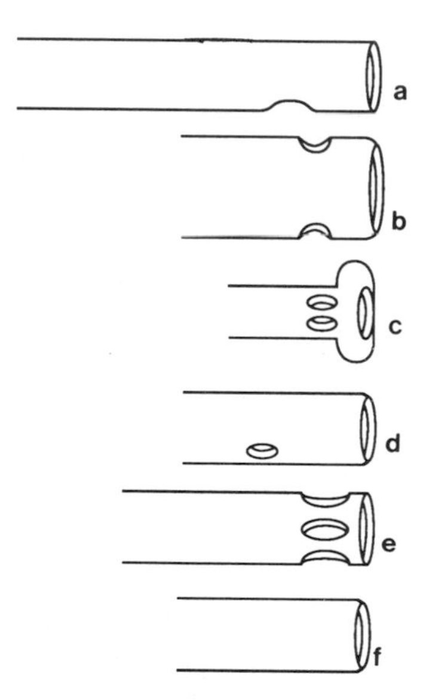

Figure 6.8 Catheter tip designs: (a) whistle tip, (b) single end hole with two small lateral eyes, (c) beaded tip, (d) single end hole with one small lateral eye, (e) single end hole with four lateral eyes and (f) single end hole with no lateral eyes.

Hypoxia

Hypoxia is a common and well documented complication of airway suction. The fall in oxygenation during suction has been shown to be greater than during apnoea (Boutros, 1970; Rindfleisch and Tyler, 1981). Several factors may contribute to the development of hypoxia during suction. The fall in oxygenation is directly related to the duration of suction time (Rosen and Hillard, 1962; Jung and Newman, 1982) and it has been suggested that the vacuum applied to the airway may remove oxygen as well as secretions from the lungs. The presuction PaO_2 is associated with the degree of subsequent hypoxia and infants with a low presuction PaO_2 seem to be at risk of developing hypoxia after suction. Thus, in a series of post cardiac surgery adult patients, greater falls in PaO_2 were found in those patients with a low PaO_2 prior to suction as compared to those who had a normal PaO_2 presuction (Taylor and Waters, 1971; Chuley, 1988a). Kelly *et al.* (1987) also demonstrated a statistically and clinically significant fall in PaO_2 following suction in patients with a presuction PaO_2 of less than 100 mmHg, but there was no correlation between inspired oxygen levels and postsuction PaO_2

Neonates are particularly vulnerable and endotracheal suction has been associated with bradycardia and hypotension (Cordero and Hon 1971; Simbruner *et al.*, 1981). In the latter study hypoxia was induced in over half of the total suction passes even if presuction levels of oxygenation were adequate. Further evidence of the adverse effect of suction on oxygenation is provided by Kerem *et al.* (1990) who, in a study of 25 haemodynamically stable and non-cyanosed paediatric patients, documented a significant fall in PaO_2 and SaO_2 following suction and concluded that severe hypoxia may occur during endotracheal suction. Reflex bronchoconstriction secondary to mechanical stimulation of the trachea has been suggested as another possible mechanism for the observation of hypoxia following suction (Naigow and Powaser, 1977).

Strenuous efforts should be made to minimize the detrimental effect of suction on oxygenation. The larger the diameter of catheter the greater the potential for evacuation of gas from the airway and therefore the greater the risk of hypoxia. Because the size of the catheter influences the degree of hypoxia, several authors suggest that the external diameter should not exceed half the internal diameter of the endotracheal tube (Rosen and Hillard, 1962; Young, 1984; Imle and Klemic, 1991). Large diameter catheters passed into similar sized segmental bronchi may lead to airway collapse due to the direct transmission of negative pressure to lung tissue (Rosen and Hillard, 1962). Despite these concerns Tolles and Stone (1990), in a survey of neonatal suction practice, reported that only 12.3% of respondents claimed to keep to the recommended ratio of catheter to tube size. In the presence of thick or viscous secretions the use of a proportionately larger catheter may be necessary, but this should be considered the exception rather than the rule.

The use of high negative pressures also increases the risk of hypoxia due to increased evacuation of gas (Rux and Powaser, 1979). Kuzenski (1978) suggested suction pressures of 70–100 mmHg and Parker (1985) suggested a level of 60–80 mmHg in neonates, although the American Society for Testing Materials reported common levels of use in clinical practice of 100 mmHg in infants and 160 mmHg in adults.

Perhaps the most effective way of reducing suction induced hypoxia is with the use of supplemental oxygen prior to suction. Crabtree Goodnough (1985) evaluated four different suction protocols in 28 adult patients who had undergone cardiac surgery and found that a protocol which used a higher inspired oxygen level presuction with hyperinflation postsuction led to a significant reduction in hypoxia during suction. In the paediatric population PaO_2 may fall significantly during suction without the use of supplemental oxygen therapy (Kerem *et al.*, 1990; Walsh *et al.*, 1989). It has been suggested that 100% oxygen should be administered for one minute prior to suction and that hyperinflation with twice the tidal volume and 100% oxygen should be used between suction passes (Kerem *et al.*, 1990). Manual rebreathing circuits can provide hyperinflation and hyperoxygenation pre and postsuction and have been used in some centres (Gold *et al.*, 1981; Chuley, 1988b). However, Stone *et al.* (1991) did not find this technique superior to hyperoxygenation via a ventilator circuit.

The use of a double lumen catheter tube enables the concurrent administration of supplemental oxygen during suction and has been recommended by some authorities (Bodai *et al.*, 1987; Graff *et al.*, 1987; Kelly *et al.*, 1987). Similarly the use of a port adaptor prevents the interruption of ventilation and oxygen supply and has also been suggested as a method of minimizing hypoxia (Jung and Newman, 1982; Bodai *et al.*, 1987; Durand *et al.*, 1989). Imle and Klemic (1991) report this to be the most useful mechanism for preventing hypoxia in their clinical practice. However, care should be taken when using these devices in low flow circuits as it is possible that the suction flow rate may exceed delivery of ventilatory flow. Studies show conclusively that some form of supplemental oxygen therapy is desirable when performing suction on those at risk from hypoxia. The choice of which method to use to deliver the supplemental oxygen is usually dependent on the clinical setting and facilities available.

Finally it has been demonstrated that the duration of suction time is significantly related to falls in PaO_2 (Boutros, 1970). Minimizing suction time may therefore be the most important factor in reducing suction induced hypoxia and most authors recommend limiting each suction pass to a maximum of 15 seconds (Imle and Klemic, 1991; Rindfleisch and Tyler, 1981; Young, 1984; Sumner, 1990). In practice, 80% of respondents to a survey on neonatal suction practice claimed to apply negative pressure for less than five seconds (Tolles and Stone, 1990).

Cardiovascular changes

Cardiovascular changes may frequently occur and may result from hypoxia or stimulation of the trachea. Cardiac arrhythmias, bradycardia and cardiac arrest have all been reported as complications during suction (Schumaker and Hampton, 1951; Rosen and Hillard, 1962; Marx *et al.*, 1968; Cordero and Hon, 1971). Significant falls in mixed venous SaO_2 with suction were reported by Walsh *et al.* (1989) which are perhaps related to changes in O_2 consumption or CO_2 production. Patients with significant intrapulmonary shunting or who have pre-existing cardiac compromise are more susceptible to these problems. Shim *et al.* (1969) reported that there was a 35% incidence of cardiac arrhythmias during suction of patients breathing room air. Cordero and Hon (1971) reported that tracheal stimulation could induce bradycardia and even cardiac arrest. This may have been due to stimulation of a vasovagal reflex resulting from increased efferent vagal activity. In a small study Winston *et al.* (1987) demonstrated a fall of at least 20% in the resting heart rate in intubated and ventilated adults during suction. Both hypotension (Winston *et al.*, 1987) and hypertension (Simbruner *et al.*, 1981) have been documented in association with suction procedures. The combination of hypertension and bradycardia in infants undergoing tracheal suction is characteristic of a hypoxic response or may partly be a response to an unpleasant experience (Simbruner *et al.*,

1981). Cardiac arrest associated with endotracheal suction has also been reported by several authors. The serious complications that may result from airway suction mean that the procedure should only be undertaken when full resuscitation facilities are available.

Atelectasis

Atelectasis following airway suction may result from the removal of air from the bronchial tree or may occur secondary to obstruction caused by tracheobronchial trauma. Nagaraj *et al.* (1980) found all infants who were ventilated for more than 20 days developed lobar/segmental atelectasis and up to 50% of preterm infants have been shown to fail attempts at extubation due to this complication (Fox *et al.*, 1977). Falls in lung compliance have been reported during suction (Brandstater and Muallen, 1969), yet Fox *et al.* (1977) found no change in lung-thorax compliance or FRC and concluded therefore that there was little evidence to support the development of postsuction atelectasis.

Changes in intracranial pressure

Endotracheal suction may alter PaO_2 and arterial carbon dioxide tension ($PaCO_2$) with a consequent profound influence on cerebral circulation, potentially subjecting patients to the risk of brain injury. During suction an increase in intrathoracic pressure, due to stimulation of a cough, impedes venous return and leads to an increase in cerebrovenous pressure. This may be responsible for the rise in blood pressure and intracranial pressure observed in ventilated preterm neonates (Durand *et al.*, 1989). Endotracheal suction may also induce an increase in cerebral blood flow and intracranial pressure and this may have a potentially dangerous effect in preterm infants at risk of intraventricular haemorrhage (Perlman and Volpe, 1983). However, in most cases elevation of intracranial pressure during suction is shortlived and a return to baseline values occurs rapidly (Durand *et al.*, 1989).

Pneumothorax

Poor suction technique may cause direct perforation of segmental bronchi (Figure 6.9) of infants with severe lung disease (Vaughan *et al.*, 1978; Alpan *et al.*, 1984). The main site of perforation is the segmental bronchus of the right lower lobe. To minimize this risk it has been suggested that the catheter should be introduced to only 1 cm below the carina by using premarked catheters according to data which relates body weight to orocarinal distance (Anderson and Chandra, 1976).

Bacterial infection

Tracheal suction may introduce bacterial contaminants into the tracheobronchial tree if strictly clean or sterile procedures are not

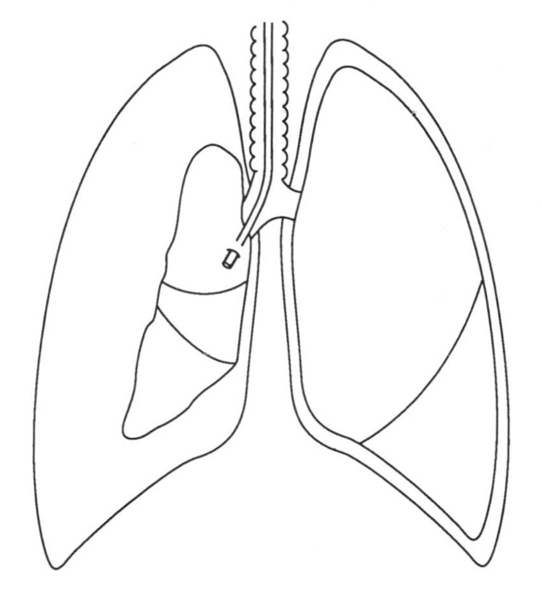

Figure 6.9 Diagrammatic representation of perforation by suction catheter into segmental bronchus. Reproduced with permission from UnoPlast (UK) Ltd.

observed. The suction equipment itself is also a potential source of contamination. Tubing and bottles should be regularly changed and a filter incorporated into the circuit to reduce the risk of infection. The clinician should always wear gloves, at least on the dominant hand. A raised vent for application of negative pressure is preferable to a flush vent which increases the risk of clinician contact with secretions.

SUGGESTED SUCTION PROCEDURE

1. explain procedure to child and parent. Ensure the infant is securely held if responsive. Wash hands.
2. increase inspired oxygen either via the ventilator circuit, manual rebreathing circuit or face mask/head box as appropriate.
3. check level of negative pressure (60–120 mmHg), attach sleeved catheter to suction tubing via Y-connection or flow control (if not integral to catheter).
4. glove dominant hand and slide catheter from sleeve avoiding contact with anything other than gloved hand.
5. disconnect patient from ventilator/oxygen source unless a port adaptor is being used. Gently introduce catheter into either the naso/oropharynx or tracheal tube without negative pressure. Do not advance the catheter if any early resistance is felt; instead withdraw slightly and attempt to reintroduce.
6. apply suction prior to withdrawal of the catheter, using either continuous vacuum in the presence of copious secretions or intermittent suction where there are few secretions. Do not apply negative pressure for more than ten seconds.
7. reconnect patient to oxygen/ventilator source.
8. return patient to presuction inspired oxygen level when baseline values have normalized.

Points to note

The procedure should be performed cleanly and carried out efficiently and effectively as it may cause significant distress.

The size of the catheter as a general rule should not exceed 50% of the airway.

Suction should not be performed at predetermined intervals and the frequency should depend on individual patient need.

NASOPHARYNGEAL SUCTION

Nasopharyngeal or tracheal suction of non-intubated infants and children is frequently necessary when other methods of stimulating an effective cough fail and a few points are worthy of mention in addition to those previously discussed. Complications of this technique may be dangerous and include a fall in SaO_2, cardiac arrhythmias, apnoea, laryngeal or bronchospasm and the possibility of vomiting and aspiration. Therefore this procedure should always be carried out with the utmost care. The patients should be well prepared. Infants and small children must be securely held or wrapped with their arms tucked in a blanket during the procedure (Figure 6.10). Ideally the patient should be in the side lying position to reduce the risk of inhalation of vomit. Slight

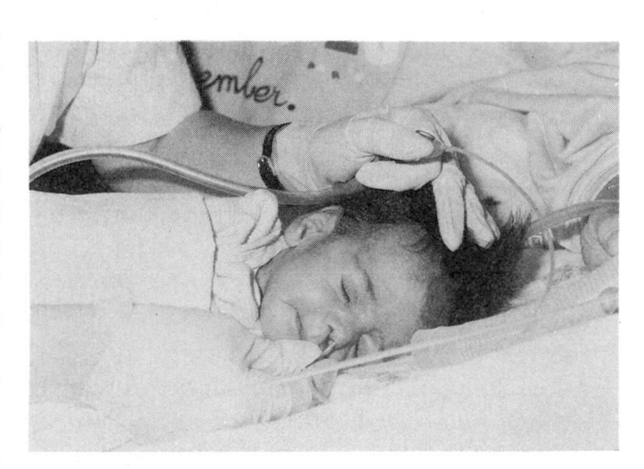

Figure 6.10 Nasopharyngeal suction, with infant securely held.

extension of the neck may facilitate the passage of the catheter through the nasopharynx. This procedure is specifically contraindicated in the presence of a cerebrospinal fluid (CSF) leak and in those with severe stridor. The procedure should not be performed without the availability of oxygen, rebreathing apparatus and full resuscitation equipment.

SELECTIVE CANNULATION OF MAINSTEM BRONCHI

In certain circumstances it may be desirable to selectively cannulate one or other mainstem bronchus, for example in cases of unilateral lobar or complete lung collapse. A variety of techniques have been suggested to facilitate selective cannulation. Anatomically the right mainstem bronchus branches from the trachea at an angle of 24° from the midline in infants and 20° in adults, whereas the left mainstem bronchus arises at a more acute angle of 44° in infants and 35° in adults. Consequently the left mainstem bronchus is more difficult to cannulate. Curved tip (Coude) catheters may improve the chances of selective cannulation of either mainstem bronchus. Kubota *et al.* (1982) were able to achieve selective cannulation in 92% of patients positioning the head in the midline and using curved tip cannulae. Placzek and Silverman (1983) reported a greater than 90% success rate in cannulating the left mainstem bronchus in neonates.

Alternative techniques include turning the head to the contralateral side or tilting the body to the same side to assist selective cannulation (Placzek and Silverman, 1983; Fewell *et al.*, 1979). Soong and Hwang (1991) passed flexible straight suction catheters through nasal ET tubes of 30 newborn infants undergoing mechanical ventilation just prior to chest radiography. With the head midline, 63% and 37% entered the right and left main bronchus respectively. With the head turned to the left or right, 87% and 73% entered the contralateral mainstem bronchus respectively and they concluded that turning the head facilitates selective cannulation of the contralateral side. Although selective cannulation during procedures such as mini bronchoalveolar lavage (see p. 88) may be achieved, care should be taken to avoid tracheal tube displacement or tracheal irritation when using this technique.

INSTILLATION OF SALINE OR IRRIGANTS

The instillation of irrigants such as 0.9% normal saline (NaCl) into artificial airways with the intent of washing out viscous secretions or mucus plugs from the airways is common clinical practice. However, there is a surprising lack of supporting literature and therefore it remains a contentious issue. Varying aliquots (0.5–10 ml) of irrigants are introduced into the airway prior to suction or chest physiotherapy and suction. The suggested benefits of this procedure are that it loosens secretions (Blodgett, 1980; Allen, 1988), suspends secretions making them easier to aspirate (Morrison, 1979; Bostick and Wendelgass, 1987), that it elicits a cough (Demers and Saklad, 1973) or that it helps to maintain patency of an artificial airway (Drew *et al.*, 1986). In a study using radioisotope labelled boluses of saline instilled into the tracheal tube, the saline was demonstrated to remain within the trachea and mainstem bronchi for up to 30 minutes following the procedure. It was concluded therefore that saline given in this manner has no effect on secretions beyond the mainstem bronchi (Hanley *et al.*, 1978). Demers and Saklad (1973) questioned the ability of such irrigants to loosen or thin secretions and reported that mucus and water in bulk form are immiscible even after vigorous shaking. This group proposed that the main advantage of saline instillation was to elicit a cough. Cough alone may not be without complications and White *et al*. (1982) reported that undesirable spasms of coughing could accompany lavage and may be associated with a rise in intracranial pressure. Indeed, endotracheal suction itself is usually enough to stimulate a cough without the use of saline. Many authorities advocate adequate patient hydration and good humidification of inspired gases rather than routine instillation of an irrigant.

Tolles and Stones' (1990) survey reported that 91% of respondents claimed to routinely use 0.9% NaCl or some other irrigant to loosen secretions prior to suction. Other irrigants which are used for this purpose include 0.45% NaCl, 0.84% sodium bicarbonate and sterile water. In spite of the differing views expressed in the literature, in our clinical experience we have found that the instillation of 0.9% NaCl and occasionally the use of mucolytic agents (Hirsch *et al*., 1969) such as Mistabron (Mesna) or N-acetyl cysteine prior to chest physiotherapy may enhance the clearance of thick viscous secretions, when other chest physiotherapy techniques have failed. However, we would not advocate the routine use of irrigants with chest physiotherapy or prior to each suction procedure.

MINI BRONCHOALVEOLAR LAVAGE

Bronchoalveolar lavage (BAL) is a technique that we have found to be of value both as a treatment and for diagnostic purposes.

ACUTE LOBAR COLLAPSE

This technique may be useful for the treatment of lobar/multilobar collapse due to mucus plugging or retention of secretions (Figure 6.11). Though a relatively simple intervention, it is essential that the patient is carefully monitored throughout the procedure. Following careful assessment and discussion with the medical and nursing team the procedure may be carried out as follows:

1. preparation of patient for procedure. If the patient is self-ventilating, anaesthetic referral is required for purposes of temporary intubation. The patient may require sedation and preoxygenation.

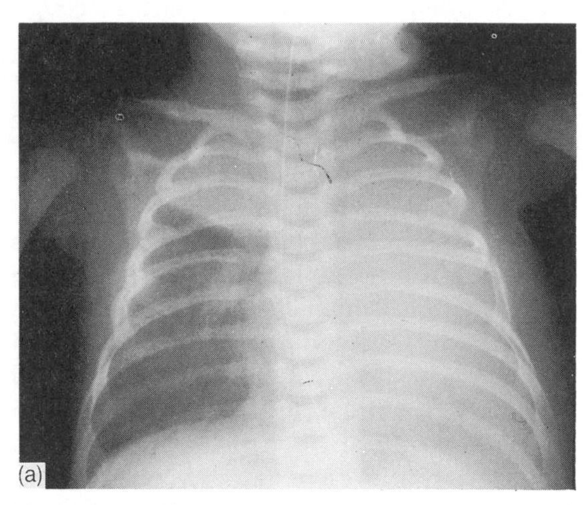

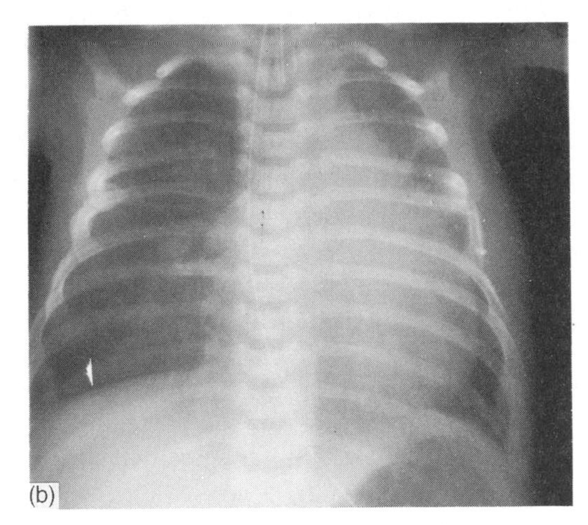

Figure 6.11 Chest X-ray: (a) showing collapse of the left lung and the right upper lobe, (b) post BAL with reinflation of collapse.

2. preparation of suction equipment, 0.9% NaCl or mucolytic for irrigation (syringe attached to a suction catheter) and manual hyperinflation circuit.
3. position patient in the 'reverse' postural drainage position (i.e. collapsed lung segment dependent), head to contralateral side (to facilitate selective cannulation of appropriate bronchus).
4. instillation of irrigant via catheter (infants 2–5 ml, older children – 10–15 ml), followed by tidal volume manual inflations.
5. reposition patient into appropriate postural drainage position and apply manual techniques with hyperinflations.
6. apply endotracheal suction.
7. evaluate efficacy of treatment and patient well-being. Repeat procedure if necessary and if patient's condition allows.

DIAGNOSTIC BAL

This procedure may be useful in the diagnosis of opportunistic infection, unresponsive pulmonary pathology without isolation of specific organisms, viral and fungal infections (e.g. *Pneumocystis carinii* pneumonia, adenovirus, cytomegalovirus, candida and aspergillus). As many of the patients requiring BAL have severe pulmonary disease and may be undergoing intensive care, the procedure does have potential complications (O'Donnel *et al.*, 1993). These include severe hypoxia which may be accompanied by bradycardia, significant bleeding from the respiratory tract and bronchospasm. Therefore we would recommend that the procedure is only conducted by experienced therapists, in the presence of a member of the medical team and with the availability of resuscitation facilities.

1. preparation of patient. This may include intubation in the self-ventilating patient, administration of paralysis/sedative agents and preoxygenation.
2. preparation of equipment using a sterile procedure. 0.9% NaCl (5–20 ml aliquots, depending on patient size) in syringes attached to suction catheters, port adaptor on endotracheal tube for suction, sputum traps and suction equipment.
3. assess patient's cardiorespiratory status and manually hyperinflate to ensure that adequate respiratory support can be maintained. Reposition patient depending on extent of radiological changes (i.e. with affected areas gravity dependent) if condition allows.
4. carefully insert catheter via port adaptor, through ETT into respiratory tract as far as possible. Instill irrigant and leave catheter in situ. Remove syringe and attach suction tubing and sputum trap to catheter (Figure 6.12).
5. manually hyperinflate and apply chest vibrations while applying suction and withdrawing catheter from ETT in order to aspirate as much of the irrigant as possible.
6. reassess patient's status and repeat procedure for further specimens if condition allows.

CONTINUOUS POSITIVE AIRWAY PRESSURE

Continuous positive airway pressure (CPAP) is a closed system which delivers a raised airway pressure throughout the respiratory cycle whilst the subject breathes spontaneously (Figure 6.13). It can be applied by face mask, nasal cannulae or prong, mouthpiece or via an artificial airway. As early as 1971 it was described as a method of elevating the airway pressure, reported to significantly decrease mortality when used in spontaneously breathing neonates suffering from respiratory distress syndrome (RDS) (Gregory *et al.*, 1971). The application

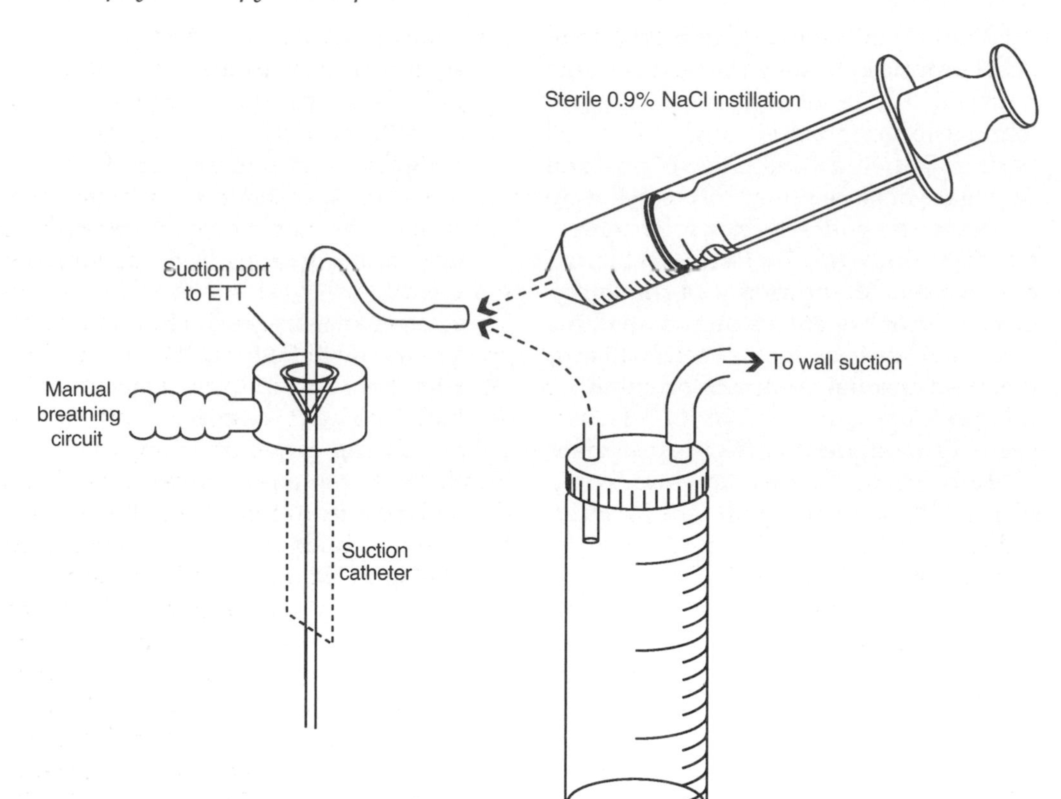

Figure 6.12 Diagram of equipment used for BAL.

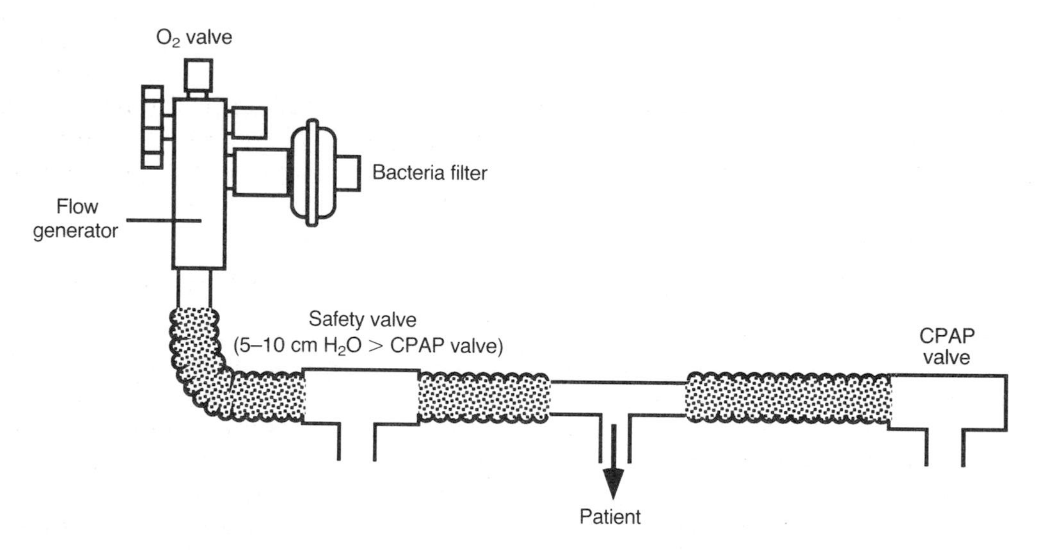

Figure 6.13 CPAP circuit, applied via face mask. Note safety CPAP valve placed between patient and flow generator which should be at least 5 cmH_2O greater than the level of CPAP being administered.

of CPAP on an intermittent basis is termed periodic continuous positive airway pressure (PCPAP).

The physiological effects of CPAP are an increase in FRC (Stock *et al.*, 1984) and an improvement in oxygenation (Dehaven *et al.*, 1985). Andersen *et al.* (1979) under experimental conditions studied the reinflation of collapsed parts of excised normal lungs which were divided into a small and a larger section. Each section was separately cannulated. By obstructing one section the lung would be ventilated through collateral channels. Five different ventilatory patterns were used for reinflation: simulated deep breathing with and without CPAP, simulated tidal breathing and mechanical ventilation with and without CPAP. The most effective way of reinflation was simulated deep breathing with CPAP. An improvement in arterial oxygen tension occurs if the normal relationship between FRC and closing volume (CV) is established. CPAP has been shown to improve hypoxaemia (Dehaven *et al.*, 1985) which was not responding to other physiotherapy modalities.

In the younger child, where collateral ventilation is poorly established, CPAP results in an increase in FRC, the application of positive pressure preventing airway closure of dependent lung regions. In the older child, once collateral ventilatory flow has been established, CPAP may lower the resistance to collateral flow, further increasing FRC and preventing closure of the terminal bronchioles during the respiratory pause. The promotion of collateral flow may also help to mobilize secretions as the pressure distal to an obstruction will increase and exceed the pressure proximally, therefore forcing secretions centrally. In this way CPAP reduces the work of breathing and increases compliance.

A period of CPAP applied via face mask postextubation in children with continued respiratory distress may prevent the need for more aggressive therapy such as reintubation. It may also be useful postoperatively (Stock *et al.*, 1985), particularly in patients with preoperative evidence of restrictive lung disease and a reduced FRC, e.g. those with structural spinal abnormalities who require major corrective surgery such as spinal fusion. Interspersing short periods of CPAP with the ACBT has been suggested in the treatment of postoperative atelectasis (Webber, 1988). In children, however, we have found it preferable to apply CPAP for at least 30–50 minutes each hour with the remaining time spent with humidified oxygen via face mask. During this period breathing exercises and airway clearance techniques can be encouraged if the child is old and well enough to cooperate. This has been successful in both postoperative patients and in those with impending respiratory failure in order to avoid more invasive support. PCPAP may also be of use in the terminal stages of respiratory disease to decrease the work of breathing (Pryor and Webber, 1992). CPAP should not be used in the presence of an undrained pneumothorax, multiple cysts or emphysematous bullae. Caution should be used in patients with low intravascular volume and in those patients unable to protect their own airway, e.g. patients with evidence of bleeding in the upper gastrointestinal tract and those who are at risk of vomiting and aspiration (Keilty and Bott, 1992).

INTERMITTENT POSITIVE PRESSURE BREATHING

Intermittent positive pressure breathing (IPPB) has been a controversial technique since its initial description by Motley *et al.* (1947). IPPB in the last few decades has changed from being frequently used to an almost discontinued mode of treatment in some centres. Although IPPB has beneficial physiological effects, there is conflicting evidence as to its efficacy in clinical practice (Gormezano and Branthwaite, 1972b; Ali *et al.*, 1984).

IPPB has been shown to increase tidal volume (Torres *et al.*, 1960; Emmanuel *et al.*, 1966). This effect is produced without increasing the work of breathing on the part of the patient. An increase in tidal volume may be desirable to both medical and surgical patients who may be hypoventilating or patients in respiratory failure who are too weak to breathe or cough effectively due to respiratory muscle fatigue, as in cases of neuromuscular disease. Patients with excessive bronchial secretions or who are unable to take deep breaths to loosen and mobilize secretions due to pain, may benefit from the larger tidal volume which in turn may help to mobilize secretions if present.

An improvement in arterial blood gases has also been demonstrated with IPPB (Starke *et al.*, 1979). The increase in tidal and therefore in minute volume causes a fall in arterial carbon dioxide tension ($PaCO_2$) and a rise in PaO_2 as long as the flow rate is sufficient to meet the individual patient's demands (Bott *et al.*, 1992). In the patient with impending coma due to CO_2 narcosis secondary to retained secretions and respiratory muscle fatigue, IPPB with chest vibrations during expiration may help to clear secretions and reduce the $PaCO_2$. Patients with chronic respiratory disease who are exhausted from an acute infection may benefit from IPPB provided it is used with caution so as not to generate excessive intrathoracic pressures which may further damage lung tissue; for example, for patients with cystic fibrosis, when maximal effort cannot be achieved with the ACBT and in the terminal stages of disease, IPPB may assist clearance of secretions (Pryor and Webber, 1992).

A reduction in the work of breathing can be successfully achieved if the patient is relaxed and is able to co-ordinate with the respirator (Sukumalchantra *et al.*, 1965). However, if the patient fights against the respirator the work of breathing may actually increase and therefore be detrimental to patient well-being. Reduction in the work of breathing by the use of IPPB may be of value in patients with acute asthmatic attacks. The efficacy of IPPB as a method of drug delivery in such patients has not been demonstrated to be superior to that of a nebulizer, but patients with severe respiratory embarrassment, unable to cope with inhalation therapy, may benefit from delivery of bronchodilator therapy via IPPB.

In selected cases, therefore, IPPB seems to be a useful adjunct to chest physiotherapy and may avoid the need for intubation and ventilation in the acutely ill patient with impending respiratory failure. However, in the paediatric age group its use is limited due to both the continuing debate over its efficacy and the concern over administration of high positive peak inspiratory pressures.

INCENTIVE SPIROMETRY

The incentive spirometer is a mechanical aid which encourages lung expansion by providing a visual stimulus and feedback during breathing exercises which emphasize inspiration. Maximal alveolar inflation can only be achieved in the spontaneously breathing patient with respiratory manoeuvres which emphasize inspiration. Incentive spirometry aims to encourage regular inflation to total lung capacity, as the active maximal inspiratory manoeuvres are performed by the patient and the device gives visual feedback of inspiratory flow or volume. In children the visual stimulus provided may encourage and motivate them to perform breathing exercises. If incentive spirometry is to be used postoperatively, careful preoperative instruction to familiarize the patient in its use is essential.

Two types of incentive spirometer are available. The Voldyne model incorporates a breath hold feature. Although this device has been reported to demonstrate a decrease in atelectasis compared to the Triflo, it is more expensive, larger and generally more difficult to use (Byrne *et al.*, 1990). The Triflo is a flow sensitive device with three chambers each containing a plastic ball. On inspiration the plastic balls rise in their chambers for as long as flow is maintained. In a UK survey it was found that incentive spirometry was used in 44% of hospitals undertaking adult cardiac surgery. This is much lower than the reported use in the USA where it is used extensively in the prevention and treatment of atelectasis (Jenkins and Soutar, 1986).

POSITIVE EXPIRATORY PRESSURE

Positive expiratory pressure (PEP) devices provide positive pressure during expiration. PEP acts on the peripheral airways and promotes collateral ventilatory flow, allowing a pressure gradient to build up behind bronchial secretions, forcing them toward central airways (Andersen *et al.*, 1979). The use of PEP as a means of clearing bronchial secretions in patients with chronic sputum production is further discussed in Chapter 11, p. 167. Postoperatively the use of PEP via face mask has been suggested as a treatment technique in patients with retained secretions (Campbell *et al.*, 1986). The treatment is performed in the sitting position using PEP of 10–20 cmH_2O during the mid expiratory phase.

INHALATION THERAPIES

HUMIDIFICATION

Under normal physiological circumstances the nose and upper respiratory tract warm, humidify and filter inspired air. In circumstances where the upper airway is bypassed (for example by a tracheal tube) and/or when a patient requires supplemental oxygen therapy it is usually necessary to administer some form of additional humidification. Appropriate humidification avoids several potential complications. Firstly, inhalation of dry gases has been associated with cilial dysfunction, mucosal drying, inflammation and ulceration and an increase in viscosity of secretions (Burton, 1962; Chalon *et al.*, 1972; Marfatia *et al.*, 1975; Tattersall, 1982). Secondly, the small calibre airways of infants and small children can be easily blocked by the resulting thick secretions; and thirdly the delivery of cool inspired gas has been associated with exacerbation of bronchospasm.

Broadly, humidification systems can be divided into two groups, maintenance or supplemental (Conway, 1992). Heat and moisture exchangers are examples of maintenance humidifiers and are designed to maintain the amount of humidity already present within the respiratory tract. In paediatric practice the use of such devices may be disadvantageous, due to the resistance they give to inspiration and a resulting increase in the work of breathing. This is particularly relevant in the infant and small child under the age of two years. Bubble-through humidifiers, which contain a reservoir of cold water through which inspired gas is bubbled and delivered to the patient usually via narrow bore tubing and face mask or nasal cannulae, are not effective. Water tends to condense within the tubing and thus may alter the oxygen delivery to the patient. Supplemental humidifiers aim either to deliver a solution in vapour form (heated water bath humidifiers) or, as a nebulizer solution, to deliver a saturated aerosol of liquid droplets.

Although some in vitro studies have shown a decrease in viscosity of sputum following humidification (Liftschitz and Denning, 1970; Richards, 1974), others have found no such decrease following water mist therapy (Rosenbluth and Chernick, 1974). More recently studies have shown an increase in sputum clearance above that of the presently optimal physiotherapy regimen for stable hypersecretory lung disease (Conway, 1992; Sutton *et al.*, 1988; Pavia *et al.*, 1978) and this effect may be due to increased periciliary hydration (Litt, 1970), increased efficiency of FET and/or coughing mechanisms (Conway, 1992).

Non-isotonic solutions such as water and hypertonic saline may induce bronchoconstriction in patients with hyperactive airways (Smith and Anderson, 1989) and therefore the use of 0.9% saline may be preferable. The use of heated humidification systems is standard practice in intubated and ventilated children and heated systems are often used in the non-intubated baby. Reported complications include bacterial colonization of warmed humidification systems and thermal injury if the humidifying solution is overheated (Shelly *et al.*, 1988). Therefore regular cleaning and replacement of humidifier chambers is essential and the temperature of inspired gas should be measured as near to the patient end of the circuit as possible.

NEBULIZER THERAPY

Compressed air or a pressurized oxygen supply can be used to produce an aerosol of a drug in solution, which can then be inhaled via a mask or preferably a mouthpiece into the airways. A variety of compressors and nebulizer systems are available. In order to achieve penetration of the inhaled drug into the lower respiratory tract the particles produced must be less than 5 microns and preferably in the region of 2 microns. To achieve optimal therapy it is therefore essential that compressors with an adequate output are provided to the patient or if using piped/cylinder gas flow, a minimal flow rate of 6 l/min is used. Patients must be taught how to administer therapy effectively and be given clear guidelines as to cleaning, replacement and maintenance of the equipment. Drug delivery in infants requires the use of a face mask, but as soon as the child is able, a mouthpiece should be used to avoid drug deposition on the face.

Bronchodilator/steroid therapy

This form of therapy does not necessitate patient co-operation and nebulized bronchodilators or steroids can be used in young patients with severe bronchoconstriction. However, it is important to note that in some infants of less than two years of age nebulizer solutions have been documented to cause an immediate, though temporary deterioration in lung function and the preferred route of delivery in these infants should be oral preparations or via metered dose inhalers (O'Callaghan *et al.*, 1986, 1989). It is also important that patients are carefully instructed in the administration of medication and given clear guidelines of safe maximal dosage. If the child's clinical status fails to improve significantly following maximal treatment immediate medical advice must be sought. Premedication with bronchodilator therapy, either via nebulizer, dry powder or aerosol, prior to chest physiotherapy is important to minimize any increase in bronchoconstriction with treatment. This may also allow for more effective clearance of secretions by dilating already constricted airways.

Mucolytic agents

Such agents may liquify viscous secretions in vitro (Brain and Valberg, 1979; Hirsch *et al.*, 1969) but there is little conclusive evidence regarding their efficacy in vivo particularly in patients with acute lung pathology (Brain, 1980). Possible adverse effects include haemorrhagic tracheitis and bronchospasm (Ratjen *et al.*, 1990). The mucolytic agents most commonly used include N-acetyl cysteine (Parvolex) and sodium-2f-mercaptoethane (Mistabron). The use of such agents has been advocated in some patients with chronic pulmonary disease such as cystic fibrosis (Weller *et al.*, 1980; Thomson *et al.*, 1975), and are thought to be most effective if administered via nebulizer prior to chest physiotherapy.

Antibiotics

In patients with chronic respiratory disease such as cystic fibrosis, antibiotics or antifungal agents delivered via nebulizer may be useful over short periods during intercurrent infection or over a long term period to reduce the need for hospitalization for treatment of acute bronchopulmonary exacerbations (Hodson *et al.*, 1981). During use of nebulized antibiotic therapy it is important to ensure the system is fitted with a one-way valve and wide bore tubing to allow the expired drug to be 'vented' out through an open window. This reduces the risk of development of multiresistant organisms. Nebulized antibiotic therapy should only be administered following chest physiotherapy sessions.

DRY POWDER/AEROSOL DEVICES

Dry powder devices release powdered drug on inspiration, but some of these devices require high inspiratory flow rates in order to achieve initiation and optimal delivery of the drug into the respiratory tract (e.g. rotohaler, diskhaler – 60 l/min). Such flow rates are usually achievable during normal health in a child of 4–5 years of age, but may be of little value in the younger age group or during times of respiratory distress (Milner, 1993). Devices such as the turbohaler, however, do allow drug delivery down to flow rates of 20 l/min, but even these may be ineffective in times of acute respiratory embarrassment. Pressurized inhalers contain suspension of active drug in a propellant. Activation of drug release needs to be co-ordinated with inhalation in most devices. Due to the co-ordination required, use of these devices may prove difficult in young children and even in the older child careful instruction is vital if optimal therapy is to be achieved. In a few newer devices inhalation itself triggers release of the drug.

Spacer devices are volume reservoirs which can be inserted between the drug delivery device and the patient. Following delivery of drug into the spacer, tidal breaths from the spacer seem to allow adequate penetration into the respiratory tract. Attachment of a sealing face mask to the patient end of the spacer allows effective drug delivery to babies and small children. Alternatively, mounting the delivery device into the base of a polystyrene cup and holding this loosely to the child's face is also an effective means of providing adequate drug delivery without requiring the co-ordination between activation and inhalation. Drugs may also be delivered to babies in the supine position by activating the delivery device and then tipping the spacer to the vertical position. The spacer valve will open and the drug will drift down the spacer into the face mask. Children above the age of two years are usually able to use the spacer device with a metered dose inhaler in the conventional manner. From approximately seven to eight years of age most children will have the ability to co-ordinate the activation of the drug with inhalation without the use of a spacer device.

GENERAL CONSIDERATIONS

PAIN

Until recently the management of pain in infancy has been suboptimal (Choonara, 1989). The inadequate recognition of pain and lack of appropriate analgesia may have a detrimental effect on the patient's condition. Although young infants and neonates may be unable to complain verbally about pain, it may be indicated by one or more of the following: an increased heart rate or blood pressure, facial grimacing or limb movements, an increase in transcutaneous CO_2 or a decrease in arterial O_2 tension. Any of these factors may lead to an increased metabolic rate and oxygen consumption. If oxygen delivery is not increased sufficiently to meet the greater demand, metabolic acidosis may result from anaerobic metabolism.

The choice and dose of analgesia involves a delicate balance between pain relief and possible detrimental side effects of the drug. For example, chest expansion can be restricted by pain, leading to a reduced FRC, hypoventilation and an increased potential for atelectasis and infection. However, the administration of opiate analgesia may itself lead to sedation and depression of the respiratory centre and potentially worsen respiratory function. It is essential that the patient should at all times receive sufficient analgesia, particularly prior to potentially uncomfortable procedures such as physiotherapy, which may necessitate the administration of bolus doses analgesia.

Analgesia is most often provided by intermittent doses of oral, intravenous or intramuscular preparations. Older children may be able to use patient controlled analgesia in the form of a continuous infusion supplemented by intermittent boluses with predetermined limits of maximum and minimum infusion. Postoperative epidural analgesia is often very effective in controlling pain. In the critically ill child analgesia may be given in the form of a continuous infusion and a sedative/paralysis agent added if appropriate.

THE EFFECTS OF HOSPITALIZATION

The adverse effects of hospitalization on children have been well described. Separation from parents or carers may lead initially to protest, then despair and finally a loss of interest (Bowlby, 1953). The importance of involving parents in both the day-to-day care of the child and in the investigative and treatment procedures cannot be overemphasized. To facilitate this degree of involvement, visiting should not be restricted and ideally provision made to allow parents to reside within the hospital. Encouraging the child to bring their own special toys to hospital and engaging in talk about siblings, pets and home will reduce the stress of being away from a familiar environment. Particular care should be taken to explain forthcoming procedures to both the parents and child. The explanation of surgical incisions and the presence of drips and drains may be best illustrated using dolls or teddies. As children grow older their understanding and awareness of their illness increases. This will inevitably have a significant impact not only on their physical well-being but also their psychological make-up. This is of particular relevance in the child suffering from a chronic disease such as cystic fibrosis. Teenagers need to come to terms with the implications of having a chronic illness and should be carefully encouraged to take responsibility for their own well-being, in order to achieve independence and lead as normal a lifestyle as possible.

The siblings of children with either acute or chronic respiratory disease may also be affected psychologically. Parents may spend much of their time at the hospital and may even be resident, leaving the siblings with relatives and friends. This disrupts the normal routine and may result in the child feeling insecure. Where regular and intensive treatment is required siblings often feel left out or jealous of the attention being paid to the affected child. It is essential therefore that they are made to feel included and are given adequate explanation of the circumstances and allowed to visit the hospital regularly.

RESEARCH IN CHEST PHYSIOTHERAPY

The scientific literature regarding the effects of chest physiotherapy is often confusing and many questions remain unanswered. In many published studies 'chest physiotherapy' is a standardized package of treatment, irrespective of the patient's clinical status (Connors *et al.*, 1980; Gormezano and Branthwaite, 1972a; Laws and McIntyre, 1969; Klein *et al.*, 1988; Finer and Boyd, 1978; Holloway *et al.*, 1969). In others a variety of techniques are incorporated, without identifying which of these interventions patients receive (Mackenzie *et al.*, 1978; Mackenzie and Shin, 1985). There is a lack of literature evaluating actual clinical practice. This is probably due to the large variety of techniques patients may receive during treatment. Clinically, techniques are rarely used in isolation and evaluating the effect of several techniques within one treatment is difficult, as is the implementation of appropriate methodologies. The randomized clinical trial (RCT) is considered the gold standard design of biomedical research, but its use in chest physiotherapy is limited. The clinical study where participants are aware of the treatment they receive (as the intervention and control treatment are distinguishable) is often more suitable.

The measurement tools dictated by the research question are often not easily used in the clinical setting. As one of the aims of treatment is the removal of tracheobronchial secretions, assessment of tracheobronchial clearance is one measurement of outcome but is difficult to measure directly. Sputum weight is often recorded but may be inaccurate as saliva may be included. This may be overcome by freeze drying but neither wet nor dry sputum weight will account for swallowed secretions. Inhalation of radionuclides tagged to aerosol particles is another measure of mucus clearance. DeCesare *et al.* (1982) questioned these methods as aerosol particles are relatively large and uniform penetration may be impeded by retained secretions and bronchial thickening. Imaging of the lung with a gaseous radionuclide (e.g. krypton 81m) has been used to evaluate regional ventilation and may be a more useful tool for future research. However, improvement of ventilation is seen through visual analysis and more objective methods of quantifying the data must be sought.

Pulmonary function tests (ranging from simple spirometry to whole body plethysmography) have also been used to evaluate treatment, particularly in long term studies (Oberwaldner *et al.*, 1986; Reisman *et al.*, 1988). However, as these tests require patient understanding and co-operation they may be difficult to perform in young children. When used, reliability of these tests must be ensured prior to data collection. Oxygen saturation as a measure of outcome has been used more recently particularly in measuring the acute effects of treatment. This is a readily available, non-invasive clinical tool and its accuracy has been demonstrated (Clayton *et al.*, 1991).

Most studies have been performed in adults and the results extrapolated to the paediatric population. This may not be appropriate due to the differences in pulmonary anatomy and physiology which may alter the response to intervention. Further research is therefore necessary in children, looking at specific patient groups and specific treatment modalities. Much of this work will need to be collaborative, but the questions to be asked should come from physiotherapists working in respiratory care who have an in-depth understanding of current clinical practice.

REFERENCES

Agostini, E. and Hyatt, R.E. (1986) Static behavior of the respiratory system, in *American Physiological Society Handbook of Physiology – The Respiratory System*, Williams and Wilkins, Baltimore.

Ali, J., Serrette, C., Wood, L.D.H. *et al.*, (1984) The effect of postoperative positive pressure breathing on lung function. *Chest*, **85**, 192–6.

Allen, D. (1988) Making sense of suctioning. *Nursing Times*, **84**, 46–7.

Alpan, G., Glick, B., Peleg, O. *et al.* (1984) Pneumothorax due to endotracheal tube suction. *American Journal of Perinatology*, **1**, 345–8.

Andersen, J.B., Qvist, J. and Kann, T. (1979) Recruiting collapsed lung through collateral channels with positive end expiratory pressure. *Scandanavian Journal of Respiratory Disease*, **60**, 260–6.

Anderson, K. and Chandra, K. (1976) Pneumothorax secondary to perforation of sequential bronchi by suction catheters. *Journal of Paediatric Surgery*, **11**, 687–93.

Bateman, J.R.M., Newman, S.P., Daunt, K.M. *et al.* (1979) Regional lung clearance of excessive bronchial secretions during chest physiotherapy in patients with stable chronic airways obstruction. *Lancet*, **1**, 294–7.

Bateman, J.R.M., Newman, S., Daunt, K.M. *et al.* (1981) Is cough as effective as chest physiotherapy in the removal of excessive tracheobronchial secretions? *Thorax*, **36**, 683–7.

Blodgett, D. (1980) *Manual of Respiratory Care Procedures*, J.B. Lippincott, Philadelphia, p. 517.

Blumenthal, I. and Lealman, G.T. (1982) Effects of posture on gastro-oesophageal reflux in the newborn. *Archives of Disease in Childhood*, **57**, 555–6.

Bodai, B.I., Walton, C.B., Briggs, S. and Goldstein, M. (1987) A clinical evaluation of an oxygen insufflation/suction catheter. *Heart Lung*, **16**, 39–46.

Bostick, J. and Wendelgass, S.T. (1987) Normal saline instillation as part of the suctioning procedure: Effects on PaO_2 and amount of secretions. *Heart Lung*, **16**, 532–7.

Bott, J., Keilty, S.E.J. and Noone, L. (1992) Intermittent positive pressure – a dying art? *Physiotherapy*, **78**, 656–60.

Boutros, A.R. (1970) Arterial blood oxygenation during and after endotracheal suctioning in the apneic patient. *Anesthesiology*, **32**, 114–18.

Bowlby, J. (1953) *Child Care and the Growth of Love*, Penguin, Middlesex.

Brackbill, Y., Douthitt, T.C. and West, H. (1973) Psychophysiologic effects in the neonate of prone versus supine placement. *Journal of Pediatrics*, **82**, 82–3.

Brain, J.D. (1980) Aerosol and humidity therapy. *American Review of Respiratory Disease*, **122**, 17–21.

Brain, J.D. and Vallberg, P.A. (1979) State of the art deposition of aerosol in the respiratory tract. *American Review of Respiratory Disease*, **120**, 1325–73.

Brandstater, B. and Muallen, M. (1969) Atelectasis following tracheal suctioning in infants. *Anesthesiology*, **31**, 468–73.

Brodsky, L., Reidy, M. and Stanievich, J. (1987) The effects of suction techniques on the distal tracheal mucosa in intubated low birth weight infants. *International Journal of Pediatric Otorhinolaryngology*, **14**, 1.

Burton, J.D.K. (1962) Effects of dry anaesthetic gases on the respiratory membrane. *Lancet*, **1**, 235–8.

Byrne, I., Geary, M. and Crawford, B. (1990) Incentive spirometry – patient compliance. *Physiotherapy Ireland*, **8**, 8–11.

Campbell, A.H., O'Connell, J.M. and Wilson, F. (1975) The effect of chest physiotherapy upon FEV1 in chronic bronchitis. *Medical Journal of Australia*, **1**, 33–5.

Campbell, T., Ferguson, N. and McKinlay, R.G.C. (1986) The use of a simple self-administered method of positive expiratory pressure (PEP) in chest physiotherapy after abdominal surgery. *Physiotherapy*, **72**, 498–500.

Chalon, L., Loew, D.A.Y. and Malebranche, J. (1972) Effects of dry anaesthetic gases on tracheobronchial ciliated epithelium. *Anesthesiology*, **37**, 338–43.

Choonara, I.A. (1989) Pain relief. *Archives of Disease in Childhood*, **64**, 1101–2.

Chuley, M. (1988a) Arterial blood gas changes with a hyperinflation and hyperoxygenation suctioning intervention in critically ill patients. *Heart Lung*, **17**, 654.

Chuley, M. (1988b) Efficacy of a hyperinflation and hyperoxygenation suctioning intervention. *Heart Lung*, **17**, 15.

Clayton, D.G., Webb, R.K., Ralston, A.C. *et al.* (1991) Pulse oximeter probes: a comparison between finger, nose, ear and forehead probes under conditions of poor perfusion. *Anaesthesia*, **46**, 260–5.

Clement, A.J. and Hubsch, S.K. (1968) Chest physiotherapy by the 'bag squeezing' method. *Physiotherapy*, **54**, 355–9.

Connors, A.F., Hammon, W.E., Martin, R.J. *et al.* (1980) Chest physical therapy. The immediate effect on oxygenation in acutely ill patients. *Chest*, **78**, 559–64.

Conway, J.H. (1992) The effects of humidification for patients with chronic airways disease. *Physiotherapy*, **78**, 97–101.

Cordero, L. and Hon, E.H. (1971) Neonatal bradycardia following nasopharyngeal stimulation. *Journal of Pediatrics*, **78**, 441–7.

Crabtree Goodnough, S.K. (1985) The effects of oxygen and hyperinflation on arterial oxygen tension after endotracheal suction. *Heart Lung*, **14**, 11–17.

Crane, L.D., Zombek, M., Krauss, A.N. and Auld, P.A.M. (1978) Comparison of chest physiotherapy techniques in infants with HMD. *Pediatric Research*, **12**, 559.

Curran, C.L. and Kachoyeanos, M .K. (1979) The effects on neonates of two methods of chest physical therapy. *American Journal of Maternal and Child Nursing*, **4**, 309–13.

Czarnik, R.E., Stone, K.S., Everhart, C.C. and Preusser, B.A. (1991) Differential effects of continuous versus intermittent suction on tracheal tissue. *Heart Lung*, **20**, 144–51.

Davies, H., Kitchman, R., Gordon, I. and Helms, P. (1985) Regional ventilation in infancy. *New England Journal of Medicine*, **313**, 1626–8.

DeCesare, J.A., Babchyck, B.M., Colten, H.R. and Treves, S. (1982) Radionuclide assessment of the effects of chest physical therapy on ventilation in cystic fibrosis. *Physical Therapy*, **62**, 820–5.

Dehaven, C.B., Hurst, J.M. and Branson, R.D. (1985) Post extubation hypoxaemia treated with continuous positive airways pressure. *Critical Care Medicine*, **13**, 46–8.

Demers, R.S. and Saklad, M. (1973) Minimising the harmful effects of mechanical aspiration. *Heart Lung*, **2**, 542.

Drew, J.H., Padoms, K. and Clabburn, S.L. (1986) Endotracheal tube management in newborn infants with hyaline membrane disease. *Australian Journal of Physiotherapy*, **32**, 3–5.

Durand, M., Sangha, B., Cabal, L.A. *et al*. (1989) Cardiopulmonary and intracranial pressure changes related to endotracheal suctioning in preterm infants. *Critical Care Medicine*, **17** 506–10.

Emmanuel, G.E., Smith, W.M. and Briscoe, W.A. (1966) The effects of intermittent positive pressure breathing and voluntary hyperventilation upon the distribution of ventilation and pulmonary blood flow to the lung in chronic obstructive lung disease. *Journal of Clinical Investigation*, **45**, 1221–33.

Etches, P.C. and Scott, B. (1978) Chest physiotherapy in the newborn; effect on secretions removed. *Pediatrics*, **62**, 713–15.

Feldman, F., Kanter, M.J., Robertson, C.S. *et al*. (1992) Effect of head elevation on intracranial pressure and cerebral blood flow in head injured patients. *Journal of Neurosurgery*, **76**, 207–11.

Fewell, J., Arrington, R. and Seibert, J. (1979) The effect of head position and angle of tracheal bifurcation on bronchus catheterisation in the intubated neonate. *Pediatrics*, **64**, 318–20.

Finer, N.N. and Boyd, J. (1978) Chest physiotherapy in the neonate: a controlled study. *Paediatrics*, **61**, 682–5.

Finer, N.N., Moriarty, R.R., Boyd, J. *et al*. (1979) Postextubation atelectasis: a retrospective review and a prospective controlled study. *Journal of Pediatrics*, **94**, 110–13.

Fisk, G.C. and Baker, W.C. (1975) Mucosal changes in the trachea and bronchi of newborn infants after nasotracheal intubation. *Anaesthesia and Intensive Care and Equipment*, **3**, 209–17.

Fox, W.W., Berman, L.S., Dinwiddie, R. *et al*. (1977) Tracheal extubation of the neonate at 2 to 3 cm H_2O continuous positive airways pressure. *Pediatrics*, **59**, 257–61.

Gallon, A. (1992) The use of percussion. *Physiotherapy*, **78**, 85–9.

Garrad, J. and Bullock, M. (1986) The effect of respiratory therapy on intracranial pressure in ventilated neurosurgical patients. *Australian Journal of Physiotherapy*, **32**, 107–11.

Gold, M., Duarte, I. and Muravchick, S. (1981) Arterial oxygenation in conscious patients after five minutes and after 30 seconds of oxygen breathing. *Anesthetic Analogues*, **60**, 313.

Gormezano, J. and Branthwaite, M.A. (1972a) Effects of physiotherapy during intermittent positive pressure ventilation. *Anaesthesia*, **27**, 258–63.

Gormezano, J. and Branthwaite, M.A. (1972b) Pulmonary physiotherapy with assisted ventilation. *Anaesthesia*, **27**, 250–7.

Graff, M., France, J., Hiatt, M. and Hegyi, T. (1987) Prevention of hypoxia and hyperoxia during endotracheal suctioning. *Critical Care Medicine*, **15**, 1133–5.

Gregory, G.A., Kitterman, J.A., Phibbs, R.H. *et al*. (1971) Treatment of the ideopathic respiratory distress syndrome with continuous positive airways pressure. *New England Journal of Medicine*, **284**, 1333–40.

Hanley, M.V., Rudd, T. and Butler, J. (1978) What happens to intratracheal saline instillations? *American Review of Respiratory Disease*, **117**, 124.

Heaf, D.P., Helms, P., Gordon, I. and Turner, H.M. (1983) Postural effects on gas exchange in infants. *New England Journal of Medicine*, **308**, 1505–8.

Hirsch, S.R., Zastrow, J.E. and Kory, R.C. (1969) Sputum liquifying agents: a comparative in vitro evaluation. *Journal of Laboratory and Clinical Medicine*, **74**, 346–53.

Hodson, M.E., Penketh, A.R.L. and Batten, J.C. (1981) Aerosol cabenicillin and gentamicin treatment for *Pseudomonas aeroginosa* infection in cystic fibrosis. *Lancet*, **2**, 1137–9.

Holloway, R., Adams, E.B., Desai, S.D. *et al.* (1969) Effect of chest physiotherapy on blood gases of neonates treated with intermittent positive pressure respiration. *Thorax*, **24**, 421–6.

Hussey, J.M. (1991) The relationship between specific chest physiotherapy techniques and oxygen saturation post paediatric cardiac surgery. MSc Thesis, University of London.

Hussey, J.M., Hayward, L.J. and Andrews, M. (1992) The effect of chest physiotherapy techniques on oxygen saturation in children post cardiac surgery. *Care of the Critically Ill*, **8**, 35.

Ibanez, J., Raurich, M., Abizanda, R. *et al.* (1981) The effect of lateral positions on gas exchange in patients with unilateral lung disease during mechanical ventilation. *Intensive Care Medicine*, **7**, 321–4.

Imle, P.C. (1989) Percussion and vibration, in *Chest Physiotherapy in the Intensive Care Unit*, 2nd edn, (eds C.F. Mackenzie, P.C. Imle and N. Ciesla), Williams and Wilkins, Baltimore, pp. 134–52.

Imle, P.C. and Klemic, N. (1991) Methods of airway clearance: coughing and suctioning, in *Chest Physiotherapy in the Intensive Care Unit*, 2nd edn, (eds C.F. Mackenzie, P.C.Imle and N. Ciesla). Williams and Wilkins, Baltimore, pp. 153–87.

Jenkins, S.C. and Soutar, S.A. (1986) A survey into the use of incentive spirometry following coronary artery bypass graft surgery. *Physiotherapy*, **72**, 492–3.

Jones, A.Y.M., Hutchinson, R.C. and Oh, T.E. (1992) Effects of bagging and percussion on total static compliance of the respiratory system. *Physiotherapy*, **78**, 661–6.

Jung, R.C. and Gottlieb, L.S. (1976) Comparison of tracheobronchial suction catheters in humans. *Chest*, **69**, 179–81.

Jung, R.C. and Newman, J. (1982) Minimising hypoxia during endotracheal airway care. *Heart Lung*, **11**, 208–12.

Keilty, S.E.J. and Bott, J. (1992) Continuous positive airways pressure. *Physiotherapy*, **78**, 90–2.

Kelly, R., Yao, F. and Artusio, J. (1987) Prevention of suction induced hypoxaemia by simultaneous oxygen insufflation. *Critical Care Medicine*, **15**, 874.

Kerem, E., Yatsiv, I. and Goitein, K.J. (1990) Effect of endotracheal suctioning on arterial blood gases in children. *Intensive Care Medicine*, **16**, 95–9.

Kigin, C.M. (1981) Chest physical therapy for the acutely ill medical patient. *Physical Therapy*, **61**, 1724–36.

Kigin, C.M. (1984) Advances in chest physical therapy, in *Current Advances in Respiratory Care*, (ed. W.J. O'Donohue), American College of Chest Physicians, Park Ridge, pp. 37–71.

Kiriloff, L.H., Owens, G.R., Rogers, R.M. *et al* (1985) Does chest physical therapy work? *Chest*, **88**, 436–44.

Kleiber, C., Krutzfield, N. and Rose, E.F. (1988) Acute histological changes in the tracheobronchial tree associated with different suction catheter insertion techniques. *Heart Lung*, **17**, 10–14.

Klein, P., Kemper, M., Weissman, C. *et al.* (1988) Attenuation of the haemodynamic response to chest physical therapy. *Chest* **93**, 38–42.

Kovnat, D.M., Rath, G.S., Anderson, W.M. and Snider, G.L. (1974) Maximal extent of visualisation of the bronchial tree by fibreoptic bronchoscopy. *American Review of Respiratory Disease*, **110**, 88–90.

Kubota, Y., Magaribuchi, T., Toyoda, Y. *et al.* (1982) Selective bronchial suctioning in the adult using a curved tip catheter with a guidemark. *Critical Care Medicine*, **10**, 767–9.

Kuzenski, B. (1978) Effect of negative pressure in tracheobronchial trauma. *Nursing Research*, **27**, 260.

Landa, J.F., Kwoka, M.A., Chapman, G.A. *et al.* (1973) Effects of suctioning on mucociliary transport. *Chest*, **77**, 202–7.

Laws, A.K. and McIntyre, R.W. (1969) Chest physiotherapy: a physiological assessment during intermittent positive pressure ventilation in respiratory failure. *Canadian Anaesthetic Society Journal*, **16**, 487–93.

Liftschitz, L.I. and Denning, C.R. (1970) Quantative interaction of water and cystic fibrosis sputum. *American Review of Respiratory Diseases*, **102**, 456–8.

Link, W.J., Spaeth, E.E., Wahle, W.M. *et al.* (1976) The influence of suction catheter tip design on tracheobronchial trauma and fluid aspiration efficiency. *Anesthetic Analogues*, **55**, 290–7.

Litt, M. (1970) Mucous rheology: relevance to mucociliary clearance. *Archives of Internal Medicine*, **126**, 417–23.

Mackenzie, C. and Shin, B. (1985) Cardiorespiratory function before and after physiotherapy in mechanically ventilated patients with post traumatic respiratory failure. *Critical Care Medicine*, **13**, 483–6.

Mackenzie, C., Shin, B. and McAslan, T.C. (1978) Chest physiotherapy; the effects on arterial oxygenation. *Anaesthesia & Analgesia*, **57**, 28–30.

Maloney, F.P., Fernandez, E. and Hudgel, D.W. (1981) Postural drainage effect after bronchial obstruction. *Archives of Physical Mecicine Rehabilitation*, **62**, 452–5.

Marfatia, S., Donahoe, P.K. and Hendren, W.H. (1975) Effect of dry and humidified gases on the respiratory epithelium in rabbits. *Journal of Pediatric Surgery*, **10**, 583–92.

Marini, J.J., Pierson, D.J. and Hudson, L.D. (1979) Acute lobar atelectasis: a prospective comparison of fibreoptic bronchoscopy and respiratory therapy. *American Review of Respiratory Disease*, **119**, 971–8.

Martin, R.J., Herrel, N., Ruben, D. and Fanaroff, A. (1979) Effect of supine and prone positions on arterial oxygen tension in the preterm infant. *Journal of Pediatrics*, **63**, 528–31.

Marx, G.F., Steen, S.N., Arkins, R.E. *et al.* (1968) Endotracheal suction and death. *New York State Journal of Medicine*, **15**, 565–6.

Mellins, R.B. (1974) Pulmonary physiotherapy in the pediatric age group. *American Review of Respiratory Disease*, **110** (supplement 2), 137–42.

Milner, A.D. (1993) Asthma in the preschool child. *Journal of Association of Chartered Physiotherapists in Respiratory Care*, **22**, 7–8.

Morrison, M.L. (1979) *Respiratory Intensive Care Nursing*, 2nd edn, Little, Brown & Co, Boston, p. 32.

Motley, H.L., Werko, L., Cournand, A. *et al.* (1947) Observations of the clinical use of intermittent positive pressure. *Journal of Aviation Medicine*, **18**, 417.

Muller, N.L. and Bryan, A.C. (1979) Chest wall mechanics and respiratory muscles in infants. *Pediatric Clinics of North America*, **26**, 503–16.

Nagaraj, H.S., Shott, R., Fellows, R. and Yacoub, U. (1980) Recurrent lobar atelectasis due to acquired bronchial stenosis in neonates. *Journal of Pediatric Surgery*, **15**, 411–15.

Naigow, D. and Powaser, M.M. (1977) The effect of different endotracheal suction procedures on arterial blood gases in a controlled experimental model. *Heart Lung*, **6**, 808–16.

Newhouse, M.T. and Rossman, C.M. (1984) Effect of chest physiotherapy on the removal of mucus in patients with cystic fibrosis. *American Review of Respiratory Disease*, **127**, 391.

Oberwaldner, B., Evans, J.C. and Zach, M.S. (1986) Forced expirations against a variable resistance: a new chest physiotherapy method in cystic fibrosis. *Pediatric Pulmonology*, **2**, 358–67.

O'Callghan, C., Milner, A. and Swarbrick, A. (1986) Paradoxical deterioration in lung function after nebulized salbutamol in wheezy infants. *Lancet*, **2**, 1424–5.

O'Callaghan, C., Milner, A. and Swarbrick, A. (1989) Paradoxical bronchospasm in wheezing infants after nebulised preservative-free iso-osmolar ipratropium bromide. *British Medical Journal*, **299**, 1433–4.

O'Donnel, D.R., Prasad, S.A., Wilkinson, K. *et al.* (1993) Nonbronchoscopic bronchoalveolar lavage: identifying groups with higher risks of complications, in *Proceedings of European Society of Paediatric Intensive Care, Madrid.*

Oldenburg, F.A., Dolovich, M.B., Montgomery, J.M. and Newhouse, M.T. (1979) Effects of postural drainage, exercise and cough on mucus clearance in chronic bronchitis. *American Review of Respiratory Disease*, **120**, 739–45.

Oppenshaw, P., Edwards, S. and Helms, P. (1984) Changes in rib cage geometry during childhood. *Thorax*, **39**, 624–7.

Paratz, J. (1992) Haemodynamic stability of the ventilated intensive care patient: a review. *Australian Journal of Physiotherapy*, **38**, 167–72.

Parker, A.E. (1985) Chest physiotherapy in the neonatal intensive care unit. *Physiotherapy*, **71**, 63–5.

Partridge, C., Pryor, J.A. and Webber, B.A. (1989) Characteristics of the forced expiration technique. *Physiotherapy*, **75**, 193–4.

Pavia, D., Thompson, M. L. and Clarke, S.W. (1978) Enhanced clearance of secretions from the human lung after the administration of hypertonic saline aerosol. *American Review of Respiratory Diseases*, **117**, 199–203.

Perlman, J.M. and Volpe. J.J. (1983) Suctioning in the preterm infant: effects on cerebral blood flow velocity, intracranial pressure and arterial blood pressure. *Pediatrics*, **72**, 329–34.

Piehl, M.A. and Brown, M.S. (1976) Use of extreme position changes in acute respiratory failure. *Critical Care Medicine*, **4**, 13–15.

Placzek, M. and Silverman, M. (1983) Selective placement of bronchial suction catheters in intubated neonates. *Archives of Disease in Childhood*, **58**, 829–31.

Pryor, J.A. and Webber, B.A. (1992) Physiotherapy for cystic fibrosis – which technique? *Physiotherapy*, **78**, 105–8.

Ratjen, F., Wonne, R., Posselt, H.G. *et al*. (1990) A double-blind placebo controlled trial with oral ambroxol and N-acetylcysteine for mucolytic treatment in cystic fibrosis. *European Journal of Pediatrics*, **144**, 374.

Reisman, J.J., Rivington-Law, B., Corey, M. *et al*. (1988) Role of conventional physiotherapy in cystic fibrosis. *Journal of Pediatrics*, **113**, 632–6.

Rhodes, L.A. (1987) A pressure regulated 'bagging' device – a pilot study. *South African Journal of Physiotherapy*, **43**, 117–20.

Richards, J.H. (1974) Effect of the relative humidity on the rheologic properties of bronchial mucous. *American Review of Respiratory Diseases*, **109**, 484–6.

Rindfleisch, S. and Tyler, M. (1981) The effects of duration of endotracheal suctioning on arterial oxygenation in anaesthetised dogs. *American Review of Respiratory Disease*, **123**, 19.

Rosen, M. and Hillard, E.K. (1962) The effects of negative pressure during tracheal suction. *Anesthetic Analogues*, **41**, 50–7.

Rosenbluth, M. and Chernick, V. (1974) Influence of mist tent therapy on sputum viscosity and water content in cystic fibrosis. *Archives of Disease in Childhood*, **49**, 606–9.

Rowe, M.L., Weinberger, M. and Poole, C.A. (1973) An experimental study on the vibration in postoperative tracheobronchial clearance. *Journal of Pediatric Surgery*, **8**, 735–8.

Rux, M.I. and Powaser, M.M. (1979) Effect of apnea and the levels of negative pressure on the fall in arterial tension produced by endotracheal suctioning in dogs. *American Review of Respiratory Disease*, **119**, 193.

Sackner, M.A., Landa, J.F., Greeneltch, N. and Robinson, M.J. (1973) Pathogenesis and prevention of tracheobronchial damage with suction procedures. *Chest*, **64**, 284–90.

Scharf, S.M., Brown, R., Saunders, N. *et al*. (1980) Hemodynamic effects of positive pressure inflation. *Journal of Applied Physiology*, **49**, 124 31.

Schwartz, F.C.M., Fenner, A. and Wolfsdorf, J. (1975) The influence of body position on pulmonary function in low birthweight babies. *South African Medical Journal*, **49**, 79–84.

Selsby, D.S., (1989) Chest physiotherpay. *British Medical Journal*, **298**, 541–2.

Shelly, M.P., Lloyd, G.M. and Park, G.R. (1988) A review of the mechanisms and methods of humidification of inspired gases. *Intensive Care*, **14**, 1–9.

Shim, C., Fernandez, R., Fine, N. and Williams, H. (1969) Cardiac arrhythmias resulting from tracheal suctioning. *American International Medicine*, **71**, 1149–53.

Shumaker, H.B. and Hampton, L.J. (1951) Sudden death occurring immediately after operation in patients with cardiac disease, with particular reference to the role of aspiration through the endotracheal tube and extubation. *Journal of Thoracic Surgery*, **21**, 48.

Simbruner, G., Coradello, H., Fodor, *et al*. (1981) Effect of tracheal suction on oxygenation, circulation and lung mechanics in newborn infants. *Archives of Disease in Childhood*, **56**, 326–30.

Smith, C.M. and Anderson, S.D. (1989) Review: inhalation provocation tests using non-isotonic aerosols. *Journal of Allergy and Clinical Immunology*, **84**, 781–90.

Soong, W.J. and Hwang, B.T. (1991) Selective placement of bronchial suction catheters in intubated full term and premature neonates. *Chung Hua I Hsueh Tsa Chih*, **48**, 45–8.

Southall, D.P. and Samuels, M.P. (1992) Reducing risks in the sudden infant death syndrome. *British Medical Journal*, **304**, 265–60.

Starke, I.D., Webber, B.A. and Branthwaite, M.A. (1979) IPPB and hypercapnoea in respiratory failure: the effect of different concentrations of inspired oxygen on arterial blood gas tensions. *Anaesthesia*, **34**, 283–7.

Stiller, K., Geake, T., Taylor, J. *et al.* (1990) Acute lobar atelectasis. A comparison of two chest physiotherapy regimes. *Chest*, **98**, 1336–40.

Stock, M.C., Downs, J.B. and Corkran, M.L. (1984) Pulmonary function before and after prolonged CPAP by mask. *Critical Care Medicine*, **12**, 973–4.

Stock, M.C., Downs, J.B., Gaver, P.K. *et al.* (1985) Prevention of postoperative pulmonary complications with CPAP, incentive spirometry and conservative therapy. *Chest*, **87**, 151–7.

Stone, K.S., Preusser, B.A., Groch, K.F. *et al.* (1991) The effect of lung hyperinflation and endotracheal suctioning on cardiopulmonary hemodynamics. *Nursing Research*, **40**, 76–9.

Sukumalchantra, Y., Park, S.S. and Williams, M.H. (1965) The effect of intermittent positive pressure breathing (IPPB) in acute ventilatory failure. *American Review of Respiratory Disease*, **92**, 885–93.

Sumner, E. (1990) Artificial ventilation of children, in *The Diagnosis and Management of Paediatric Respiratory Disease*, (ed. R. Dinwiddie), Churchill Livingstone, London, pp. 267–87.

Sutton, P.P., Parker, R.A. and Webber, B.A. (1983) Assessment of the forced expiration technique, postural drainage and directed coughing in chest physiotherapy. *European Journal of Respiratory Disease*, **64**, 62–8.

Sutton, P.P., Lopez-Vidriero, M.T., Pavia, D. *et al.* (1985) Assessment of percussion, vibratory shaking and breathing exercises in chest physiotherapy. *European Journal of Respiratory Disease*, **66**, 147–52.

Sutton, P.P., Gemmell, H.G., Innes, N. *et al.* (1988) Use of nebulised saline and nebulised terbutaline as an adjunct to chest physiotherapy. *Thorax*, **43**, 57–60.

Tattersall, M. (1982) Should we humidify our anaesthetic gases? A review. *Anaesthesia Points West*, **15**, 17–19.

Taylor, P. and Waters, H. (1971) Arterial Oxygen tensions following endotracheal suctioning on IPPV. *Anaesthesia*, **26**, 289.

Thomson, M.L., Pavier, D., Jones, C.J. *et al.* (1975) No demonstrable effect of S-carboxymethylcysteine on clearance of secretions from the human lung. *Thorax*, **30**, 669–73.

Tolles, C.L. and Stone, K.S. (1990) National survey of neonatal endotracheal suctioning practices. *Neonatal Network*, **9**, 7–14.

Torres, G., Lyons, H.A. and Emerson, P. (1960) The effects of intermittent positive pressure breathing on the interpulmonary distribution of inspired air. *American Journal of Medicine*, **29**, 946–54.

Tudehope, D.I. and Bagley, C. (1980) Techniques of physiotherapy in intubated babies with the respiratory distress syndrome. *Australian Paediatric Journal*, **16**, 226–8.

Vaughan, R.S., Menke, J.A. and Giacoia, G.P. (1978) Pneumothorax: a complication of endotracheal tube suction. *Journal of Pediatrics*, **92**, 633–4.

Wagaman, M.J., Shutack, J.G., Moomjian, A.S. *et al.* (1979) Improved oxygenation and lung compliance with prone positioning in neonates. *Journal of Pediatrics*, **94**, 787–91.

Walsh, J.M., Vanderwarf, C., Hoscheit, D. *et al.* (1989) Unsuspected hemodynamic alterations during endotracheal suction. *Chest*, **95**, 162–5.

Webber, B.A. (1988) Adjuncts to physiotherapy, in *The Brompton Hospital Guide to Chest Physiotherapy*, 5th edn (ed. B.A. Webber), Blackwell Scientific Publications, Oxford, pp. 120–45.

Weller, P.H., Ingram, D., Preece, M.A. and Matthew, D.J. (1980) Controlled trial of intermittent aerosol therapy with sodium 2-mercaptoethane sulphonate in cystic fibrosis. *Thorax*, **35**, 42–6.

White, P.F., Schlobohm, R.M., Pitts, L.H. *et al.* (1982) A randomised study of drugs for preventing increases in intracranial pressure during endotracheal suction. *Anesthesiology*, **57**, 242–4.

Windsor, H.M., Harrison, G.A. and Nicholson, T.J. (1972) 'Bag squeezing', a physiotherapeutic technique. *Medical Journal of Australia*, **2**, 829–32.

Winston, S.J., Gravelyn, T.R. and Sitrin, R.G. (1987) Prevention of bradycardic responses to endotracheal suctioning by prior administration of nebulized atropine. *Critical Care Medicine*, **15**, 1009–11.

Wollmer, P., Ursing, K., Midgren, B. and Eriksson, L. (1985) Inefficiency of chest percussion in the physical therapy of chronic bronchitis. *European Journal of Respiratory Disease*, **66**, 233–9.

Wong, J.W., Keens, T.G., Wannamaker, E.M. *et al.* (1977) Effects of gravity on tracheal transport rates in normal subjects and patients with cystic fibrosis. *Pediatrics*, **60**, 146–52.

Young, C.S. (1984) Recommended guidelines for suction. *Physiotherapy*, **70**, 106–8.
Young, C.S. (1988) Airway suctioning: a study of paediatric physiotherapy practice. *Physiotherapy*, **74**, 13–16.
Zack, M.B., Pontoppidan, H. and Kazemi, H. (1974) The effect of lateral positions on gas exchange in pulmonary disease. *American Review of Respiratory Disease*, **110**, 49–55.
Zausmer, E. (1968) Bronchial drainage, evidence supporting the procedures. *Physical Therapy*, **48**, 586–91.
Zinman, R. (1984) Cough versus chest physiotherapy, a comparison of the acute effects on pulmonary function in patients with cystic fibrosis. *American Review of Respiratory Disease*, **129**, 182–4.

COMMON NEONATAL DISORDERS 7

Anne Greenough and Annette Parker

INTRODUCTION

Approximately 7% of babies each year are born prematurely, that is, prior to 37 weeks of completed gestation. About two thirds of these infants will be of an appropriate weight for their gestational age and the other third small for gestational age (SGA) (their birthweight will be less than the 10th centile of that expected for gestational age). Premature infants may be further classified according to their birthweight: low birthweight (LBW) less than 2500g: very low birthweight (VLBW) less than 1500g: extremely low birthweight (ELBW) less than 1000g and incredibly low birthweight (ILBW) less than 750g.

PROBLEMS RELATED TO PREMATURITY

The premature infants' problems may be simply attributed to immaturity of various systems. In addition, a proportion of infants will be SGA or growth retarded and will also suffer problems due to reduced reserves. The major problem of prematurity is respiratory insufficiency and this will be dealt with separately later in the chapter.

TEMPERATURE REGULATION

Premature infants have a large surface area to body weight ratio, not an ideal combination to conserve heat and in addition, they are further handicapped by immature central heat controlling mechanisms. In all babies, changing their environmental temperature alters oxygen consumption; in a term baby a 2° fall in the environmental temperature will double the oxygen consumption. As a consequence, it is essential to nurse premature infants in their thermal neutral range, that is, where their oxygen consumption is minimal. As the preterm infant is particularly poor at conserving heat, appropriate artificial means must be used to cut down convective and conductive losses. In practice, this means nursing infants in incubators which are also extremely useful in creating a barrier between the baby and the outside world. This reminds staff that the premature baby is extremely fragile and at high risk of nosocomial infections (Thompson *et al.*, 1992) so a minimal handling rule must be observed.

INFECTION

Approximately 1% of premature infants suffer a congenital infection (Greenough *et al.*, 1991b). The premature infant has very inadequate defence mechanisms against infection: only one type of immunoglobulin, IgG, can cross the placenta and the premature infant's white cells are functionally immature. This means the premature infant is an easy prey to nosocomial infections, which occur in approximately 17% of infants (Thompson *et al.*, 1992). It is therefore mandatory to exercise preventative measures; for example, scrupulous attention to hand washing is essential for all carers and use of communal equipment must be avoided.

JAUNDICE

Premature infants may become jaundiced because of overproduction of bilirubin due to excessive breakdown of red blood cells. They may also have impaired hepatic clearance of bilirubin and be further compromised by postnatal sepsis or neonatal hepatitis. Unfortunately, the majority of the bilirubin in a premature infant is unconjugated and fat soluble and can enter the brain. In large quantities, this will cause an encephalopathy (kernicterus) leading to chorioathetoid cerebral palsy and high frequency deafness. Manoeuvres are performed to prevent the bilirubin reaching such a level; phototherapy is used to convert the bilirubin into a water-soluble, non-neurotoxic product or, in emergencies, exchange transfusion is necessary. Neither procedure is without complication.

FEEDING

Premature infants are usually initially unable to suck and have a very poor cough reflex. They therefore require feeding nasogastrically or initially intravenously when they are intolerant of enteral feeding. Many premature infants suffer from gastro-oesophageal reflux and are at increased risk of aspiration pneumonia and this will be exacerbated by handling and procedures such as physiotherapy.

HYPOGLYCAEMIA

This results from inadequate or depleted glycogen stores and may be exacerbated by intrapartum asphyxia and septicaemia. Certain premature infants will have high levels of insulin, for example, those born to diabetic mothers or who suffer from haemolytic disease. The premature infant's symptoms of hypoglycaemia are those of 'end organ failure', bradycardia and heart failure, apnoea with convulsions. Symptomatic hypoglycaemia is associated with an unfavourable outcome but 'asymptomatic' premature infants who have had blood glucose levels less than 2.5 mmol/l perform less well at follow-up (Lucas *et al.*, 1988). Appropriate treatment of hypoglycaemia, therefore, is avoidance, by regular monitoring of blood sugar in high risk groups and prompt response to any low blood sugar demonstrated.

APNOEA

Apnoea may be central in origin, in part due to immaturity of the respiratory centre or obstructive apnoea which can be due to upper airway incoordination (Ruggins, 1991). Apnoea can be a sign of other problems which include overheating, infection, intraventricular haemorrhage (IVH) and anaemia. Thus infants who develop apnoea should be fully investigated and once pathological causes are excluded, treated with an aminophylline derivative and/or continuous positive airway pressure (CPAP).

COMPLICATIONS OF PREMATURITY

Premature infants suffer a number of complications (Chan *et al.*, 1992). Necrotizing enterocolitis (NEC), a bowel disorder due to hypoxic damage and infection, may be managed conservatively but some infants do require surgery because of stricture formation or perforation. This condition carries a mortality and long term morbidity due to lactose intolerance and the development of further stricture formation.

The ductus arteriosus frequently remains patent in a premature infant. This relates to the severity of the lung disease but also to the use of exogenous surfactant replacement therapy. The presence of a patent ductus arteriosus (PDA) worsens respiratory status and may require treatment with fluid restriction and a prostaglandin synthetase inhibitor such as indomethacin or even surgical ligation.

The increased survival of ILBW infants has seen a re-emergence of retinopathy of prematurity. This condition was initially thought due to high levels of arterial oxygen but has now been demonstrated to have a multifactorial aetiology (Editorial, 1992). Fortunately, few infants develop severe retinopathy and require cryotherapy. Preterm infants are at high risk of developing intraventricular/intracerebral haemorrhage and periventricular leucomalacia which are all associated with handicap at follow-up. The more severe the haemorrhage, the more likely this will lead to mortality and morbidity and in addition there may be blockage of cerebrospinal fluid (CSF) flow leading to posthaemorrhagic hydrocephalus. Periventricular leucomalacia, which is neuronal loss and gliosis in the periventricular regions of the brain, results from hypotensive insults which can occur postnatally or antenatally (in the early stages ultrasound examination of the brain reveals bright lesions which later resolve to give a classic cystic appearance).

RESPIRATORY PROBLEMS OF THE NEWBORN

RESPIRATORY DISTRESS SYNDROME

Aetiology

Respiratory distress syndrome (RDS) is due to surfactant deficiency or abnormality. The major cause of surfactant deficiency is prematurity; the earlier the infant is born, the more likely it is to have RDS (excluding those less than 24 weeks gestation). Surfactant abnormality is seen in infants of diabetic mothers and those who have suffered form rhesus isoimmunization. The condition is made more severe by perinatal asphyxia. Elective caesarean section will also be associated with worse respiratory failure due to delayed clearance of lung liquid. Rarely, RDS seen at term is familial.

The major components of surfactant are phospholipids, particularly dipalmitoyl phosphatidyl choline (lecithin) and phosphatidyl glycerol. Surfactant reduces the surface tension at the alveolar air/fluid interface and thus reduces the work of breathing (La Place's law). It promotes alveolar stability and protection of the epithelial surfaces. The absence of a normal amount of functioning surfactant results in atelectasis. This causes a deterioration in blood gas status with a reduction in pulmonary blood flow and right to left shunting which exacerbates hypoxia.

Presentation

Infants with RDS are obviously working hard to breathe. The infant relies heavily on diaphragmatic contraction and with a very compliant chest wall, this results in sternal wall retraction. Infants use their accessory muscles of respiration - nasal flaring. The most typical feature, however, is grunting which may be a sign of atelectasis and is caused by expiration against a closed glottis, in an attempt to self-generate positive end expiratory pressure. The chest radiograph is uniformly abnormal (Figure 7.1), with an alveolar atelectasis leading to a diffuse symmetrical reticular granular pattern and air in the bronchi against unaerated alveoli standing out as air bronchograms.

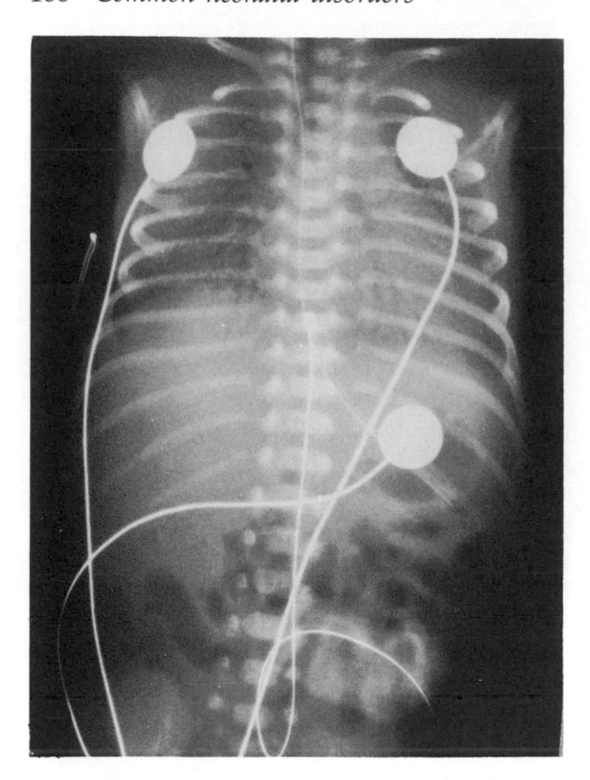

Figure 7.1 Chest radiograph of a neonate with respiratory distress syndrome.

Surfactant deficiency or abnormality is present from birth and thus clinical signs are present within four hours of birth. Regardless of the immaturity of the infant, surfactant will start to be produced at about 48 hours of age. The condition, therefore, persists beyond 24 hours, reaches a maximum severity at 48 hours and is self-limiting.

Treatment

Until the advent of exogenous surfactant replacement therapy, treatment of RDS was supportive. The infant was maintained in the thermoneutral range as below 34°C surfactant ceases to function. Antibiotics, usually penicillin and gentamicin, are given as it is not possible to distinguish the clinical signs and chest radiograph appearance of RDS from those of group B streptococcal septicaemia. Antibiotics are administered for at least 48 hours until the culture results are known to be negative. Many infants with RDS will need some form of respiratory support, an increased inspired oxygen concentration, CPAP or even mechanical ventilation.

Prevention

Despite optimization of these supportive forms of therapy, RDS still carries a significant mortality and morbidity. Therefore, over recent years attention has been focused on preventative measures.

a) Estimation of fetal lung maturity

Antenatally lung maturity may be estimated by measurement of the lecithin:sphingomyelin (L:S) ratio from amniotic fluid obtained by amniocentesis, an L:S ratio greater than 2 indicating lung maturity. Unfortunately, however, an L:S ratio less than 2 has only a 50% ability to predict RDS.

b) Antenatal therapy

A variety of drugs have been given to mothers to stimulate surfactant production. These include beta-2 stimulants, such as aminophylline, steroids, thyroxin and thyrotropic releasing hormone (TRH). Meta-analysis of 23 trials which have examined the effect of maternal steroids demonstrate that therapy is associated with a 50% reduction in mortality and a 70% reduction in the likelihood of developing RDS if administered between 24 hours and seven days prior to birth (Crowley *et al.*, 1990). Outside that period a 30% reduction is achieved. Although the majority of the trials have recruited infants between 30 and 34 weeks' gestation, seven trials have shown significant reduction in RDS in infants less than 30 weeks' gestation. The efficacy of TRH is at present being tested, but preliminary results suggest it is synergistic with glucocorticoids and is effective after only six hours of administration.

c) Exogenous surfactant

Since the early 1980s, postnatal exogenous surfactant replacement therapy has been available. Numerous trials have demonstrated that this form of therapy reduces mortality by approximately 50% and it also reduces IVH, but the effect on chronic lung disease is variable (Morley, 1991). Many surfactant preparations are available. There are natural surfactants obtained from homogenized cow's lungs (surfactant TA or Survanta); calf lung surfactant extract (CLSE); minced pig's lungs (Curosurf); extracted cow lung lavage (Alveofact); and human surfactant from amniotic fluid. A variety of artifical surfactants are also available; a mixture of dipalmitoyl phosphatidyl choline and phosphatidyl glycerol (ALEC or Pumactant) and dipalmitoyl phosphatidyl choline, tyloxapol and hexadecanol (Exosurf). There have been very few comparative studies of the different types of surfactant. It is, however, noticeable that the natural surfactant works more rapidly than an artificial surfactant, causing immediate changes in oxygenation. As yet, there are a number of unanswered questions about surfactant replacement therapy regarding type of preparation, dosage regimen, prophylaxis or rescue and which patients benefit most. Surfactant replacement therapy seems to be effective even in very small babies and, equally excitingly, it may have a place in respiratory conditions other than RDS.

CHRONIC LUNG DISEASE

Infants who remain oxygen dependent at one month of age are now defined as having neonatal chronic lung disease (CLD type I). Their chest radiograph usually shows small volume hazy lung fields. A small proportion of those infants have cystic abnormalities on their chest radiograph and are described as suffering from bronchpulmonary dysplasia or CLD type II (BPD), this being the most severe form of chronic lung disease (Greenough, 1990). Approximately 20% of very low birthweight infants, ventilated in the neonatal period, develop chronic lung disease. The majority will only be oxygen dependent for a few weeks, but those with BPD remain oxygen dependent for many months and may even require home oxygen therapy (Greenough *et al.*, 1991a). BPD has a high mortality and, once discharged, infants have a higher incidence of sudden infant death syndrome.

Aetiology

Chronic lung disease has a multifactorial aetiology which includes prematurity, a genetic predisposition and low antioxidant status. Infants at highest risk are those who have severe respiratory failure necessitating high inspired oxygen concentrations and ventilator pressures. The condition is also significantly associated with the development of a PDA and certain infections, such as cytomegalovirus, have been incriminated.

Prevention

Although CLD is most likely in infants who require mechanical ventilation in the neonatal period, there is no evidence to date that the newer forms of ventilation, high frequency positive pressure ventilation, patient triggered ventilation or high frequency jet ventilation reduce the incidence of chronic lung disease (Greenough and Milner, 1993). Preliminary study, however, suggests that high frequency oscillation may be more useful. High inspired oxygen concentrations are also toxic to the lung, generating oxygen free radicals. The premature infant is deficient in antioxidants but supplementation with vitamin E does not reduce CLD and superoxide dismustase may increase the risk of infection. It is controversial whether vitamin A supplementation will influence the incidence of CLD.

Management

It is important to reduce mechanical ventilation to a minimum and wean infants from respiratory support as soon as possible. Theophylline and steroids assist weaning and if the latter form of therapy is given as a prolonged course from two weeks of age, it has also been claimed to improve neurological outcome at follow-up. Steroid treatment unfortunately is associated with numerous side effects, particularly hypertension (Greenough *et al.*, 1992). Some infants with CLD are wheezy even while remaining on the neonatal intensive care unit. Fortunately preterm infants, even in the first year of life, are sensitive to bronchodilators (Greenough and Milner, 1991). Nebulized therapy, however, should be given with caution as, prior to bronchodilation, this can cause an initial paradoxical deterioration in lung function associated with a drop in oxygen saturation. An equally effective method of administration, which does not have such an adverse effect, is a metered dose inhaler and spacer device (Yuksel and Greenough, 1994). Diuretic therapy is also associated with short term improvements in lung function in ventilator dependent infants. Long term administration of frusemide should, however, be avoided as this is associated with renal calcification.

PERSISTENT FETAL CIRCULATION

Persistent fetal circulation (also known as persistent pulmonary vascular obstruction, pulmonary hypertension, transitional circulation, fetal cardiopulmonary circulation) is a clinical syndrome consisting of pulmonary hypertension and right–left shunting through the patent ductus arteriosis and/or foramen ovale (Editorial, 1988). Infants present with hypoxia, tachypnoea and tricuspid or mitral regurgitation. There is hypovascularity on the chest radiograph and if the ductus arteriosus is closed the electrocardiogram shows changes of myocardial ischaemia. The condition may be idiopathic or associated with lung disease, aspiration syndromes, congenital malformation or polycythaemia with hyperviscosity. Minimal handling of affected infants is of great importance as a slight disturbance, for example, turning the baby for physiotherapy, can precipitate severe hypoxaemia. Endotracheal tube suctioning should be carried out only when indicated and chest physiotherapy is contraindicated. Treatment is of the usual supportive nature. Hyperventilation has been used in the past, but has been demonstrated to cause unnecessary barotrauma of the lungs. High frequency oscillation supports the infant with PFC and effective oxygenation can be achieved without hyperventilation. Vasodilator drugs are used, most commonly tolazoline. Unfortunately these drugs are not specific pulmonary vasodilators and may cause significant hypotension. In addition, gastrointestinal haemorrhage is a common side effect. There has been recent enthusiasm for magnesium sulphate, although early reports of this drug's success have not been confirmed in clinical practice. Nitric oxide may be a useful option for the 1990s. Infants who fail to respond to all these manoeuvres may respond to extracorporeal membrane oxygenation.

MECONIUM ASPIRATION SYNDROME

This illness follows inhalation of meconium before, during or immediately after delivery. The incidence of meconium aspiration syndrome is very low in the United Kingdom, probably less than 0.2%,but is up to ten times more common in the United States. In utero, infants pass meconium in response to acute or chronic hypoxia. If the hypoxia continues, the infant gasps and inhales meconium during the delivery process. Premature infants rarely pass meconium in utero unless they are infected, usually with either group B streptococcal or listeria infection (Editorial, 1988).

Presentation

Once meconium is inhaled it causes chemical irritation resulting in atelectasis and surfactant inhibition, mechanical obstruction with air trapping and predisposes the infant to infection. The infant develops ventilation/perfusion mismatch and is at high risk of developing pneumothoraces. If severe hypoxia and hypercarbia develop, this results in persistent fetal circulation. Infants who suffer meconium aspiration syndrome are usually mature or postmature and have a dry skin with staining of the fingernails and umbilical cord. The infants are tachypnoeic, use their accessory muscles of respiration and may have an overdistended chest. On examination, crepitations and occasional rhonchi can be heard. The chest radiograph demonstrates patchy infiltrates and overexpansion in the early stage. Later as the disease progresses the appearance changes to that of diffuse and homogeneous opacification, which is the result of pneumonitis and interstitial oedema.

Prevention

A paediatrician should attend all deliveries associated with fetal distress. At delivery the infant's airway must be immediately cleared, if necessary, under direct vision. The aim is to remove as much meconium as possible prior to the initiation of respiration or ventilation.

Management

Physiotherapy is of paramount importance to these infants to try and dislodge meconium from the lungs. As the meconium predisposes the infant to infection prophylactic antibiotics should be used. Infants usually require some form of respiratory support. Mechanical ventilation increases the risk of pneumothorax. Slow rates with a long expiratory time and low levels of positive end expiratory pressure (PEEP) are used to reduce the likelihood of airtrapping. The infant will usually require a neuromuscular blocking agent if ventilated conventionally or patient triggered ventilation may be a useful alternative. Many infants have pulmonary hypertension and require a pulmonary vasodilator. Some infants will develop very severe respiratory failure and in these infants there is a preliminary success with high frequency oscillation, but extracorporeal membrane oxygenation may be necessary. Recent studies have demonstrated that patients with meconium aspiration syndrome have an increased prevalence of respiratory problems and lung function abormalities, suggestive of asthma, at follow-up (MacFarlane and Heaf, 1988).

PULMONARY AIR LEAK

Pulmonary air leak, particularly pneumothorax and pulmonary interstitial emphysema, are common the newborn.

Pneumothorax

Approximately 1% of infants develop a pneumothorax at birth, but only 10% of these are symptomatic. The incidence of pneumothorax increases proportional to the level of respiratory support used, being particularly common in ventilated infants. Small pneumothoraces may be asymptomatic, but ventilated babies may develop large tension pneumothoraces and present dramatically with pallor and shock, hypotension and very abnormal blood gases. Unfortunately there is a frequent association of intraventricular haemorrhage (IVH). The chest radiograph (Figure 7.2) is diagnostic but pneumothoraces may also be identified by transillumination.

a) Prevention

Optimization of methods of ventilation reduces the incidence of pneumothoraces, fast rates mimicking the infants' spontaneous respiratory rate and promoting synchronous respiration (Greenough and Milner, 1993). Selective paralysis of infants fighting the ventilator also prevents air leak (Greenough *et al.*, 1984).

b) Management

Asymptomatic pneumothoraces need no treatment. Ventilated infants and non-ventilated infants with tension pneumothoraces require treatment with underwater sealed drains and suction. The drain should remain in situ for at least 24 hours after the pneumothorax has drained.

Pulmonary interstitial emphysema

Pulmonary interstitial emphysema (PIE) is due to gas trapping within the perivascular sheaves of the lung. Its incidence is inversely proportional to gestational age. It usually

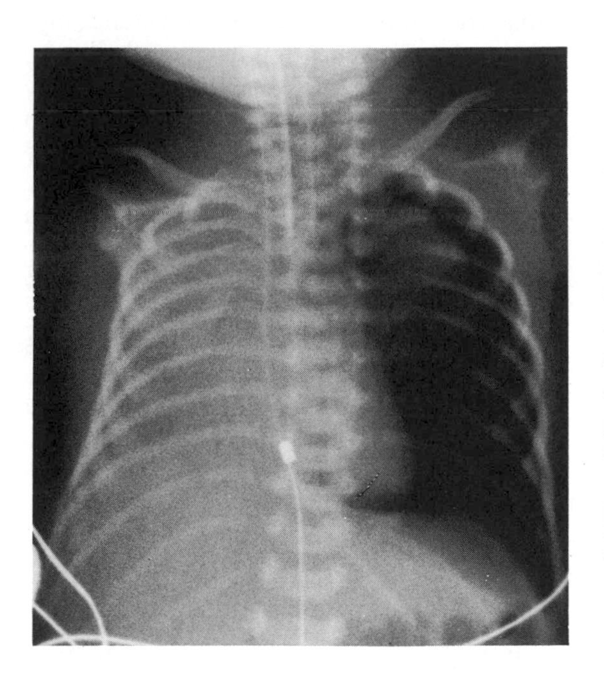

Figure 7.2 Chest radiograph showing a pneumothorax.

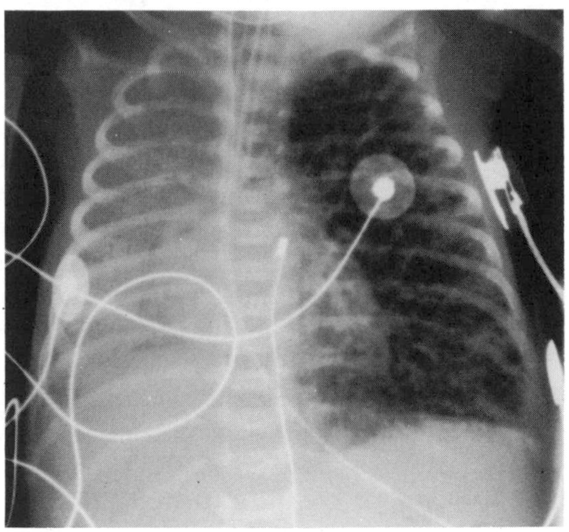

Figure 7.3 Pulmonary interstitial emphysema in a preterm infant.

presents when a chest radiograph is taken in a severely ill infant whose condition is deteriorating (Figure 7.3).

a) Management

Infants with localized interstitial emphysema should be positioned with the affected side lowermost. Vigorous physiotherapy has been claimed to improve the condition by disruption of the emphysematous bullae, although this is not considered safe practice. If localized interstitial emphysema persists, selective bronchial intubation may be useful or selective obstruction of the main bronchus of the affected area. If all else fails, surgical resection is necessary. If the interstitial emphysema is generalized, linear pleurotomies are performed to create an artificial pneumothorax. Peak pressures and PEEP need to be reduced to try and decompress the interstitial emphysema. Fast rate ventilation can reduce the incidence of pneumothorax.

SURGICAL CONDITIONS

Numerous surgical conditions cause respiratory problems in the neonatal period. The most common are congenital diaphragmatic hernia (CDH) and oesophageal atresia with tracheo-oesophageal fistula.

Congenital diaphragmatic hernia

Infants with CDH have a hypoplastic ipsilateral lung and the contralateral lung may also be affected. In the labour ward it is essential to avoid resuscitation using a face mask, face mask T piece or bag and mask system which will cause distension of the bowel in the chest. Infants usually require resuscitation and many surgeons favour ventilation and immediate paralysis to prevent swallowing and hence gas filling of the bowel within the chest (Figure 7.4). The infant should be stabilized prior to being sent to theatre as this improves their outlook. Surgical closure of the diaphragm and restoration of the bowel into the abdomen is associated with a deterioration in lung function. Infants also suffer from an element of persistent fetal circulation but, in addition, have an abnormality of pulmonary vasculature. Infants who have a severe degree of pulmonary hypoplasia usually do very badly from birth. Neither antenatal diagnosis nor extracorporeal membrane oxygenation has improved their outcome. The mortality of infants who survive the first 24 hours is as low as 10%. In the long term the infants do have persisting problems with lung function and ventilation/perfusion abnormalities.

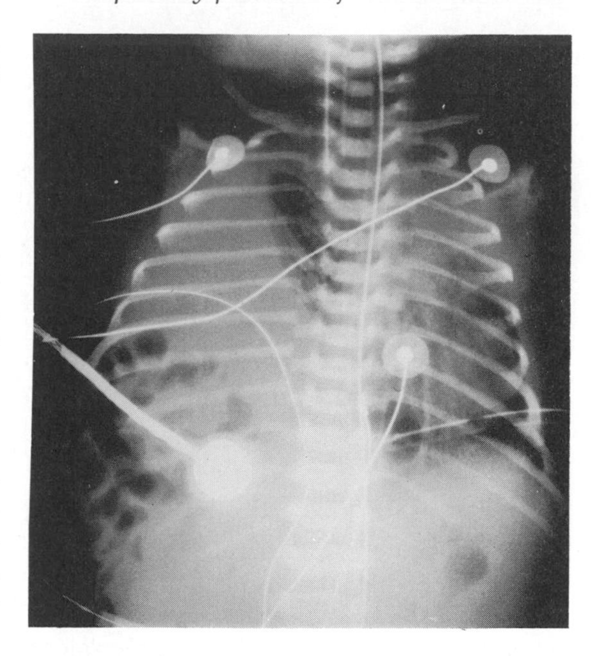

Figure 7.4 Congenital diaphragmatic hernia prior to surgical correction.

Oesophageal atresia

Oesophageal atresia occurs in one in 3000

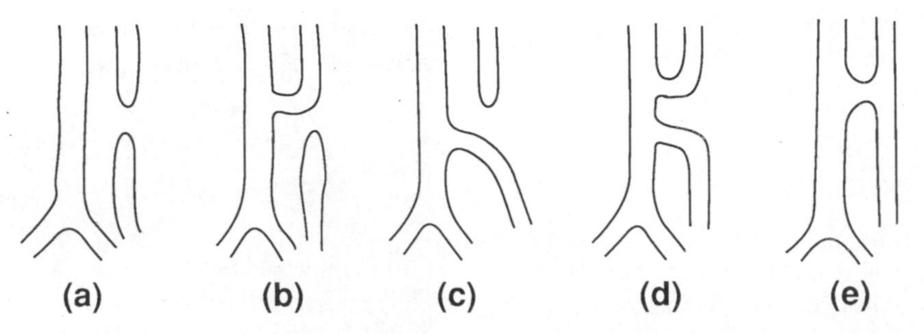

Figure 7.5 Oesophageal atresia (OA) with tracheo-oesophageal fistula (TOF): (a) isolated OA, (b) OA with proximal TOF, (c) OA with distal TOF, (d) OA with proximal and distal TOF and (e) TOF without OA or 'H-type fistula'.

births. In 80% of cases there is a blind proximal pouch and fistula between the trachea and distal oesophagus and 10% of patients have oesophageal atresia without a fistula (Figure 7.5). Polyhydramnios alerts the physician to the possibility of the diagnosis. The infant presents postnatally with saliva or mucus dribbling from the mouth with episodes of choking, cyanosis and coughing due to overflow of secretions into the larynx and trachea. The condition can be diagnosed by hold-up of the nasogastric tube, usually about 10 cm from the lips. Initially management is aimed at maintaining the airway free of secretions and once the infant is stable he or she should be transferred to a unit specialized in repairing the anomaly.

Tracheo-oesophageal fistula without oesophageal atresia is much more uncommon than oesophageal atresia. These infants do not have polyhydramnios in pregnancy and may not present even in the neonatal period. Respiratory symptoms, particularly on feeding, however, are common and the infants may have a right upper lobe pneumonia due to aspiration of material through the fistula. They also have gaseous distension of the abdominal content due to air passing through the fistula into the oesophagus and down the alimentary tract. These infants are more likely to have 13 pairs of ribs than non-affected infants. Treatment is surgical division of the fistula.

Gastroschisis and omphalocele

Anterior abdominal wall defects are relatively uncommon, occurring in one in 3500 live births. Exomphalos has been the term used for protrusions at and around the umbilicus. Infants so affected can be divided into three groups: those with a hernia into the cord, an omphalocele or a gastroschisis. The omphalocele usually contains liver as well as bowel and affected infants frequently have other major anomalies and chromosomal abnormalities. Omphaloceles may be managed conservatively by treating the covering sac with dessicating agents, but more commonly surgical closure is performed. Either a primary closure is undertaken or alternatively a silastic pouch is sutured to the abdominal wall followed by gradual reduction of the bowel contents into the abdomen with closure after 10–14 days. Infants with a gastroschisis have a defect of the anterior abdominal wall which occurs to the right of the umbilicus and through the defect prolapses the midgut. In some patients the exposed bowel becomes densely matted antenatally and is meconium stained. Postnatally treatment is directed

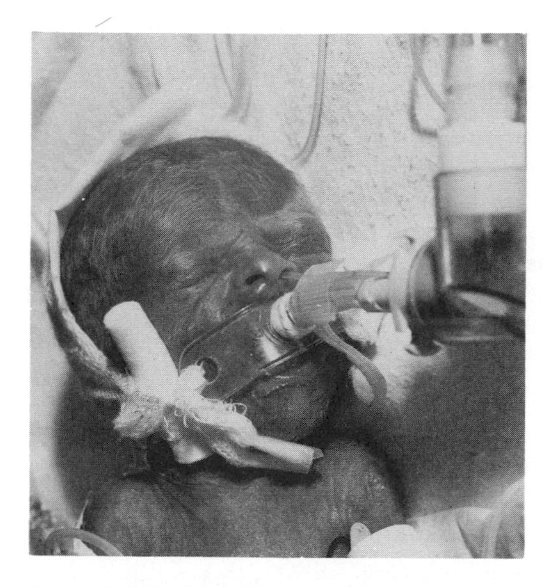

Figure 7.6 Oral intubation in a preterm infant.

as with an omphalocele, at repair and reduction of the bowel into the abdominal cavity.

Following surgical repair the infants experience respiratory insufficiency due to the increased intra-abdominal pressure – this effect is limited to the immediate post-operative period. Some infants, however, have impaired antenatal lung growth and follow-up studies (Thompson *et al.*, 1993) have demonstrated a proportion having persistent abnormal lung function during infancy.

PHYSIOTHERAPY MANAGEMENT OF THE NEONATE

The management of the acutely ill neonate is directed towards minimal handling. Respiratory physiotherapy with its known detrimental effects should not, therefore, be carried out routinely. Each infant should be assessed by experienced and qualified staff and techniques should be chosen as appropriate for each individual, prior to any intervention. Frequently preterm infants and neonates are intubated with oral endotracheal tubes (Figure 7.6).

INDICATIONS FOR PHYSIOTHERAPY

Retention of secretions and lobar collapse due to mucus plugging are the main indications for physiotherapy in the neonate. Lobar collapse due to other reasons, e.g. pulmonary interstitial emphysema in adjacent lung tissue is not an indication for physiotherapy.

Meconium aspiration

If initial attempts to remove meconium at delivery have been unsuccessful then physiotherapy treatment is essential (Parker, 1985; Crane, 1981). Appropriate positioning and percussion should be performed within one hour of delivery, if possible (Parker, 1993). Treatment is usually well tolerated as these are, most commonly, full term infants.

If early treatment is not given areas of pneumonitis and hyperinflation develop and the infant is often very ill. Physiotherapy techniques are not indicated at this stage. Later, resolution of consolidated areas may produce excessive secretions and physiotherapy techniques may help in their removal if secretions are not cleared by suction alone.

Aspiration of feed or vomit

Infants who have aspirated feed or vomit should be suctioned immediately to clear the airway. Positioning and percussion should be performed as soon as possible if suctioning has not fully removed the aspirate. Following aspiration a chemical pneumonitis and consolidation will occur if the aspirate is not removed quickly. Physiotherapy management would then follow as for meconium aspiration.

In patients with recurrent aspiration due to gastro-oesophageal reflux physiotherapy may not be appropriate. Techniques of head down positioning, percussion and vibrations exacerbate existing gastro-oesophageal reflux. To avoid this, treatment, if it is indicated, should not be performed in the horizontal or head down positions and nasal rather than oropharyngeal suction should be used (Demont *et al.*, 1991). Treatment should be given before feeds or at least one hour after a feed has finished. In some infants the benefits of physiotherapy are outweighed by increased reflux and aspiration.

Chronic lung disease

Infants with chronic lung disease show variable patterns of wheeze, airway collapse and sometimes retention of secretions. Careful assessment of the effects of treatment will determine whether physiotherapy is appropriate for individual patients.

Postoperatively

The effects of immobility and anaesthesia are the same in infants as in older children.

a) Congenital diaphragmatic hernia

Infants with this condition are often very unwell postoperatively. It is important to keep the contralateral lung clear of secretions as the ipsilateral lung is usually hypoplastic. Manual hyperinflation is contraindicated because of the pulmonary hypoplasia as high inspiratory pressures should be avoided.

b) Oesophageal atresia and tracheo-oesophageal fistula

Preoperatively some patients may require physiotherapy if there is collapse and increased secretions due to reflux of gastric contents. The infant will be nursed head up both pre and postoperatively and if treatment is indicated it should be undertaken in this position due to the risk of reflux. Care must be taken not to extend the neck which may strain the anastomosis site. In the non-intubated patient great caution must be taken with pharyngeal suction to avoid passing the catheter into the oesophagus and damaging the anastomosis.

CONTRAINDICATIONS TO PHYSIOTHERAPY

Unstable infant

Although there are rarely absolute contraindications to physiotherapy the very unstable acutely ill infant should not be treated unless absolutely necessary.

Pulmonary haemorrhage

Pulmonary haemorrhage can occur spontaneously in preterm infants and has been associated with surfactant therapy. Physiotherapy techniques such as percussion and vibrations are liable to exacerbate the haemorrhage, so are contraindicated. Careful positioning and gentle suctioning should be given as necessary to maintain a clear airway. When the secretions aspirated become brown and tenacious rather than fresh blood, then manual techniques such as percussion and vibrations may aid secretion removal. Treatment should be discontinued if fresh bleeding recurs.

Respiratory distress syndrome

Physiotherapy is not indicated in early uncomplicated RDS as the main problem is lack of surfactant. One study has linked routine chest physiotherapy in the first 24 hours of life with an increased incidence of

IVH when compared with suction alone (Raval *et al.*, 1987). Infrequent suctioning, i.e. 12 hourly, has been shown to be sufficient to maintain a clear airway in early RDS (Wilson *et al.*, 1991).

ASSESSMENT

Many aspects of respiratory assessment of the neonate are the same as in older children. When assessing the neonate the following points are relevant:

1. history of pregnancy, labour and delivery.
2. apgar scores – these grade five clinical features (respiratory effort, heart rate, muscle tone, reflex irritability and colour) which are measured at one minute and five minutes postdelivery to give an indication of the degree of asphyxiation at delivery.
3. gestational age and weight.
4. how well the infant tolerates handling and how long has elapsed since the last handling episode. It is important for neonates to have long periods of rest.
5. if the infant's temperature is 36.5°C or below then non-essential handling should be left until the temperature has risen.
6. apnoeic spells, self-limiting bradycardias and bradycardias requiring stimulation may be due to retention of secretions, although they can also be due to other causes.
7. the oxygen disassociation curve is shifted to the left in a newborn infant. This is due to the amount of fetal haemoglobin present in the blood in the first 3–4 weeks of life. Fetal haemoglobin has a higher affinity for oxygen than adult haemoglobin.
8. auscultation is difficult to interpret in the very preterm, extremely low birthweight infant due to the easy transmission of sounds. It is often impossible to hear any breath sounds at all in the spontaneously breathing infant.

PHYSIOTHERAPY TECHNIQUES

Most techniques used in children can be applied to the neonate. It is crucial to try and maintain cardiovascular stability during treatment of the preterm, particularly in the first week of life. During this time large swings in arterial oxygen and carbon dioxide levels, heart rate and blood pressure increase the risk of IVH which may have long term neurological sequelae.

Positioning and postural drainage

In most neonatal units infants are nursed tilted head up. This position has been shown to increase the transcutaneous arterial oxygen tension in spontaneously breathing infants (Thoresen *et al.*, 1988). The prone position also increases arterial oxygen levels whilst supine is the least beneficial position (Dean, 1985). Young children and neonates preferentially ventilate the uppermost areas of lung in side lying (Davies *et al.*, 1985). All these documented effects are less important in infants who are paralysed and fully ventilated.

Gravity assisted positioning (postural drainage) of the lower and middle lobes which requires a head down tip should be avoided or used with great caution, particularly in spontaneously breathing preterm infants. The head down position causes arterial oxygen levels to drop (Thoresen *et al.*, 1988) and increases the risk of IVH and gastro-oesophageal reflux. This position is poorly tolerated by infants with abdominal distension. Preterm infants with unilateral lung disease may not tolerate their affected lung being turned uppermost for physiotherapy as a rapid desaturation may occur. These infants may tolerate treatment in prone and, if very unstable, may need to be nursed with the unaffected lung uppermost in order to optimize gas exchange. Specific gravity assisted positions are, therefore, not so useful in sick neonates, particularly the preterm. Treatment is often given in situ with the infant remaining tilted head up. It is important, however, that there are regular changes of position from prone to alternate side lying in those infants who can tolerate it.

As preterm infants are hypotonic and have soft, easily moulded bones, it is important to position them carefully in order to avoid future postural deformity (Downs *et al.*, 1991).

Chest percussion (clapping) and vibrations

In full term infants over 3.0 kg percussion can be carried out using the cupped hand. In smaller infants percussion with cup shaped objects, tenting or contact heel percussion as previously described in Chapter 6, p. 74 can be used. Percussion with a face mask has been shown to be well tolerated (Tudehope and Bagley, 1980) and contact heel percussion is a technique that uses the thenar and hypothenar eminences, used by physiotherapists in Australia and Canada but not widely taught or practised in the UK.

The very soft and compliant chest wall of the preterm infant means that vibrations can be very effective. However, vibrations seem to be less well tolerated than percussion. Vibrations to the left side of the chest can mimic external cardiac massage. They are less useful in infants whose respiratory or ventilator rate is very fast because of the short expiratory time.

Great care should be taken when using both percussion or vibrations in very preterm infants as the skin is extremely fragile and easily damaged. Osteoporosis can be a problem in preterm infants and chest physiotherapy has been implicated as the cause of rib fracture (Geggel *et al.*, 1978) and periosteal new bone formation (Wood, 1987). The techniques of physiotherapy were not fully described in these studies and one of the infants also had femoral and fibular fractures. However, percussion and vibrations should be avoided or given with great caution in infants with osteoporosis.

Manual hyperinflation

Manual hyperinflation as a physiotherapy technique is less useful in infants than in children and adults. All contraindications and precautions that apply to children also apply to infants. In addition collateral ventilation is not well developed in the newborn (Hussey, 1992) so diffusion of air between bronchioles and alveoli does not occur. Gas under positive pressure takes the line of least resistance so inflated areas of lung will become hyperinflated whilst atelectatic areas will remain collapsed. Manual hyperinflation also increases the risks of barotrauma leading to the development of pulmonary interstitial emphysema or pneumothorax. As a physiotherapy technique manual hyperinflation should probably not be used for preterm infants. It can be used with caution in full term infants using a peak inspiratory pressure (PIP) of no more than 20% above the PIP of the ventilator. Pressure should always be monitored using a manometer in the circuit (Howard-Glenn and Koniak-Griffin, 1990).

Airway suction

The hazards of suctioning are well recognized and have been previously described (Chapter 6, p. 80). The following points are particularly related to neonates.

Nasopharyngeal suction is important in non-intubated preterm infants to clear upper airway secretions which may be a cause of apnoeic spells (Pickens *et al.*, 1988). However, nasopharyngeal suction has also been cited as a cause of apnoea and bradycardia in the newborn after delivery (Cordero and Hon, 1971). Preoxygenation should be used cautiously in preterm infants to avoid hyperoxia which may contribute to the development of retinopathy of prematurity and IVH. Inspired oxygen (FiO_2) should be carefully increased in hypoxic infants to bring the arterial oxygenation (PaO_2) up to a satisfactory level. The PaO_2 should be maintained between 7.0–9.5 kPa (50–70 mmHg) and the arterial carbon dioxide level ($PaCO_2$) between 4.5–7.0 kPa (35–50 mmHg). Oxygen saturation levels are kept between 90% and 95%. Preterm infants who have a normal PaO_2 should only have the FiO_2 increased by 10% (i.e. 30%–40%) immediately prior to passing the suction catheter. Following suction the FiO_2 can again be increased if the infant remains hypoxic. In the very unstable infant the ventilator rate can be temporarily increased to avoid severe hypoxia. Once recovery begins the inspired oxygen should be slowly reduced to the pretreatment level to avoid a swing to hyperoxia.

Pneumothorax secondary to perforation of a segmental bronchus by a suction catheter has been reported (Anderson and Chandra, 1976; Vaughan *et al.*, 1978; Alpan *et al.*, 1984). The infants at greatest risk are those with severe lung disease, although poor suctioning technique is also implicated. The risk of perforation and mucosal trauma can be reduced by only passing catheters to 1 cm past the end of the endotracheal tube (Kleiber *et al.*, 1988; Bailey *et al.*, 1988). A catheter precut to the correct length can be attached to the side of the incubator as a guide. Suction catheters are also available which have centimetre markings corresponding with those on endotracheal tubes.

Saline instillation

In many neonatal units suctioning is preceded by a lavage with a diluent or mucolytic. Drew *et al.*, (1986) conducted a random trial of saline or no saline in 86 intubated infants. They concluded that routine saline instillation was necessary when the size of the endotracheal tube was 2.5 mm or less. When size 3.0 mm or greater was used routine instillation of saline was only necessary after 36 hours of intubation. Routine instillation of a diluent or mucolytic is less important if an infant is systematically well hydrated and there is efficient humidification of inspired gases (Ackerman, 1985).

ADJUNCTS TO PHYSIOTHERAPY

Humidification

The narrow diameter of endotracheal tubes used in preterm infants means that these can easily be blocked by even a small amount of thick mucus. Efficient humidification is therefore extremely important in small infants. The amount of humidity received by the infant is dependent upon the temperature of the humidifier, the ambient room/incubator temperature, the level of water in the humidifier chamber, the length of ventilator tubing, the gas flow rate and the position of the temperature probe in the ventilator circuit (Tarnow-Mordi *et al.*, 1989). Although no study has determined the optimum temperature of the humidifier these authors reported a reduction in the incidence of pneumothorax and chronic lung disease in infants weighing less than 1500g when the humidifier temperature was greater than 36.5°C. Possible dangers of overhumidification include pyrexia and fluid overload (Tarnow-Mordi *et al.*, 1986).

REFERENCES

Ackerman, M.H. (1985) The use of bolus normal saline instillation in artificial airways: is it useful or necessary? *Heart Lung*, **14**, 505–6.

Alpan, G., Glick, B., Peleg, O. *et al.* (1984) Pneumothorax due to endotracheal tube suction. *American Journal of Perinatology*, **1**, 345–8.

Anderson, K. and Chandra, K. (1976) Pneumothorax secondary to perforation of sequential bronchi by suction catheters. *Journal of Pediatric Surgery*, **11**, 687–93.

Bailey, C., Kattwinkle, J., Teia, K. and Buckley, T. (1988) Shallow versus deep endotracheal suctioning in young rabbits: effects on the tracheobronchial wall. *Pediatrics*, **82**, 746–51.

Chan, V., Greenough, A. and Gamsu, H.R. (1992) Neonatal complications of mechanical ventilation in extremely preterm infants. *European Journal of Pediatrics*, **151**, 693–6.

Cordero, L. and Hon, E. (1971) Neonatal bradycardia following nasopharyngeal stimulation. *Journal of Pediatrics*, **78**, 441–7.

Crane, L. (1981) Physical therapy for neonates with respiratory dysfunction. *Physical Therapy*, **61**, 1764–73.

Crowley, P., Chalmers, I. and Keirse, M.J.N.C. (1990) The effects of corticosteroid administration before preterm delivery: an overview of evidence from controlled trials. *British Journal of Obstetrics and Gynaecology*, **97**, 11–25.

Davies, H., Kitchman, R., Gordon, I. and Helms, P. (1985) Regional ventilation in infancy. *New England Journal of Medicine*, **313**, 1626–8.

Dean, E. (1985) Effects of body position on pulmonary function. *Physical Therapy*, **65**, 613–18.

Demont, B., Escorrou, P., Vincon, D. *et al.* (1991) Effects of respiratory physical therapy and nasopharyngeal suction on gastrooesophageal reflux in infants less than a year of age with or without abnormal reflux. *Archives Françaises de Pediatric (Paris)*, **48**, 621–5.

Downs, J., Edwards, A.D., McCormick, D.C. *et al.* (1991) Effect of intervention on development of hip posture in very preterm babies. *Archives of Disease in Childhood*, **66**, 797–801.

Drew, J., Padoms, K. and Clabburn, S.L. (1986) Endotracheal management in newborn infants with hyaline membrane disease. *Australian Journal of Physiotherapy*, **32**, 3–5.

Editorial (1988) Persistent fetal circulation and extracorporeal membrane oxygenation. *Lancet*, **ii**, 1289–91.

Editorial (1992) Oxygen restriction and retinopathy of prematurity. *Lancet*, **ii**, 961–3.

Geggel, R., Pereira, G. and Spackman, T. (1978) Fractured ribs: unusual presentation of rickets in premature infants. *Journal of Pediatrics*, **93**, 680–2.

Greenough, A. (1990) Personal practice – bronchopulmonary dyspalasia – early diagnosis, prophylaxis and treatment. *Archives of Disease in Childhood*, **65**, 1082–8.

Greenough, A., Emery, E.F. and Gamsu, H.R. (1992) Dexamethasone and hypertension in preterm infants. *European Journal of Pediatrics*, **152**, 134–5.

Greenough, A., Hird, M.F. and Gamsu, H.R. (1991a) Home oxygen therapy following neonatal intensive care. *Early Human Development*, **26**, 29–35.

Greenough, A. and Milner, A.D. (1991) Prematurity and asthma – is there a link? *Current Medical Literature – Paediatrics*, **4**, 87–91.

Greenough, A. and Milner, A.D. (1993) Recent advances in neonatal ventilation. *Care of the Critically Ill*, **9**, 154–7.

Greenough, A., Osborne, J. and Sutherland, S. (eds) (1991b) *Congenital, Perinatal and Neonatal Infections*, Churchill Livingstone, Edinburgh.

Greenough, A., Wood, S., Morley, C.J. and Davis, J.A. (1984) Pancuronium prevents pneumothoraces in ventilated premature infants who actively expire against positive pressure ventilation. Lancet, **i**, 1–3.

Howard-Glenn, L., and Koniak-Griffin, O. (1990) Evaluation of manometer use in manual ventilation of infants in neonatal intensive care units. *Heart Lung*, **19**, 620–7.

Hussey, J. (1992) Effects of chest physiotherapy for children in intensive care after surgery. *Physiotherapy*, **78**, 109–13.

Kleiber, T., Krutzfield, N. and Rose E. (1988) Acute histologic changes in the tracheobronchial tree associated with different catheter insertion techniques. *Heart Lung*, **17**, 10–14.

Lucas, A., Morley, R. and Cole, T.J. (1988) Adverse neurodevelopmental outcome of moderate hypoglycaemia. *British Medical Journal*, **297**, 1304–8.

Macfarlane, P.I. and Heaf, D.P. (1988) Pulmonary function in children after neonatal meconium aspiration syndrome. *Archives of Disease in Childhood*, **63**, 368–72.

Morley, C.J. (1991) Surfactant treatment for premature babies – a review of clinical trials. *Archives of Disease in Childhood*, **66**, 445–50.

Parker, A.E. (1985) Chest physiotherapy in the neonatal intensive care unit. *Physiotherapy*, **71**, 63–5.

Parker A.E. (1993) Paediatrics, in *Physiotherapy for Respiratory and Cardiac Problems*, (eds B. Webber and J. Pryor), Churchill Livingstone, Edinburgh, pp. 281–318.

Pickens, D., Schesst, G. and Thach, B. (1988) Prolonged apnoea associated with upper airway protective reflexes in apnoea of prematurity. *American Review of Respiratory Disease*, **137**, 113–18.

Raval, D., Yeh, T.F., Mora, A. *et al.* (1987) Chest physiotherapy in preterm infants with respiratory distress syndrome in the first 24 hours of life. *Journal of Perinatology*, **7**, 301–4.

Ruggins, N. (1991) Pathophysiology of apnoea in preterm infants: current problem. *Archives of Disease in Childhood*, **66**, 70–3.

Tarnow-Mordi, W.O., Fletcher, M., Sutton, P. and Wilkinson, A.D. (1986) Evidence of inadequate humidification of inspired gas during artificial ventilation of newborn infants in the British Isles. *Lancet*, **ii**, 909–10.

Tarnow-Mordi, W.O., Reid, E., Griffiths, P. and Wilkinson, A.R. (1989) Inspired gas temperature and respiratory complications in very low birthweight infants. *Journal of Pediatrics*, **114**, 438–42.

Thompson, P.J., Greenough, A., Hird, M.F. *et al.* (1992) Nosocomial bacterial infections in very low birthweight infants. *European Journal of Paediatrics*, **151**, 451–4.

Thompson, P.J., Greenough, A., Nicolaides, K.H. and Dykes, E. (1993) Impaired respiratory function in infants with anterior abdominal wall defects. *Journal of Pediatric Surgery*, **28**, 664–6.

Thoreson, M., Cavan, F. and Whitelaw, A. (1988) Effect of tilting on oxygenation in newborn infants. *Archives of Disease in Childhood*, **63**, 315–17.

Tudehope, D. and Bagley, C. (1980) Techniques of physiotherapy in intubated babies with the respiratory distress syndrome. *Australian Paediatric Journal*, **16**, 226–8.

Vaughan, R., Menke, J. and Giacoia, G. (1978) Pneumothorax: a complication of endotracheal tube suctioning. *Journal of Pediatrics*, **92**, 633–4.

Wilson, G., Hughes, G., Rennie, J. and Morley, C. (1991) Evaluation of two endotracheal suction regimes in babies ventilated for respiratory distress syndrome. *Early Human Development*, **25**, 87–90.

Wood, B. (1987) Infant ribs: generalized periosteal reaction resulting from vibrator chest physiotherapy. *Radiology*, **162**, 811–12.

Yuksel, B. and Greenough, A. (1994) Comparison of the effects on lung function of different methods of bronchodilator administration. *Respiratory Medicine*, **88**, 229–33.

PAEDIATRIC CARDIAC SURGERY 8

Martin Elliott and Juliette Hussey

INTRODUCTION

The diagnosis of congenital heart defects can now be made largely non-invasively and almost all conditions can now be considered amenable to surgery. Overall mortality has fallen to less than 5% in the best units and the majority of operations are performed in the first year of life. Each aspect of the child's care is an integrated process merging the skills of surgeons, nurses, physicians, technicians and, of course, respiratory physiotherapists. Care must be carried out in specialist institutions - the more cases done, the better the results.

Anderson and Becker (1994) defined a system of 'sequential analysis' which allows for a logical description of the defects and this terminology will be used throughout the chapter. The incidence of congenital heart disease is about 8:1000 live births. However, only about a third of these require any kind of surgical intervention, the remainder either resolving spontaneously or not being haemodynamically significant enough to require intervention.

DIAGNOSIS AND REFERRAL

The age at which patients present varies with the severity of the condition and the screening facilities available. There have been very important improvements in ultrasonic diagnosis of fetal abnormalities and now it is possible for experienced operators to diagnose significant cardiac anomalies in the fetus in utero as early as 18 weeks for some abnormalities. This service is far from widespread or uniform in quality, but when diagnoses are made it provides the additional option of termination of pregnancy. Many parents do take this option and as the service of prenatal diagnosis extends the number of children who present for surgery may fall. However, prenatal diagnosis offers a number of other options to the families and carers. The mother and her uterus may be regarded as a highly efficient transport incubator and be used to transfer the child with congenital heart disease to a specialist centre for both delivery and subsequent surgery on the newborn infant.

Some workers have used the ability to diagnose CHD prenatally to develop techniques of prenatal in utero intervention. There have been several reports of prenatal transcatheter interventions designed to dilate stenosed valves or open obstructed outflow tracts from the ventricles. Other researchers are evolving methods of performing open heart surgery on the fetus.

In Great Britain, most babies with significant congenital heart disease are diagnosed relatively early in life by paediatricians, health visitors or general practitioners. Telephone discussions take place with a specialist centre, allowing refinement of diagnosis and establishment of appropriate immediate care (Franklin *et al.*, 1991). Once a child has been transferred to a specialist unit it will be seen immediately by paediatric cardiologists. With modern, two-dimensional echocardiography virtually all congenital heart defects can be accurately diagnosed and the images recorded for later study, analysis and decision making. The development of pulsed and continuous wave Doppler techniques has also enhanced the importance of echocardiography as a diagnostic modality both in accuracy and scope. If a diagnosis cannot be firmly established using these techniques or if more detailed physiological information is needed, then cardiac catheterization with or without angiography may be required. Cardiac catheterization is also used as a therapeutic procedure in a number of conditions in order to avoid an operation. These circumstances will be discussed in relevant sections of the chapter.

Once the diagnosis is made, the process of educating the family can begin. Decisions to carry out any intervention to a child's heart must be well informed, open, meticulous and documented. The management should be agreed between at least the cardiologist, the surgeon and the family and as the child grows he or she must be brought into the decision making process.

STAGING OR PALLIATION

The current preference is to perform an early complete repair wherever possible. In those defects which do not allow such an approach, a palliative or staging procedure must be introduced. There are three main reasons why such a procedure might be indicated:

1. excessive blood flow to the lungs;
2. inadequate blood flow to the lungs;
3. inadequate mixing.

EXCESSIVE PULMONARY BLOOD FLOW

This occurs whenever there is a systemic to pulmonary shunt associated with intracardiac communications. Excessive pulmonary blood flow usually presents with heart failure, tachypnoea and poor feeding and is seen in the presence of large ventricular septal defects (especially those with coarctation of the aorta), atrioventricular septal defects, double inlet or outlet ventricles and truncus arteriosus. Wherever possible a corrective repair should be performed, but if it is decided that this is too dangerous then the blood flow to the lungs must be limited to prevent pulmonary arteriolar muscle hypertrophy. This involves banding the pulmonary artery (PA) (using a nylon tape or a silk ligature) through a left thoracotomy incision, ligating it to such an extent that the distal pulmonary artery pressure is reduced to around 30% of the aortic pressure and the systemic arterial oxygen saturation is reduced to around 80–85%. Banding is now performed rarely and only in patients who are considered at high risk or in preparation for right heart bypass operations. In earlier years PA banding carried a risk of 13–53%, but the main determinant is the severity of the underlying condition. In a recent series of 145 patients banded between 1985–1991 at the Great Ormond Street Hospital for Children NHS Trust, there was an 8% mortality for pulmonary banding (12 patients).

INADEQUATE PULMONARY BLOOD FLOW

If there is inadequate flow of blood to the lungs, then insufficient oxygen can be transferred to the circulating red cells. Central cyanosis is seen in tetralogy of Fallot, pulmonary or tricuspid atresia and in any complex ventricular morphology with pulmonary or subpulmonary stenosis. Complete repair should be the primary option. If this is judged unsafe, then something must be done to provide more blood flow to the lungs in order to improve tissue oxygenation. This can usually be achieved by the creation of a shunt (an artificial communication between the systemic and pulmonary circulations), most commonly a modified Blalock–Taussig shunt. This type of shunt involves the interposition of a piece of thin walled polytetrafluoroethylene (PTFE) between the subclavian artery and the ipsilateral PA.

These shunts are inserted via a thoracotomy and will usually result in an increase in the oxygen saturation to around 80–85%. Dangers of this kind of shunt include distortion of the pulmonary arteries and the provision of excess pulmonary blood flow to the lungs. In later life the shunt has to be taken down, although it may usually simply be ligated at the time of definitive repair.

INADEQUATE MIXING

In transposition of the great arteries the pathophysiology is characterized by inadequate mixing of red and blue blood within the heart. Without some form of intracardiac communication, red blood never crosses the septum to meet the metabolic demands of the systemic circulation. To create such a communication, it is possible to enlarge the foramen ovale. In the neonate this can be achieved using a catheter (a Rashkind balloon atrial septostomy) or in older children surgically using a Blalock–Hanlon septectomy. The Rashkind balloon atrial septostomy is a technique in which a catheter with a balloon on its tip is passed through the atrial septum into the left atrium, inflated and pulled firmly back through the atrial septum tearing the fossa ovales and enlarging the atrial communication. As the child ages, the septum becomes tougher and the balloon is incapable of tearing the septum without major damage to the heart.

The ability to perform a good definitive repair or correction is entirely dependent upon the quality of the previous palliative procedure. A poorly performed shunt may lead to distorted pulmonary arteries; an inadequately positioned band may lead to the development of pulmonary vascular disease. Palliative procedures have to be carried out with meticulous technique and an awareness that the child's future is at stake. The postoperative complications of the palliative procedures largely relate again to those of thoracotomy, but specific mention must be made of the risk to the phrenic nerve in all these approaches.

CORRECTIVE PROCEDURES

Corrective cardiac surgery may be divided into closed procedures not requiring cardiopulmonary bypass (CPB) and open surgery, requiring CPB.

CLOSED SURGERY

Patent ductus arteriosus

The ductus arteriosus connects the main pulmonary trunk with the aorta, usually distal to the origin of the left subclavian artery. The arterial duct normally closes at birth but can be maintained patent for some time under the influence of the drugs prostaglandin E1 and E2. In the pathological situation in which the duct remains patent without these agents, the left to right shunt which follows from the aorta to the pulmonary artery may be associated in the long term with the development of pulmonary hypertension and subsequent pulmonary vascular disease. Thus it is widely considered that a patent ductus arteriosus (PDA) should be closed.

Surgery to a PDA is usually carried out via a left thoracotomy and the ductus can be closed by ligation using a silk ligature or a liga clip. Alternatively closure may be achieved using a cardiac catheter and a double umbrella device (Porstmann *et al.*, 1971; Rashkind and Cuaso, 1979) and produces good results. The results of surgery for closure of PDA are excellent. Mortality in the older child approaches zero and for the preterm infant less than 2%. Recently, a promising thoracoscopic technique of closing the ductus arteriosus has been developed which is minimally invasive and may have a place in the future.

Coarctation of the aorta

Coarctation of the aorta is a congenital narrowing of the aorta, usually situated between the origin of the left subclavian artery proximally and the junction of the aorta and the ductus arteriosus distally. Coarctation can occur in other sites of the aorta, but this is rare. Presentation can take two forms:

1. in the neonatal period when children are admitted to hospital with the symptoms of congestive heart failure;
2. in older children coarctation rarely produces symptoms and is often first recognized during a routine examination on entry to school. There may be hypertension, absent or reduced femoral pulses and, occasionally, a murmur.

Appropriate surgical treatment depends upon age. For symptomatic neonates surgical repair is mandatory. Two principal techniques are employed:

1. resection and end-to-end anastomosis. The duct is ligated, the coarctation resected and the two ends approximated using a very fine prolene suture. In the presence of hypoplasia of the aortic arch, a more extensive procedure called the extended aortic arch angioplasty is performed. This has produced excellent results in our institution, carries a very low mortality and has a 95% freedom from reoperation at five years (Elliott, 1987; Van Heurn *et al.*, 1994).
2. the second procedure is the subclavian flap angioplasty. This operation has had good results, but is not suitable for a hypoplastic aortic arch. It has the further disadvantage of reducing forward flow into the appropriate limb and whilst ischaemia of a limb is extremely rare, it can occur.

Repair of simple coarctation with either of the methods should be achievable with an almost zero mortality at any age. However, if there is a serious intracardiac abnormality the outcome is more influenced by the severity of that lesion than the presence of a coarctation. A particularly severe form of coarctation is interruption of the aortic arch in which the upper and lower arches are completely separate, with the lower descending aorta being supplied by the arterial duct. One-stage correction of this anomaly is now the preferred treatment and this carries an operative mortality of less than 10% (Monro *et al.*, 1989).

The most worrying specific complication of coarctation repair is paraplegia. This is extremely rare, but very distressing and expensive. The estimated incidence in 1972 was 0.41% (Brewer *et al.*, 1972). It is widely accepted amongst paediatric cardiac surgeons that if the aortic cross clamp time can be kept below 30 minutes in a neonate, the chances of having paraplegia are very remote. In the older child or in the adult, it is sometimes necessary to insert some form of temporary shunt between the upper and lower parts of the body before the aortic cross clamps are applied. Other complications include abdominal pain with ileus and postoperative hypertension which may occur in up to 30% of patients (Pennington *et al.*, 1979).

It has been suggested that the long term results of coarctation repair are disappointing. One study suggested that only 20% of patients were alive without a complication 25 years after coarctation repair. However, it should be noted that these data all relate to an era in which neonatal repair was quite unusual. Late hypertension after neonatal repair seems to be rare and other complications few.

Vascular ring

Vascular ring is the term given to the anatomical state in which the trachea and oesophagus are compressed by the abnormal course of certain mediastinal vessels. There are certain patterns of lesion which cause a vascular ring:

1. a right aortic arch with a left arterial duct or ligament;
2. a double aortic arch;
3. abnormal position of the inominate artery;
4. an anomalous subclavian artery;
5. a pulmonary artery sling in which the left pulmonary artery leaves the main pulmonary artery, but crosses behind the trachea heading leftward, thus compressing it. This can result in severe tracheal compression and occasionally, complete tracheal ring abnormality known as stove pipe trachea.

Details of the surgical management of this condition are beyond the scope of this book, but in (1) and (2) it is necessary only to separate either the ductus or ligamentum arteriosum or the anterior arch in order to relieve the vascular ring. Treatment for (3) and (4) varies depending on the exact anatomy, but for (5) the management is dictated by the severity of the tracheal abnormality. If there is marked tracheal stenosis, the preferred treatment is to perform surgery on cardiopulmonary bypass to resect the stenosed trachea and effect a primary anastomosis behind the pulmonary artery bifurcation. This operation is very successful for stenoses of limited length and, in neonates, may have a place when the whole trachea is stenosed. However, in more complicated or older patients a combination of therapies up to and including an anterior tracheoplasty with the implantation of cartilage or pericardium may also be indicated. The postoperative management of these patients can be extremely difficult and specialized, requiring close co-operation between the cardiac surgeon, the ENT surgeon and the physiotherapist. Long term ventilation or intubation via a tracheostomy are often required (Murphy *et al.*, 1990).

OPEN CORRECTIVE SURGERY

Performing direct surgery on the heart requires cardiopulmonary bypass. This technique requires important modifications to practice in children. These include scale (all the equipment has to be much smaller), flow rate, perfusion temperature and the use of certain drugs.

Cardiopulmonary bypass in children may necessitate a reduction in blood flow to the left atrium, compromising oxygen delivery to the tissues. Hypothermia (less than 25°C) or deep hypothermia (less than 20°C) is used to reduce the metabolic rate and consequent oxygen demand in the body and, particularly important, in the brain. Certain operations require the use of circulatory arrest in which flow to the body is completely ceased. The safe duration of a period of circulatory arrest is unknown but recent data suggest that periods of 30 minutes are fairly safe. As the temperature of blood is reduced its viscosity rises. Accordingly it is necessary to introduce some form of haemodilution, using either an electrolyte solution or fresh frozen plasma. During rewarming from hypothermia the metabolic rate of the body rises and there may be an inadequate oxygen delivery to the rewarming tissues if the haemodilution is too severe. The oxygen requirement in a child per unit mass of tissue may be twice that of an adult. The management of cardiopulmonary bypass remains controversial, but there is consensus amongst most paediatric cardiac surgeons on the need for haemodilution and hypothermia (Elliott, 1994; Jonas and Elliott, 1994).

Atrial septal defect

Atrial septal defect (ASD) is one of the most common congenital heart defects and was among the first to be successfully treated surgically. Several methods have been developed for its closure, most recent of which is the development of devices which can be placed via a cardiac catheter. Most children with a secundum atrial septal defect are asymptomatic. However, they are often discovered at a school examination when a murmur is found or when a chest X-ray is taken demonstrating a large heart with pulmonary plethora. The natural history of atrial septal defect is progression of the symptoms with a rise in pulmonary artery pressure culminating in pulmonary hypertensive disease. Right ventricular failure can result. There are several types of atrial septal defect ranging from a patent foramen ovale through an ostium secundum ASD to the sinus venosus defects which occur close to the superior vena caval orifice. Occasionally the atrial septal defect is associated with the anomalous return of a pulmonary vein to part of the right side of the atrium or one of its attached systemic veins, for example, the SVC.

The atrial septum can be approached via a median sternotomy, a bilateral submammary incision with an ordinary median sternotomy being performed below the created skin flap to provide a more cosmetically acceptable scar in girls (Brutel de la Riviere *et al.*, 1981) or a right thoracotomy (Rosengart and Stark, 1993). Most ASDs can be closed by direct suture and it is rare to require a patch. However, if there is an anomalous pulmonary venous return then this should be deviated to the left atrium utilizing a patch to close the atrial septum anterior to the anomalous veins. The operative mortality should approach zero and the long term quality of life is excellent.

Ventricular septal defect

The ventricular septum is curved in three dimensions and has been defined as having an inlet, a trabecular and an outlet portion. This allows ventricular septal defects (VSD) to be described in relation to these three components of the septum. More than 60% of VSDs will close spontaneously and can be followed up by echocardiography as they become smaller. Large VSDs, particularly in the outlet or subarterial position, require surgery. The operation can be performed at any age, but our preference is to perform surgery when the child presents. All VSDs require cardiopulmonary bypass for closure. Most perimembranous inlet and trabecular inlets can be closed from a right atrial approach. This has the advantage of avoiding both incisions in, and traction to, the ventricle which may severely disturb the ventricular function in the immediate postoperative period. All defects are closed with a patch, the most common types of which are Gore-tex, Dacron and bovine pericardium. When suturing the patch care must be taken to avoid the bundle of Hiss and damage to the tricuspid valve.

Results for surgery to VSDs are excellent if the indications for surgery are well defined. For repair of isolated VSDs in infancy the mortality approaches zero, but for multiple VSDs, so called 'Swiss cheese' defects, the mortality may reach 8%. The risks of surgery rise with the PA pressure, which itself rises with age. Thus, it is probably preferable to operate on defects in infancy wherever possible. The conduction system is vulnerable at the time of surgery. However, as knowledge of the anatomy has improved, the incidence of this has now approached zero.

Atrioventricular septal defect

Atrioventricular septal defects (AVSD) comprise a spectrum of anomalies characterized by varying degrees of incomplete development of the inferior portion of the atrial septum, the inflow portion of the ventricular septum and the atrioventricular (AV) valves. AVSDs are conventionally described as partial, in which there is an interatrial communication, or complete in which, as well as a defect in the inferior atrial septum, there is a VSD in the inflow portion of the septum. These two extremes of partial and complete forms of AV septal defect represent two ends of a spectrum. There may be a wide variation in severity within that spectrum and there may be associated anomalies such as small ventricles to complicate the issue.

There is a strong association between AVSD and Down's syndrome, but this should not modify the therapy. The severity of symptoms and the indication for surgery depend on the size of the shunt from left to right, the severity of the regurgitation through the AV valves and the presence or absence of elevated pulmonary vascular resistance.

a) Partial AVSD

Complete open repair is the method of choice. A patch is utilized to close the AVSD, stitching the patch around the inferior rim of the atrial septum and along the crest of the ventricular septum, placing the sutures through the valve. Care must be taken around the inferior margin of the crest of the septum because it is at this position that the AV node and bundle penetrate through into the ventricle.

b) Complete AVSD

Repair of complete AVSD can be carried out using either a single or two patch technique. In the former a single patch is placed between the margins of the AVSD. In the two patch technique one patch is inserted to close the ventricular septal defect component and a second patch can then be placed to close the atrial component.

The long term survival after partial AVSD repair is now 98% and 95% after complete AVSD repair. Among the most important recent advances in the management of this condition have been the trend towards early complete repair. Severe AV valve regurgitation and poor preoperative condition are risk factors for a worse prognosis. Approximately 10–15% of patients will require further surgery to the leftsided AV valve.

Truncus arteriosus

Persistent truncus arteriosus is rare, accounting for about 3% of all congenital heart defects. In this condition there is a single arterial trunk which arises from the base of both ventricles through a single valve, under which is a high ventricular septal defect. The pulmonary arteries arise from the single truncal artery rather than from the right ventricle. The truncal valve is often abnormal and a significant proportion of the patients have Di George's syndrome which consists of either complete or partial absence of the thymus and parathyroid glands associated with T-cell deficiency and hypocalcaemia. These children frequently present in severe heart failure and the disease rapidly progresses to pulmonary vascular disease.

Primary complete repair is indicated. The pulmonary arteries must be separated from the truncal artery, the resultant defect patched and the VSD closed to divert left ventricular blood to the single truncal valve. Following this a conduit must be inserted between the right ventricle and the pulmonary artery. The mortality for primary repair varies between 11% and 17%. However, the mortality may be reduced further if the operation is performed in the first 2–3 weeks of life (Bove *et al.*, 1993; Castaneda *et al.*, 1993).

Tetralogy of Fallot

In tetralogy of Fallot there is a ventricular

septal defect above which the infundibular septum is deviated anteriorly. This produces narrowing of the right ventricular outflow tract, pulmonary valve and, sometimes, the pulmonary artery and is associated with hypertrophy of muscle bundles in the right ventricular outflow tract. Thus there is a reduction of flow of blood to the pulmonary circulation and preferential flow of blue blood to the aorta, causing cyanosis. Despite the relative frequency of this condition, there has been considerable controversy over its management. Several surgeons advocate complete repair at any age including neonatal presentation. Others adopt a more conservative approach and prefer to use a shunt between the systemic and pulmonary circulations (usually a modified Blalock–Taussig shunt) to increase the size of small pulmonary arteries, to allow repair at a later age. The basic principles inherent in the repair are a complete patch closure of the ventricular septal defect, relief of right ventricular outflow tract obstruction and relief of pulmonary arterial abnormalities.

The operative mortality for tetralogy of Fallot should be less than 3%. If the operation is postponed until after the neonatal period mortality in the order of 1% should be achievable (Castaneda and Mayer, 1994). Long term results are also good. The 15 year actuarial survival is in the order of 93% and the quality of life seems excellent.

Pulmonary atresia

Pulmonary atresia can occur with and without a ventricular septal defect. The pathophysiological consequences of the presence of a VSD are highly significant.

a) Pulmonary atresia with VSD

The presentation of this condition and the intracardiac anatomy are very similar to those of tetralogy of Fallot. However, the subpulmonary outflow tract may be either greatly hypoplastic or even absent. The pulmonary valve is always atretic and there may be absence of the supravalvular pulmonary arteries either centrally or into the branch vessels. In order for the child to survive some form of alternative blood supply to the lungs must exist. This usually takes the form of either a ductus supplying distal pulmonary arteries or major aorto-pulmonary collateral arteries (MAPCAs) which occur during part of the failure of the normal maturation of the segmental blood supply to the lung. Occasionally these MAPCAs may be unrestrictive and result in excessive pulmonary blood flow to a particular area of lung causing localized pulmonary vascular disease. In assessing children with pulmonary atresia, ventricular septal defects and MAPCAs detailed angiographic assessment of the distribution of the blood supply to all segments of the lung is mandatory. Planning therapy in these patients can be difficult and requires close co-operation between cardiologist and surgeon.

The eventual aim of treatment is to link up all the segments of the lung with a vascular supply taking origin from the right ventricle and a staged approach to the management is usually necessary. The VSD must be closed in the long term and, usually, connection of the right ventricle to the arteries to the lungs requires the insertion of a conduit between the right ventricle and neopulmonary arteries. The staging of palliative treatments may be required for the following reasons:

1. to increase the pulmonary blood flow in a child with severe cyanosis;
2. to decrease the pulmonary blood flow in a child in heart failure in whom the MAPCAs are unrestricted;
3. to prepare the distal pulmonary circulation in such a way that it can receive a conduit from the right ventricle at a later stage.

The anatomy of this condition is so variable that each child's situation must be taken on its own merit. In some cases a complete repair may be possible using similar principles to those used for tetralogy of Fallot. The only real difference is that a conduit is required between RV and PA. Each bronchopleural segment must be linked up centrally to this conduit in order that the ventricular septal defect may be closed. If there is high resistance peripherally then the ventricular septal defect may be left open or the patch perforated to reduce right ventricular workload. The results are dictated by the severity of the anatomy. In a large series reported by Kirklin *et al.* in 1988, the overall operative mortality was 15%, with only a 58% survival at 20 years. Recently more radical approaches involving multiple procedures are being proposed and the long term results of these are awaited (Sawatari *et al.*, 1989).

b) Pulmonary atresia with intact septum (and critical pulmonary stenosis)

The presentation and management of this anatomical subset of anomalies depend on the size of the right ventricle and tricuspid valve. These can be judged fairly accurately by echocardiography, but despite this, there remains considerable controversy about the appropriate management. If the right ventricle is considered to be salvable in any way then the preferred option would be a pulmonary valvotomy (if the ventricle was large and the pulmonary valve adequate) or a transannular patch together with a small modified Blalock–Taussig shunt (if the right ventricle is smaller). This can be performed in one stage via a median sternotomy. It is anticipated that the ventricle will grow as the flow through it increases and that the only treatment required in due course will be closure of the ASD and division of the shunt.

If the right ventricle is considered too small to be salvable at primary operation, then a shunt should be performed and a long term plan to perform a Fontan or total cavopulmonary connection operation (see p.133) adopted (de Leval *et al.*, 1988).

This remains a particularly disappointing subset of patients. The overall survival rate of 147 patients operated on at Great Ormond Street between 1970 and 1992 was 41%. The impact of the newer approaches (particularly transannular patching and shunting) on long term results has yet to be determined.

Transposition of the great vessels

In transposition of the great arteries (TGA) the aorta arises from the right ventricle and the pulmonary artery from the left ventricle. Children therefore present in the first day of life with severe cyanosis, unless there is either a large interatrial communication, a VSD or a persistent patent ductus arteriosus. Without such a connection survival is impossible. Thus the primary therapy of these children is aimed at maintaining some communication between the systemic and pulmonay circuits. Initially this can be in the form of prostaglandin, which keeps the arterial duct patent, allowing for safe transfer of the child to a specialist institution where the second line of management, a balloon atrial septostomy, can be performed. Thereafter, the management of transposition will depend on the associated defects if present.

The management of simple transposition, or of transposition with only VSD, is the arterial switch procedure (anatomic repair of transposition of great arteries). It is performed in the first 2–3 weeks of life, although some workers are extending the deadline until 4–8 weeks. The reason for the surgery having to be done so early after birth is that, during this time, the pulmonary vascular resistance is high and thus the left ventricle is pumping into a high resistance circuit. Accordingly, if the switch is performed during this time then the left ventricle is trained, ready to receive the systemic workload. The operation consists of transection of the aorta and pulmonary arteries and their transfer to the opposite base vessel. The transection takes place above the level of the coronary arteries which themselves must be transferred. The most successful method of performing the arterial switch is to use a trapdoor type incision into the old pulmonary artery/new aorta to receive the coronary arteries, thus reducing their rotation to a minimum (Mee, 1994). The distal pulmonary arteries can then be mobilized and the duct divided to allow the former anteriorly placed aorta to be repositioned below the bifurcation of the pulmonary artery.

Prior to the successful evolution of the arterial switch procedure during the last decade, the most common form of treatment was an atrial switch in which the inflow to the ventricles was reversed. Two operations were utilized for this physiological manipulation. One was the Mustard operation, in which a patch was manufactured to divert the SVC and IVC blood to the mitral valve, allowing the red pulmonary venous blood to pass over the roof of the tunnel and down into the tricuspid valve. An alternative approach was the Senning operation, in which the child's own atrial wall is utilized to create this tunnel. This allows for the blood flow to be redirected without the use of synthetic material and reduces the risk of subsequent obstruction to the pathways.

The operative mortality for both the Senning and the switch should be less than 2%. It is in the long term results that the difference between the two procedures is most relevant. In the arterial switch the left ventricle supplies the systemic circulation, whereas after the Senning, it is the right ventricle that supplies the systemic circulation. It is well established that the Senning-type repair is associated with gradual right ventricle failure. It is thought that all the right ventricles of patients with Senning procedures will gradually fail and either they must be converted to an arterial switch or else a transplant undertaken in later life. The long term results of the arterial switch procedure, however, have been very encouraging indeed, with excellent ventricular function, no loss of sinus rhythm and good preservation of right ventricular performance. However, more time is required to give a clearer picture of the long term future.

TGA with VSD

This group is also managed by the arterial switch procedure with simultaneous closure of the ventricular septal defect. There is no increased risk associated with the operation and the mortality should now approach zero.

TGA, VSD and left ventricular outflow tract obstruction

Patients with this condition are usually cyanosed due to inadequate pulmonary blood flow. The obstruction is usually subvalvular. For many years the treatment has been palliative in the form of a shunt, followed by the Rastelli procedure in which the VSD is closed such that the left ventricular blood passes to the aorta and a conduit is placed between the right ventricle and pulmonary artery. Mortality should be in the order of 10–20%, but there is the risk, as with all extracardiac conduits, that the conduit may obstruct in later life and require replacement.

Total anomalous pulmonary venous connection

Total anomalous pulmonary venous connection (TAPVC) is a rare congenital heart defect accounting for 1.5% of congenital heart defects. Again, it covers a spectrum of disorders:

1. supracardiac – the pulmonary venous drainage is via a vertical vein to an innominate vein and thence to the right atrium.
2. cardiac – there is direct connection of the pulmonary veins to either the right atrium or the coronary sinus.
3. infracardiac – the pulmonary veins drain into a descending vein which passes below the diaphragm to a portal vein or inferior vena cava, before passing to the right atrium through the normal IVC pathway.
4. mixed – any of these variants may be combined.

Children with this anomaly usually present in early infancy unless the pulmonary venous drainage is completely unobstructive. Once diagnosed, treatment is surgical. For supra and infracardiac lesions repair requires cardiopulmonary bypass with deep hypothermia and circulatory arrest. The pulmonary venous confluence and the back of the left atrium are anastomosed. These anastomoses seem to grow normally without obstruction in the vast majority of patients. The principle of correcting the cardiac defects is to maintain an atrial septal defect large enough to permit adequate pulmonary flow. During the last five years the overall mortality at Great Ormond Street in 44 patients operated on with TAPVC has been 11%. Patients who are severely ill preoperatively are at risk of pulmonary hypertensive crises in the postoperative period.

Abnormalities of the cardiac valves

a) Aortic and pulmonary valve

Critical aortic and pulmonary stenosis in the neonatal period require urgent treatment. Critical pulmonary stenosis can be managed along similar lines to pulmonary atresia (with intact septum), but the management of critical aortic stenosis remains controversial. Results of all forms of surgery have been disappointing with a mortality of approximately 10%. The options available are:

1. open aortic valvotomy on cardiopulmonary bypass;
2. closed aortic valvotomy on inflow occlusion, in which the vena cava are temporarily occluded whilst the aorta is cross clamped and the aorta opened under direct vision without cardiopulmonary bypass;
3. transventricular blunt Hagar dilatation of the aortic valve.

b) Mitral valve

Congenital anomalies of the mitral valve may present as either stenotic or incompetent lesions. They are usually associated with other intracardiac anomalies and, although the basic principle of 'repair is better than replacement' applies, sometimes in the neonate our ability to perform a repair is very limited and replacement remains the only option. If the valve is replaced in the early months of life then the mortality remains high, in the order of 20%.

c) Tricuspid valve

The most important condition presenting with a tricuspid valve is Epstein's anomaly. This occurs in only 0.5% of patients with congenital heart disease and again covers a wide spectrum of anatomical variants. Characteristically, however, the tricuspid valve is displaced downwards into the right ventricle, leaving a dysplastic and obstructive valve with very little functional right ventricle beyond.

Patients can present in severe heart failure, with cyanosis or, quite commonly, with dysrhythmia. Surgery in the neonatal period or early infancy carries an extremely high risk and palliative approach, leading to a Fontan operation, may be preferable. However, in the older child, either an annuloplasty or a more complicated repair of the Epstein's anomaly can be achieved and if all these fail, tricuspid valve replacement should be undertaken. In conjunction with a wide spectrum of anatomy, there is a wide spectrum of results in literature, ranging from 5% to 60%. Early age is thought to be a risk factor.

Tricuspid atresia and right heart bypass operations

a) Tricuspid atresia

This condition accounts for 2% of congenital heart disease. There is absence of rightsided atrioventricular connection and thus a shunt at atrial level with blue blood flowing to the left. There may or may not be associated pulmonary stenosis and the presence or absence of this stenosis will dictate whether this child will present with cyanosis or in heart failure because of excess pulmonary blood flow. The ultimate treatment will be to bypass the right side of the heart altogether and thus any operation performed must be designed to restrict distortion of the pulmonary arteries and to maintain a low pulmonary vascular resistance. The child presenting with cyanosis should have a modified Blalock–Taussig shunt performed in the first instance and the child presenting in heart failure should have a pulmonary artery band performed as soon as possible.

b) Right heart bypass operation

When the right side of the heart is hypoplastic or atretic, then some means must be found to deliver deoxygenated blood to the lungs. A number of operations have been designed under the loose generic term of the Fontan operation. The original Fontan operation was described to treat tricuspid atresia and involved the insertion of a conduit between the right atrium and the right ventricle jumping across the atretic valve. Various modifications have subsequently been created, allowing direct connection of the right atrium to the pulmonary artery. The most recent and most successful modification of these procedures has been the total cavopulmonary connection (TCPC) (de Leval *et al.*, 1988). The operation can be performed either in one or two stages, the first stage of which is a procedure called the bidirectional Glenn shunt in which the superior vena cava is transected at a separate operation and anastomosed to the superior surface of the pulmonary artery.

Recently a considerable improvement in the quality of results of the TCPC has been obtained by leaving a small hole in the Goretex tube which is used to divert the IVC blood to the SVC blood (Mayer *et al.*, 1992). The presence of the small hole will allow some blood to be shunted across the atrial septum to provide the left ventricle with some blood to eject. As the situation improves, gradually more flow will pass forward through the lungs restricting the flow through the ASD. In our experience of 152 Fontan-type opertions, 88 had total cavopulmonary connection with an 8% mortality and 64 had atriopulmonary connection with a 22% mortality. Our most recent results, however, demonstrate that a total cavopulmonary anastomosis can be performed in appropriately selected patients with a risk of less than 5%.

Hypoplastic left heart syndrome

Another condition in which the Fontan-type operation may be required in later life is the hypoplastic left heart syndrome. This is currently rarely seen by surgeons in the United Kingdom since cardiologists attending women both prenatally and postnatally usually advise against surgical intervention. However, the current results for surgery in the United States suggest 95% survival of a first stage operation (a Norwood procedure) and perhaps as much as a 70% survival of a second stage Fontan procedure (Norwood and Jacobs, 1994).

CARDIAC TRANSPLANTATION

The indications for transplantation in childhood are similar to those in adults – namely terminal failure of the affected organ. We have undertaken heart and heart/lung transplantation in our unit since 1988 for both congenital and acquired cardiac disease, the acquired disease being largely cardiomyopathy. The results are similar to those seen in adults, with a 65% five year survival and good quality of life. However, after heart/lung transplantation the five year survival is in the order of 45% and only 13% of patients are free of the dreadful complication of obliterative bronchiolitis at five years. Heart/lung transplantation thus is restricted to those with severe cystic fibrosis or congenital heart disease with terminal pulmonary hypertension .

The donor supply which makes these organs possible is becoming progressively limited as, fortunately, safety in cars and in the home is receiving more publicity. If the strategy of transplantation is to be developed further, work has to be carried out with long term preservation of organs, the use of cadaver organs or the development of xenograft transplantation from non-alike species.

POSTOPERATIVE MANAGEMENT

The postoperative care of children after surgery for congenital heart disease must be carried out in a specialized unit, usually in intensive care. Most children require ventilation to reduce the cardiac workload and careful cardiovascular monitoring is vital. Respiratory care is required after all operations for congenital heart defects because the lungs are undoubtedly affected by that surgery and by the underlying condition. After simple open or closed operations there may only be a need for an increased inspired oxygen, together with humidification of that inspired oxygen and regular physiotherapy. However, the majority of patients after open procedures require mechanical ventilation and careful attention to respiratory care during their management. Chest physiotherapy is crucial to the treatment of patients with congenital heart defects, both before and after surgery. A variety of techniques are employed and these are covered elsewhere but the importance of physiotherapy is mentioned to confirm the role which we feel it has in the management of children with heart disease.

PULMONARY HYPERTENSIVE CRISES

In pulmonary hypertensive crises there is acute elevation of the PA pressure as pulmonary arteriolar musculature contracts. This restricts the flow of blood through the lungs, is associated with a fall in left atrial pressure and a dramatic fall in cardiac output with a fall in systemic blood pressure. A variety of stimuli for the development of this condition have been described, but underlying all of them is the presence of hypertrophic reactive arteriolar muscle in the lungs. Thus it is particularly common in those patients who have had significant left to right shunts (VSD, AVSD and truncus arteriosus) and prevention is the key to its management. Early surgery seems to reduce the risk of pulmonary hypertensive crises.

A number of stimuli have been said to trigger the acute constriction of the pulmonary arterioles and amongst those is physiotherapy. Perhaps the reason for this is that there may be a fall in oxygen saturation during physiotherapy and hypoxia is a known and potent stimulus for pulmonary arteriolar vasoconstriction. The management of a pulmonary hypertensive crisis is thus by provision of an FiO_2 of 1.0, usually administered by handbagging; hyperventilation to reduce the $PaCO_2$, since an elevated $PaCO_2$ may also precipitate pulmonary arteriolar vasoconstriction; acidosis should be reversed and excessive pulmonary vasoconstricting drugs (adrenaline, etc.) should be restricted to minimum dosage. In the resistant case, prostacycline or glycerine trinitrate infusions are useful, but more recently we have adopted a policy of utilizing nitric oxide by inhalation in cases when pulmonary arterial pressure begins to rise. Nitric oxide can be given through the ventilator and, in a dose of 5–10 parts/million, is relatively safe. Nitric oxide is rapidly deactivated on contact with haemoglobin and thus the action of the agent is almost confined to the lung, making it unique as an almost specific pulmonary vasodilator when given through the ventilator.

PHYSIOTHERAPY FOLLOWING PAEDIATRIC CARDIC SURGERY

ASSESSMENT

Chest physiotherapy is frequently required for the child post cardiac surgery. Open heart surgery induces changes in pulmonary function many of which are seen after any general anaesthetic. In addition, the lungs may be compressed intraoperatively leading to atelectasis and the incision and chest drains cause pain and splinting of the chest wall, which in self-ventilating patients results in shallow breathing and a decrease in chest wall compliance (Schleien *et al.*, 1992). Immobility and the use of muscle relaxants, which prevent sighs and cause a fall in FRC, add to the above problems and the end result is a reduction in secretion clearance, leading to atelectasis and loss of lung volume. This is particularly seen in children because of their small terminal airways and lack of collateral ventilation. Prolonged ventilation is often necessary postoperatively especially in those of younger age who have undergone lengthy cardiopulmonary bypass times, a long aortic cross clamp time or who suffer adverse postoperative haemodynamics (Kanter *et al.*, 1986). Weaning of ventilation should only be commenced after the patient's inotropic requirement has decreased.

Both assisted and controlled ventilation have disadvantages particularly in the very young patient. They may increase PA pressures, impede venous return and decrease cardiac output. If pulmonary hypertension exists, satisfactory ventilation and oxygenation are especially important as high pulmonary artery pressures may exacerbate hypoxaemia (Tahran *et al.*, 1977). Patients with pulmonary arterial hypertension and pulmonary vascular disease represent high surgical risks and require special postoperative management. Because of the marked degree of pulmonary arterial smooth muscle hypertrophy present there is danger of pulmonary arteriospasm with a sudden decrease in cardiac output rapidly leading to cardiac arrest. Patients with pulmonary vascular disease are extremely sensitive to hypoxia, hypercarbia and acidosis. Haemodynamic stability is imperative for a successful outcome post cardiac surgery.

Continuous close observation is essential throughout the postoperative course. Prior to chest physiotherapy a complete assessment of the haemodynamic state of the patient is required (Table 8.1). Cardiac output is dependent on heart rate and stroke volume. Heart rate is a particularly important determinant of cardiac output in infants whose ventricles are less compliant and therefore less responsive to changes in filling pressures. Bradycardia in infants and children can severely compromise cardiac output. Continuous pulse oximetry is particularly helpful in patients with reactive

Table 8.1 Haemodynamic status assessment prior to physiotherapy

Heart rate and rhythm
Oxygen saturation
Urine output
Temperature
core
peripheral
Blood pressure
Central venous pressure (CVP)
Pulmonary artery pressure (PAP)
Left atrial pressure (LAP)
Chest drainage

pulmonary hypertension where a small decrease in saturation may be the first sign of increased pulmonary artery pressure and right to left shunting.

The hourly rate of urine output should be noted as this is an excellent indicator of renal perfusion. The urine output should exceed 0.5 ml/kg/hr. Central and peripheral temperatures are closely monitored in the postoperative period. Central temperature is usually measured rectally and peripheral temperature is measured on the skin of the big toe. A difference between core and peripheral temperature of more than 2°C is associated with a compromised cardiac output (Schleien *et al.*, 1992). Poor peripheral perfusion postoperatively may impede the accurate measurement of cuff blood pressure. Intra-arterial blood pressure monitoring is essential to observe minute to minute medication adjustments. The presence of an arterial catheter also allows frequent blood gas measurements. The central venous pressure (CVP) reflects the rightsided filling pressures and is of great benefit in postoperative management. By infusing volume and observing the CVP along with blood pressure and heart rate the optimal filling pressures can be determined.

Pulmonary artery pressure monitoring can be measured via a catheter placed through the wall of the right atrium into the pulmonary artery during surgery. This allows measurement of pulmonary vascular resistance and can therefore guide the management of pulmonary hypertension. Pulmonary capillary wedge pressure can be determined by occlusion of pulmonary blood flow providing information on left atrial filling pressure.

Mediastinal and pleural chest tubes are routinely used for thoracic drainage following cardiac surgery. Chest tube drainage needs to be monitored very closely in the early postoperative period. Blood loss greater than 10 ml/kg/hr or bright red drainage usually warrants a return to the operating theatre for exploration and control of bleeding. Generally tubes can be removed when the drainage is less than 3 ml/kg/day. Fresh blood in the drains at any time should prompt a thorough investigation of possible causes. Physiotherapy should not be performed in the presence of uncontrolled bleeding as the patient may rapidly become hypovolaemic.

CHEST PHYSIOTHERAPY TECHNIQUES

The indications for chest physiotherapy have been discussed in Chapter 5, p.56. Where possible the child should be assessed preoperatively with regard to both respiratory and developmental status. Preoperative physiotherapy involves giving both the child and parents an outline of the planned procedure, an explanation of physiotherapy and the reasons why it is necessary postoperatively. An understanding of the need for postoperative chest physiotherapy will hopefully enhance patient co-operation.

To prevent the separation distress that may be experienced by the child when admitted to hospital adequate preparation and facilities for one or both parents to be with the child should be ensured. Preoperative chest clearance may be indicated. In the older child breathing exercises, huffing and supported coughing may be taught. A preoperative visit will help establish a relationship that will be built on in the postoperative period.

All patients should be assessed with regard to respiratory status postoperatively and haemodynamic stability ensured prior to treatment. Pain may be a cause of respiratory difficulty and relief from it may greatly assist clearance of retained secretions. Chest movement can also be restricted by pain, leading to a reduction in FRC. Postoperatively deep breathing, coughing and manual techniques may increase the pain experienced by the patient. Generally morphine given by continuous infusion is the analgesic and method of delivery of choice. In the older child patient controlled analgesic systems can be used. In the patient who is not on continuous infusions of analgesia pain relief should be given when required. This should occur prior to chest physiotherapy with sufficient time allowed for the analgesic effect to occur.

Positioning and postural drainage

Children immediately post cardiac surgery are usually nursed in the supine position. As soon as the child is relatively stable it may be feasible to quarter turn the child to side lying. Extreme care must be taken not to kink or disrupt lines, wires or infusions. When turning the head care must be taken to ensure that neck lines do not become occluded as the delivery of inotropic drugs may be temporarily ceased. The prone position is not usually possible in the early postoperative period due to the presence of mediastinal drains. The head down position is generally contraindicated until the patient is haemodynamically stable as in this position myocardial oxygen demand is greater. Hussey (1991) demonstrated a greater fall in oxygen saturation in patients who were turned as part of treatment. It may therefore be advisable to treat the child in situ, or to turn, wait and treat after 20–30 minutes.

Percussion and vibrations

Percussion and vibrations may be carried out postoperatively to aid mucociliary clearance. In cases where the child is bleeding excessively manual techniques should be avoided as they may increase bleeding. Care must be taken to avoid performing manual techniques too close to incision and drain sites.

Manual hyperinflation

Manual hyperinflation may be indicated post cardiac surgery if the child has secretion retention and/or areas of collapse. Hussey *et al*. (1992) demonstrated a negligible mean maximum fall in oxygen saturation when chest physiotherapy post cardiac surgery involved manual hyperinflation, vibrations and suction. Care must be taken in the child with a borderline blood pressure as positive intrathoracic pressure may decrease venous return, leading to a fall in stroke volume and therefore cardiac output. Excessive positive pressure may also decrease pulmonary blood flow and therefore should be avoided in children with conditions causing a low pulmonary blood flow (e.g. tetralogy of Fallot or pulmonary atresia).

SPECIFIC PROBLEMS PRESENTING POST PAEDIATRIC CARDIAC SURGERY

Pulmonary hypertension

Suctioning, handling and physiotherapy may precipitate a pulmonary hypertensive crisis. A child presenting with respiratory signs will require chest physiotherapy as secretion retention may cause a fall in PaO_2 which may in turn cause a crisis. Chest physiotherapy in these patients must not be associated with a fall in oxygenation. Treatment should always involve additional oxygen either by manual hyperinflation/ hyperventilation or by increasing the inspired oxygen. It should be kept as short as possible and preferably without a change in position. The child should be fully sedated and chest physiotherapy must not be performed after other potentially destabilizing manoeuvres but after the child has been stable for a period of at least 30 minutes. The physiotherapist must continually observe the blood pressure, pulmonary artery pressure and oxygen saturation so that any changes can guide treatment.

Delayed sternal closure

The technique of delayed sternal closure has facilitated the management of the immediate postoperative period in neonates and infants in whom there is resultant pulmonary, myocardial and chest wall oedema due to prolonged cardiopulmonary bypass times because of particularly complicated intracardiac repairs (Odim *et al.*, 1989). Closing the sternum can cause a constrictive effect on cardiopulmonary function and can lead to life threatening respiratory or haemodynamic complications. These patients can present the physiotherapist with problems as the child is preferentially nursed in the supine position often for prolonged periods of time. Physiotherapy for patients with unsplinted sternums may involve gentle manual hyperinflation with vibrations applied to the posterior chest wall with the patient in supine. If the patient is haemodynamically stable physiotherapy may involve a quarter turn towards side lying. If the child's sternum is splinted, by a surgical stent or chest drain pieces sutured between the sternal edges, side lying and manual techniques may be performed. Vigorous treatment must be avoided, as should the prone position.

Phrenic nerve damage

Phrenic nerve damage is well recognized post paediatric cardiac surgery and is associated with morbidity and mortality (Wantabe *et al.*, 1987; Ross-Russell *et al.*, 1991). It occurs most frequently after operations requiring dissection close to the phrenic nerve or following secondary procedures in which the phrenic nerve can be obscured by fibrous adhesions (Mickwell *et al.*, 1978). Much of the increased morbidity is associated with the complications of prolonged ventilation. Phrenic nerve damage results in the diaphragm on the affected side being elevated and moving upwards on inspiration. This will compress particularly the lower lobes, there will be loss of lung volume and persistent collapse may become a problem. These patients often require frequent physiotherapy to help remove retained secretions. However, the problem will recur until the underlying problem is treated. Positioning the child in sitting will increase vital capacity and is advised for periods of time.

The management of unilateral phrenic nerve palsy (PNP) is influenced by the age of the patient. Older children often require little more than attention to postoperative atelectasis as significant respiratory distress is not usual because the accessory muscles of respiration can compensate for the loss of diaphragmatic function. In infants with PNP weak intercostal musculature, horizontal lie of the ribs, a mobile mediastinum and the fact that the infant is usually recumbent can all result in the need for prolonged mechanical ventilation. In these patients diaphragmatic plication is of most value (Wantabe *et al.*, 1987).

HEART/LUNG TRANSPLANTATION

Physiotherapy is an integral part of the pre- and postoperative management of children undergoing heart/lung transplantation. Initial assessment and preparation usually take 4–5 days at the hospital to which the child is referred and comprises a multidisciplinary team approach. The physiotherapist at this stage needs to assess the patient's respiratory status and exercise tolerance, build up a relationship with the child and family and explain the postoperative regime. Children undergoing heart/lung transplantation are prone to respiratory problems in the early postoperative period. As well as the problems of anaesthesia, immobility and pain the child post heart/lung transplantation has additional complications. There is loss of sensation below the level of the tracheal anastomosis which causes loss of the normal cough reflex below that level. There is loss of cilia around the tracheal anastomosis which may lead to secretion retention. The lymphatic drainage is interrupted in the implanted lungs and the child is fluid restricted in order to prevent pulmonary oedema, but this may result in thick bronchial secretions. In children with cystic fibrosis (CF) the upper airways may still be infected with secretions which may drip down to the larger airways particularly until the child is up and moving about (Andrews, 1993).

Preoperatively these problems must be explained to the child and family so that they understand the need for postoperative treatment. Children with CF will have been having regular physiotherapy all their life and therefore need little introduction to methods of airway clearance. The methods may differ, but many will be doing the ACBT. Their technique should be assessed and revised as necessary. Communication with the local physiotherapy team is important to inform them of decisions made during the assessment period and to enable them to reinforce any advice regarding treatment and regularly review the patient's airway clearance technique. The reason the ACBT is so important is that postoperatively the child will find it extremely difficult to cough as the normal reflex stimulated by the presence of secretions is absent. To clear secretions effectively the patient must be able to huff. This cannot be easily taught postoperatively due to pain, drowsiness, etc. If unfamiliar with airway clearance techniques such as the ACBT, the child and family should be taught them during the assessment period. Liaison with the local therapist can again permit reinforcement of the teaching and regular review of technique.

If there are indications for treatment prior to extubation then care must be taken when:

1. performing airway suction, as the tip of the endotracheal tube lies above the level of the tracheal anastomosis and the anastomotic site is easily traumatized by suction procedures;
2. using manual hyperinflation, as the patient is prone to pneumothoraces in the donor lungs. The therapist should ensure that the pleural drains are functioning correctly (Andrews, 1993).

Once extubated and off inotropic support mobilization is encouraged and exercise is gradually increased. It may take considerable time before the child has a reasonable exercise tolerance as many of these children will have been doing extremely little or no exercise for some months/years prior to transplant. At this stage the physiotherapist must encourage exercise as much as possible and in many forms to allow the child to return to as normal a lifestyle as possible. The ultimate aim for the physiotherapist is to provide the individual with the opportunity to maximize the benefits of the operation and enable the patient to achieve a good level of rehabilitation and a better quality of life.

CONCLUSION

Surgery for congenital heart disease has progressed rapily over the last 30 years and the mortality for most conditions now approaches zero. It is the awareness of all aspects of cardiorespiratory physiology and the integrated nature of the team approach to care which has resulted in this progressive improvement. Respiratory management is fundamental to success and an understanding of the underlying procedures, anatomy and pathophysiology is critical.

REFERENCES

Anderson, R.H. and Becker, A.E. (1994) Surgical anatomy, in *Surgery for Congenital Heart Defects*, 2nd edn, (eds J. Stark and M. de Leval), W.B. Saunders, Philadelphia, pp. 13–36.

Andrews, M. (1993) Respiratory management of children following heart-lung transplantation. *Association of Chartered Physiotherapists in Respiratory Care Journal*, **22**, 12–13.

Bove, E., Lupenetti, F., Fridjian, A. *et al.* (1993) Results of a protocol of early repair for truncus arteriosus. *Journal of Thoracic and Cardiovascular Surgery*, **105**, 1057.

Brewer, L.A., Fosburg, R.G., Mulder, G.A. and Verska, J.J. (1972) Spinal cord complications following surgery for coarctation of the aorta. A study of 66 cases. *Journal of Thoracic and Cardiovascular Surgery*, **64**, 368.

Brutel de la Riviere, A., Brom, G.H.M. and Brom, A.G. (1981) Horizontal submammary skin incision for medium stenotomy. *Annals of Thoracic Surgery*, **32**, 101.

Castaneda, A., Hanley, F., Mayer, J. and Jonas, R. (1993) Repair of truncus arteriosus in the neonate. *Journal of Thoracic and Cardiovascular Surgery*, **105**, 1047.

Castaneda, A.R. and Mayer, J. (1994) Tetralogy of Fallot, in *Surgery for Congenital Heart Defects*, 2nd edn, (eds J. Stark and M. de Leval), W.B. Saunders, Philadelphia, pp. 405–16.

De Leval, M., Kilner, P., Gewillig, M. and Bull, C. (1988) Total cavo-pulmonary connection: a logical alternative to atrio-pulmonary connection for complex Fontan operations. *Journal of Thoracic and Cardiovascular Surgery*, **96**, 682.

Elliott, M.J. (1987) Coarctation of the aorta with arch hypoplasia: improvements on a new technique. *Annals of Thoracic Surgery*, **44**, 321.

Elliott, M.J. (1994) Perfusion techniques, in *Surgery for Congenital Heart Defects*, 2nd edn, (eds J. Stark and M. de Leval), W.B. Saunders, Philadelphia, pp. 155–74.

Franklin, R.C.G., Spiegelhalter, D.G.A., Macartney, F.J. and Bull, K. (1991) Evaluation of a diagnostic algorithm for heart disease in neonates. *British Medical Journal*, **302**, 935.

Hussey, J. (1991) The relationship between specific chest physiotherapy techniques and oxygen saturation in children post cardiac surgery. MSc Thesis, University of London.

Hussey, J., Hayward, L. and Andrews, M. (1992) The effect of chest physiotherapy techniques on oxygen saturation in children post cardiac surgery. *Care of the Critically Ill*, **8**, 35.

Jonas, R.A. and Elliott, M. (eds) (1994) *Cardiopulmonary Bypass for Neonates, Infants and Children*, Heinemann, London.

Kanter, R.K., Bove, E.L., Tobin, J.R. *et al.* (1986) Prolonged mechanical ventilation of infants after open heart surgery. *Critical Care Medicine*, **14**, 211–14.

Kirklin, J.W., Blackstone, E.H., Shimazaki, Y. *et al.* (1988) Survival, functional status and reoperations after repair of tetralogy of Fallot with pulmonary atresia. *Journal of Thoracic and Cardiovascular Surgery*, **96**, 102.

Mayer, J.E.J.R., Bridges, N.D., Lock, L.E. *et al.* (1992) Factors associated with marked reduction in mortality for Fontan operations in patients with single ventricle. *Journal of Thoracic and Cardiovascular Surgery*, **103**, 444.

Mee, R. (1994) The arterial switch operation in *Surgery for Congenital Heart Defects*, 2nd edn, (eds J. Stark and M. de Leval), W.B. Saunders, Philadelphia, pp. 483–500.

Mickwell, J.J., Oh, K.S., Siewers, R.D. *et al.* (1978) Clinical implications of post operative unilateral phrenic nerve paralysis. *Journal of Thoracic and Cardiovascular Surgery*, **76**, 297–304.

Monro, J.L., Bunton, R.W., Sutherland, G.G. and Keaton, B.R. (1989) Correction of interrupted aortic arch. *Journal of Thoracic and Cardiovascular Surgery*, **98**, 421.

Murphy, R., Lloyd-Thomas, A. and Elliott, M. (1990) Management of congenital tracheal stenosis in infants. *British Journal of Hospital Medicine*, **44**, 266.

Norwood, W.I. and Jacobs, M.L. (1994) Hypoplastic left heart syndrome, in *Surgery for Congenital Heart Defects*, 2nd edn, (eds J. Stark and M. de Leval), W.B. Saunders, Philadelphia, pp. 587–98.

Odim, J.N.K., Tchervenkov, C.I. and Pobell, R.C. (1989) Delayed sternal closure: a life saving manoeuvre after early operation for complex congenital heart disease in the neonate. *Journal of Thoracic and Cardiovascular Surgery*, **98**, 413–16.

Pennington, D.G., Liberthson, R.R., Jacobs, M. *et al.* (1979) Critical review of experience with surgical repair of coarctation of the aorta. *Journal of Thoracic and Cardiovascular Surgery*, **77**, 219.

Porstmann, W., Wierny, L., Warnke, H. *et al.* (1971) Catheter closure of patent ductus arteriosus. 62 cases treated without thoracotomy. *Radiological Clinics of North America*, **9**, 203.

Rashkind, R.J. and Cuaso, C.C. (1979) Transcatheter closure of patent ductus arteriosus: successful use in 3.5 kilogram infant. *Pediatric Cardiology*, **1**, 3.

Rosengart, T.K. and Stark, J. (1993) Repair of atrial septal defect through a right thoracotomy. *Annals of Thoracic Surgery*, **55**, 1138.

Ross-Russell, R.I., Mulvey, D., Laroche, C. *et al.* (1991) Bedside assessment of phrenic nerve function in infants and children. *Journal of Thoracic and Cardiovascular Surgery*, **101**, 143–7.

Sawatari, K., Imai, Y., Kurosawa, H. *et al.* (1989) Staged operation for pulmonary atresia and ventricular septal defect with major aortopulmonary collateral arteries. *Journal of Thoracic and Cardiovascular Surgery*, **98**, 738.

Schleien, C.L., Setzer, M.A., McLaughlin, G.E. *et al.* (1992) Post operative management of the cardiac surgical patient, in *Textbook of Pediatric Intensive Care*, Vol 1, 2nd edn, (ed. M. Rogers), Williams and Wilkins, Baltimore, pp. 467–523.

Tahran, S., White, R.D. and Moffit, E.A. (1977) Anaesthesia and post operative care for cardiac operations. *Annals of Thoracic Surgery*, **23**, 173–93.

Van Heurn, L.W.E., Wong, C.M., Spiegelhalter, D.J. *et al.* (1994) Surgical treatment of aortic coarctation in infants aged < 3 months; 1985–1990; the extended end-to-end arch aortoplasties are successful in almost all arch morphologies. *Journal of Thoracic and Cardiovascular Surgery*, (in press).

Wantabe, T., Trusler, G.A., Williams, W.G. *et al.* (1987) Phrenic nerve paralysis after pediatric cardiac surgery. *Journal of Thoracic and Cardiovascular Surgery*, **94**, 383–8.

NEUROLOGICAL INTENSIVE CARE 9

Robert C. Tasker and S. Ammani Prasad

INTRODUCTION

Appropriate management of the child with primarily an acute neurological insult requires a working knowledge of the underlying basic pathophysiology. For the purpose of this chapter, head injury will be used to illustrate many of these points, with particular emphasis on their implications in chest management.

BRAIN INJURY AND HEAD TRAUMA

In the acutely brain injured child, the term 'primary brain injury' refers to the damage sustained at the time of trauma and consists of three components of varying severity: bleeding, contusion and neuronal shearing. Bleeding may be into the brain (e.g. intracerebral, intraventricular) or on the surface of the brain (e.g. extradural, subdural, subarachnoid). Severe contusion causes focal cerebral cortical damage, but does not result in an altered level of consciousness. Shearing of nerve cell fibres from their bodies in the deeper and more superficial parts of the brain results in 'concussion' and potentially permanent neurological deficits. After the period of the acute insult, secondary (or subsequent) brain injury results from complicating events or processes, which can be attributed to intracranial or systemic factors (Table 9.1).

Table 9.1 Events and processes leading to 'secondary' brain injury

Intracranial	*Systemic*
Bleeding	Hypoxia
Brain swelling	Hypercarbia
Seizures	Hypotension
Infection	Hypertension
Raised ICP	Hyper- or hyponatraemia
	Hyper- or hypoglycaemia
	Fever

HAEMORRHAGE AND BRAIN SWELLING

Even after the seemingly most trivial of head injuries, continued intracranial bleeding into the extradural compartment may result in a deteriorating level of consciousness and death from cerebral compression. Generally, most children with an acute extradural or subdural clot develop symptoms and signs of cerebral decompensation within 12 hours of the initial injury. In hospital these patients can be monitored with a modification of the Glasgow Coma Scale (Teasdale and Jennett, 1974; Reilly *et al.*, 1988) (Table 9.2) which assigns scores for clinical findings that develop in the course of progressive deterioration. When of clinical significance, such haemorrhages are treated surgically.

Brain swelling may either be focal or generalized and is due to an intracellular accumulation of water (cytotoxic oedema). Focal swelling occurs in areas of contusion and may appear or increase over a period of 2–5 days. Generalized swelling with a resultant increase

Table 9.2 Paediatric Glasgow coma scale

Activity	*Best response*	*Score*
Eye opening	Spontaneous	4
	To speech	3
	To pain	2
	None	1
Verbal (words) orientated		5
	Words	3
	Vocal sounds	3
	Cries	2
	None	1
Motor	Obeying	5
	Localizing	4
	Flexing to pain	3
	Extending	2
	None	1

The normal aggregate score for children is: birth to six months, 9; six months to one year, 11; one year to two years, 12; two years to five years, 13; older than five years, 14.

in intracranial pressure (ICP) can cause a more rapid and progressive deterioration, for which a variety of medical measures are often used to limit this process (see below).

MANAGEMENT OF RAISED INTRACRANIAL PRESSURE

Increased ICP represents an increase in the volume of the intracranial contents due to a focal or diffuse cerebral process (e.g. focal haemorrhage and contusion, generalized swelling) and in the normal state should be below 15 mmHg. Cerebral perfusion pressure (CPP) is defined as the difference between mean arterial blood pressure and mean ICP and is the 'driving pressure' for brain perfusion and relates to cerebral blood flow. CPP is therefore a crucial parameter and should in the normal state be in the range of 50–70 mmHg. Hence the importance of maintaining an adequate blood pressure.

When medical management of raised ICP is considered, the range of treatments available can only be safely orchestrated with reference to a least invasive monitoring of the ICP and arterial pressure. Before such monitoring is established (see below), 'first-line' treatments need to be started. This

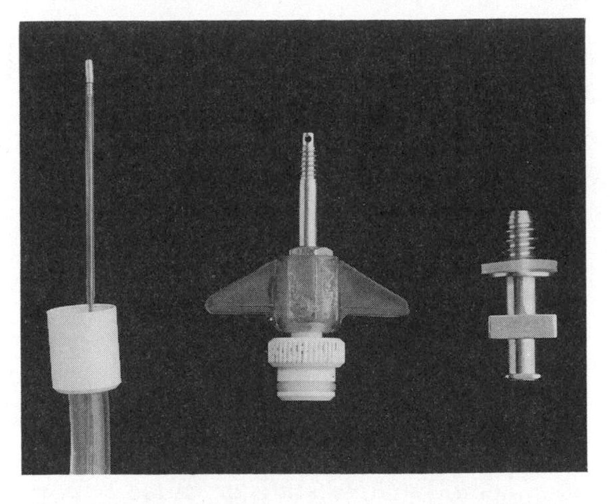

Figure 9.1 Monitors used in measuring ICP.

includes using appropriate precautions and drugs at the time of endotracheal intubation, hyperventilation, bolus doses of mannitol and specific nursing care: at all times there should be an adequate blood pressure.

A variety of ICP monitoring systems are available and include monitoring from the intraventricular, intraparenchymal, subdural and subarachnoid spaces (Figure 9.1). The respective advantages and disadvantages of each of these methods along with the technical and nursing details are reviewed elsewhere (Allen, 1986). Although the 'gold standard' is the intraventricular measurement, choice of particular monitoring is often based on local availability, expertise and relative complication rates for infection and haemorrhage.

The treatment protocol adopted by most units for controlling raised ICP includes: mechanical hyperventilation ($PaCO_2$ 25–30 mmHg, 3.3–4.0 kPa), sedation, paralysis and osmotherapy (Morriss and Cook, 1984) (Figure 9.2). Known precipitants of acute rises in ICP should either be avoided or limited. This involves preventing the sensation of painful stimuli with adequate sedation and analgesia, avoiding a kinked neck position, controlling any fever and limiting 'routine' endotracheal tube suction. Fluid restriction (50–75% of maintenance), although often

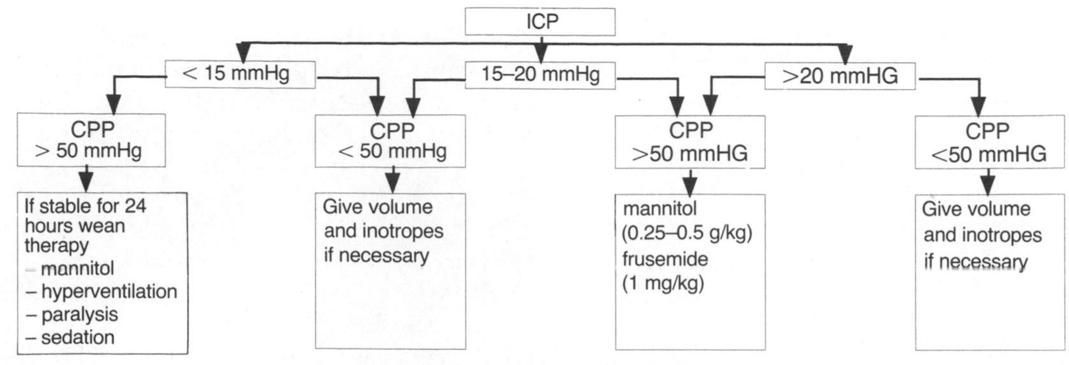

Figure 9.2 Guidelines to medical management of raised ICP.

used, should not be allowed to compromise the haemodynamic state or cause hyperosmolality (greater than 310 mosm/l).

Once these 'first-line' measures have been started, the majority of patients will be controlled with normal ICP and CPP. Patients who remain with an ICP below 15 mmHg for 24 hours can be gradually weaned from treatment and if the ICP remains normal, monitoring can be discontinued. Those patients who do not respond to this therapy may require regular as well as intermittent doses of mannitol (0.25–0.5 g/kg) and frusemide (1 mg/kg). Failing this, intravenous thiopentone can be used as a bolus dose (1–2 mg/kg) or alternatively intravenous lignocaine (1 mg/kg) may be used. At this stage the actual measures undertaken vary between centres.

When treatment is no longer considered necessary, gradual weaning of each therapy (which may take a number of days) should be carefully monitored to ensure that ICP and CPP remain normal.

SEIZURES

In the young infant or child suffering an acute brain insult, seizures are a frequent problem. Within the first few hours of a head injury they do not necessarily indicate the presence of focal haemorrhage or injury. However, in those patients with raised ICP, they can be responsible for deteriorating neurological function, because of acute changes in intracranial dynamics due to secondary hypoxia, hypercarbia, increased intrathoracic pressure and increased cerebral metabolism.

Generally, most seizures are self-limiting and therefore the aim of drug therapy is not just acute control, but also the prevention of further seizures. The commonly used anticonvulsants include: phenobarbitone, phenytoin and diazepam. When given repeatedly or in high doses, they have the potential for worsening mucociliary clearance and impairing cough (see below).

INFECTION

Infection is the bane of any child requiring intensive care, not least for those with head injury. Altough this may take the form of complicating meningitis or brain abscess, of particular concern to pulmonary management is the development of nosocomial pneumonia.

The frequency of pneumonia in severely head injured patients who require prolonged ventilatory support varies between 35% and 70%, with mortality rates approaching 50% (Demling and Riessen, 1993). The most common organisms involved are staphylococcus, enterobacter and pseudomonas, with oropharyngeal colonization and subsequent aspiration of infected secretions being considered to be the major cause. The principle of pulmonary care in the head injured patient is therefore prevention against developing infection. This should include warming the humidified inspired gas to 37°C and the institution of aggressive pulmonary toilet and the avoidance of measures such as steroids, prophylactic antibiotics and antacids, since these may merely promote bacterial colonization.

GENERAL THERAPY

In contrast to the normal brain, the injured brain is not able to tolerate swings in blood pressure, pulse rate, serum electrolytes, PaO_2 and $PaCO_2$ levels. These often result in a worsening of any brain swelling and therefore are closely monitored and aggressively treated. This usually includes: attending to the airway with prompt treatment of atelectasis and pulmonary dysfunction; rapid treatment of hypotension, agitation and discomfort; avoidance of fluid overload, 'water intoxication', hyper- or hypoglycaemia and hypomagnesaemia (Figure 9.2).

PHYSIOTHERAPY TREATMENT

The supine position is often considered to be the most convenient position in which to nurse the critically ill, ventilated, unstable child. However, although monitoring and management are often made easier by this position, lung volume is at its lowest (Muller and Bryan, 1979). In addition, in the supine position, the respiratory state is further compromised during intermittent positive pressure ventilation because passive movement of the diaphragm results in less excursion posteriorly, where opposing pressure from the viscera is greatest (Agostini and Hyatt, 1986). Furthermore pooling of secretions occurs in the dependent areas, which in the supine position are posteriorly in both upper and lower lung zones.

Drugs used for muscle relaxation, analgesia and sedation, as well as endotracheal intubation alone can also impair lung function during the course of intensive care. Contributory factors include immobility, a reduced or absent cough reflex (Ciesla, 1981), poor cough due to immobilization of the glottis, depression of the respiratory centre and pain. Respiratory airway mucociliary function may also be affected by the delivery of dry gases, anaesthetic agents, paralysis and lower body temperatures (Gamsu *et al*., 1976; Mann and Punt (1986). This may further increase the likelihood of pooled secretions in the respiratory tract.

As well as these general factors responsible for compromising respiratory function, other factors related to the underlying injury or its management can have marked effects which may influence prognosis (Warren, 1983), e.g. primary lung or thoracic cage damage (such as rib fractures and lung contusions), neurogenic pulmonary oedema and prolonged immobility.

Safe physiotherapy of children with raised ICP should therefore be based on an understanding of the treatment aims, careful assessment and judicious use of appropriate (sometimes modified) physiotherapy techniques (Prasad and Tasker, 1990). Since clinical studies in this field are scarce, the following is a guideline to the approaches which can be applied in treatment.

POSTURAL DRAINAGE

Since the head down position impairs venous return from the head and results in ICP elevation, it is generally considered to be contraindicated. A 30° head up tilt with the head in the midline position has therefore been recommended (Durward *et al*., 1983). A recent study (Feldman *et al*., 1992) of 22 head injured adults found that head elevation to 30° significantly reduced ICP in the majority of patients, without compromising CPP or cerebral blood flow. This position aids venous drainage, which when impaired can exacerbate a raised level of ICP. Modified postural drainage, maintaining careful positioning of the head in relation to the body (Shalit and Umanski, 1977), and 'log-rolling' procedures can, however, be used as soon as the patient's condition and monitoring allow. Although movement may affect the ICP, provided any positioning does not involve neck compression, the ICP changes will usually return quickly to baseline. In some instances head down positioning may be necessary. Imle *et al.* (1988) reported that such manoeuvring was not detrimental in causing low levels of CPP despite increases in ICP. It should be remembered, though, that this procedure should be attempted only when it is known that the CPP is not being compromised and the necessary recalibration of monitoring equipment has been performed (Whitelaw and Kaiser, 1984).

PERCUSSION, VIBRATIONS AND MANUAL HYPERINFLATION

Percussion is not usually associated with elevations in the level of ICP (Ciesla, 1981; Shapiro, 1975), and in fact prolonged percussion has even been reported to lower the ICP (Garrad and Bullock, 1986). Repeated vibrations can increase intrathoracic pressure and therefore indirectly increase ICP (Hough, 1986, 1991). The severity of any acute change depends on the overall stability of the patient and how vigorously the vibrations are performed.

Manual hyperinflation (bag squeezing) is not routinely used in paediatric practice. The induced increase in intrathoracic pressure not only causes a rise in ICP (Garrad and Bullock, 1986) by compromising cerebral venous return but also, by reducing systemic venous return and therefore lowering cardiac output (Laws and McIntyre, 1969), it may result in a fall in blood pressure, which may cause a further decrease in CPP. However, in many patients with raised ICP and respiratory problems, bag squeezing seems to be a necessary and indeed a more effective means of clearing bronchial secretions in the shortest period. For such patients alternating 'hand-bagging' hyperventilation (fractional inspired oxygen 1.0) with single large volume breaths augmented by chest compression seems to be an effective means of treatment without compromising CPP. Monitoring of end tidal carbon dioxide, which reflects arterial carbon dioxide gas tension ($PaCO_2$), is essential while performing manual hyperinflation. This prevents dangerously compromising cerebral blood flow with extreme hypocapnia. The $PaCO_2$ should be kept between 25–30 mmHg (3.3–4.0 kPa). The reliability of the monitoring can be intermittently reviewed by comparing the end tidal monitor readings with arterial blood gas values.

ENDOTRACHEAL TUBE SUCTION

The hazardous effects of endotracheal suction in patients with raised ICP are well recognized (Garrad and Bullock, 1986; Rudy *et al.*, 1986; Oriot *et al.*, 1987). Significant changes can be seen in the partial pressure of carbon dioxide and oxygen, both of which are known to have profound and sometimes prolonged effects on the cerebral circulation and ICP (Pascucci, 1988). In addition, part of the ICP response may be related to tracheal stimulation (Fisher *et al.*, 1982), pain or changes in intrathoracic pressure due to coughing. Hence it is important that endotracheal suction is carried out with care and skill. Hypoxia can be prevented or limited by good oxygenation before suction as well as by ensuring that this procedure is carried out as quickly as possible. High suction pressures and the use of large diameter catheters should be avoided, since the high negative pressures generated have been reported to cause falls in arterial oxygen (Young, 1984). Finally, manual hyperventilation before

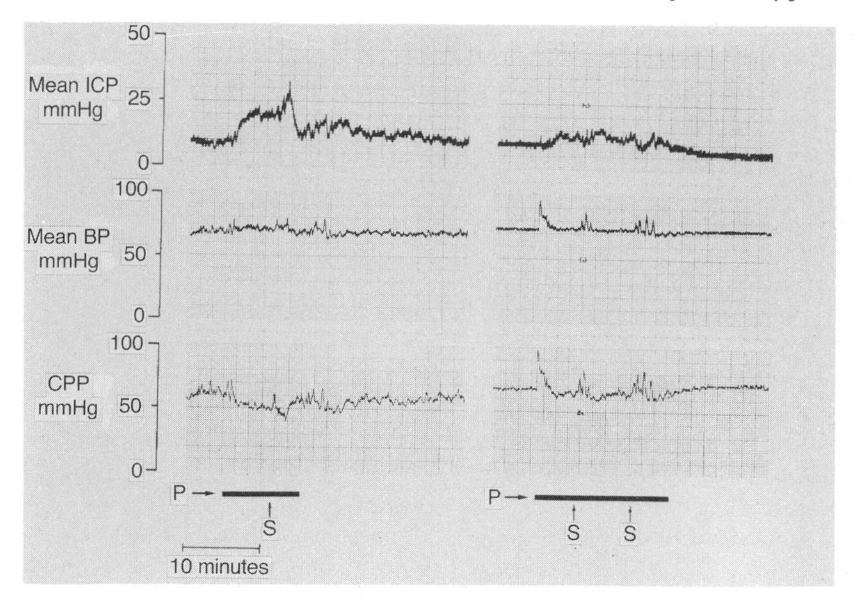

Figure 9.3 Two sections each of 35 minutes duration taken 16 hours apart showing recording of mean ICP, mean BP and CPP during physiotherapy. P denotes the period of chest physiotherapy and S endotracheal suction. In the first tracing (left) the baseline ICP of 10 mmHg increased to 15–20 mmHg with physiotherapy. Endotracheal suction resulted in a further rise in ICP to greater than 25 mmHg. During this period the CPP fell from 60 mmHg to below 50 mmHg. In the second tracing (right) taken 16 hours after the first, the baseline ICP of 10 mmHg increased to 10–15 mmHg with physiotherapy. Neither of the two episodes of endotracheal suction was associated with a rise in ICP above 15 mmHg and at all times the CPP was above 60 mmHg. Reproduced with permission from S.A. Prasad and R.C. Tasker, Guidelines for the physiotherapy management of critically ill children with raised intracranial pressure, *Physiotherapy*, 1990.

suction may reduce the propensity to develop an acute elevation in ICP

PRACTICAL CONSIDERATIONS

During individual treatments changes in ICP and CPP precipitated by physiotherapy are not always predictable (Figure 9.3). Irrespective of the technique used (see p. 146), other factors should be considered. The total treatment time is said to be a crucial factor in the level of ICP, with longer treatment times being more likely to produce potentially more dangerous ICP elevations (Garrad and Bullock, 1986). Therefore, if necessary more frequent but shorter periods of treatment are advisable. Time should be allowed for acute increases in ICP to recover to acceptable baseline values (15–20 mmHg) both between general procedures such as change of position and between individual manoeuvres, which should ensure that sustained increases in ICP during cumulative procedures are avoided (Mitchel *et al.*, 1981).

An ICP above 20 mmHg for longer than three minutes requires immediate medical intervention. However, acute elevations that occur with stimulation and return to baseline within 30 seconds are usually well tolerated and, if indicated, physiotherapy should not be restricted. In those patients with a high baseline ICP but well maintained CPP, treatment, if necessary, should be performed

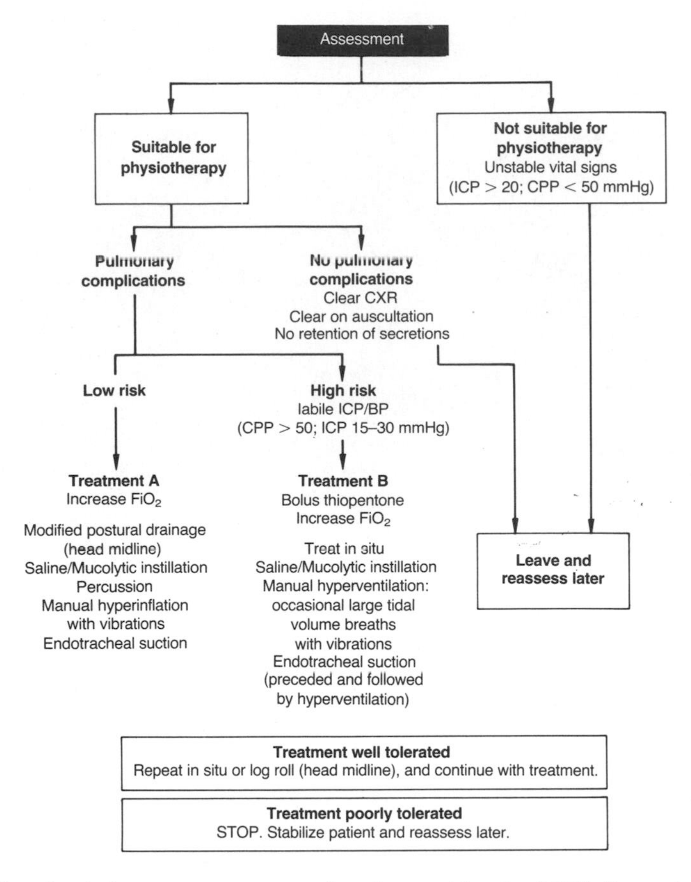

Figure 9.4 Protocol for physiotherapy assessment of patients with raised ICP. Reproduced with permission from S.A. Prasad and R.C. Tasker, Guidelines for the physiotherapy management of critically ill children with raised intracranial pressure, *Physiotherapy*, 1990.

carefully. In such patients, if adequate sedation and analgesia with a benzodiazepine and opiate combination (e.g. midazolam 0.1–0.2 mg/kg and morphine 0.1 mg/kg) is not effective in limiting expected rises in ICP, then an intravenous bolus dose of thiopentone (1–2 mg/kg) or lignocaine (1 mg/kg) can be given before therapy. However, there are disadvantages in such therapy, particularly when repeated bolus doses of barbiturates are used, since the drug effects are invariably cumulative and may make clinical neurological evaluation impossible. A protocol for patient assessment is outlined in Figure 9.4. In our experience we apply this in the context of joint consultation between physiotherapists and medical and nursing attendants, which provides a multidisciplinary assessment of individual problems and enables informed decision making about physiotherapy treatment priorities and objectives. In this setting we have found that chest physiotherapy can be carried out to the advantage of overall patient care.

REFERENCES

Allen, R. (1986) Intracranial pressure: a review of clinical problems, measurement techniques and monitoring methods. *Journal of Medical Engineering Technology*, **10**, 299–320.

Agostini, E. and Hyatt, R.E. (1986) Static behaviour of the respiratory system, in *Handbook of Physiology – The Respiratory System III*, (The American Physiological Society), Williams and Wilkins, London.

Ciesla, N. (1981) Chest physiotherapy for special patients, in *Chest Physiotherapy in the Intensive Care Unit*, (ed. C.M. McKenzie), Williams and Wilkins, London.

Demling, R.H. and Riessen, R. (1993) Respiratory failure after cerebral injury. *Critical Care Medicine*, **1**, 440–6.

Durward, Q.J., Amacher, L., Del Maestro, R.F. and Sibbald, W.J. (1983) Cerebral and cardiovascular responses to changes in head elevation in patients with intracranial hypertension. *Journal of Neurosurgery*, **59**, 938–44.

Feldman, Z., Kanter, M.J., Robertson, C.S. *et al*. (1992) Effect of head elevation on intracranial pressure and cerbral blood flow in head injured patients. *Journal of Neurosurgery*, **76**, 206–11.

Fisher, D.M., Frewent, T. and Swedlow, B.D. (1982) Increase in intracranial pressure during suctioning – stimulation vs rise in $PaCO_2$. *Anesthesiology*, **57**, 416.

Gamsu, G., Morley, M., Singer, H. *et al*. (1976) Post-operative impairment of mucous transport in the lung. *American Review of Respiratory Diseases*, **114**, 673–9.

Garrad, J. and Bullock, M. (1986) The effect of respiratory therapy on intracranial pressure in ventilated neurosurgical patients. *Australian Journal of Physiotherapy*, **32**, 107–11.

Hough, A. (1986) How does head injury influence the physiotherapy management of the ventilated patient? *Association of Chartered Physiotherapists in Respiratory Care Newsletter*, **9**, 25–33.

Hough, A. (1991) Physiotherapy in intensive care, in *Physiotherapy in Respiratory Care*, Chapman & Hall, London, pp. 166–93.

Imle, C., Mars, M.P., Eppinghaus, C. *et al*. (1988) Effect of chest physiotherapy (CPT) positioning on intracranial (ICP) and cerebral perfusion pressure (CPP). *Critical Care Medicine*, **16**, 3823.

Laws, A.K. and McIntyre, R.W. (1969) Chest physiotherapy: the physiological assessment during IPPV in respiratory failure. *Canadian Anaesthetists Society Journal*, **16**, 487–93.

Mann, N. and Punt, J. (1986) Intracranial pressure monitoring in children. *Care of the Critically ill*, **2**, 143–50.

Mitchel, P.H., Ozuma, J. and Lipe, H.P. (1981) Moving the patient in bed: effects on intracranial pressure. *Nursing Research*, **30**, 212–18.

Morriss, F.C. and Cook, J.D. (1984) Increased intracranial pressure, in *A Practical Guide to Pediatric Intensive Care*, 2nd edn, (eds F.C. Morriss and G.C. Moor), C.V. Mosby, Toronto, pp. 47–53.

Muller, N.L. and Bryan, A.C. (1979) Chest wall mechanics and respiratory muscles in infants. *Pediatric Clinics of North America*, **26**(3), 39–52.

Oriot, D., Fausser, C., Wood, C. *et al*. (1987) Intracranial pressure and physiotherapy in comatose children. *Intensive Care Medicine*, **13**, 457.

Pascucci, R.C. (1988) Head trauma in the child. *Intensive Care Medicine*, **14**, 185–95.

Prasad, S.A. and Tasker, R.C. (1990) Guidelines for physiotherapy management of critically ill children with acutely raised intracranial pressure. *Physiotherapy*, **76**(4), 248–50.

Reilly, P.L., Simpson, D.A., Sprod, R. and Thomas, L. (1988) Assessing the conscious level in infants and young children: a paediatric version of the Glasgow coma scale. *Child's Nervous System*, **4**, 30–3.

Rudy, E.B., Baun, M., Stone, K. *et al*. (1986) The relationship between endotracheal suctioning and changes in intracranial pressure – a review of the literature. *Reviews in Critical Care*, **15**, 488–94.

Shalit, M.N. and Umanski, F. (1977) Effect of routine bedside procedures on intracranial pressure. *Israel Journal of Medical Science*, **13**, 881–6.

Shapiro, H.M. (1975) Intracranial hypertension; therapeutic and anaesthetic considerations. *Anesthesiology*, **54**, 496–503.

Teasdale, G. and Jennett, B. (1974) Assessment of coma and impaired consciousness.

A practical scale. *Lancet*, **ii**, 81–4.
Warren, J.B. (1983) Pulmonary complications associated with severe head injury. *Journal of Neurosurgical Nursing*, **15**, 194–200.
Whitelaw, A. and Kaiser, A. (1984) Head position affects intracranial pressure in newborn infants. *Journal of Pediatrics*, **105**, 506.
Young, C.S. (1984) The adverse effects of airway suction. *Physiotherapy*, **70**, 104–8.

RESPIRATORY TRACT DISORDERS 10

Robert Dinwiddie

INTRODUCTION

Respiratory tract infections are the commonest cause of illness in children and occur due to infection with a wide variety of organisms whose pathogenicity varies from time to time (Editorial, 1985). The child's age and state of immune response are also important. The immune response may be inhibited by age related immaturity or underlying disease processes such as primary or secondary immune deficiency, for example, HIV infection. The respiratory system also has a number of intrinsic defence mechanisms which are important including the anatomy of the upper and lower airway, mucociliary clearance, particularly the cilia themselves which line the respiratory tract, and reflex mechanisms inhibiting invasion of the lower respiratory tract such as the cough reflex and bronchoconstriction in the small airways. Other more general factors which affect the severity of infection include the environment where dust, air pollution and tobacco smoke are important. Lung damage due to previous infections or congenital malformations such as lung cysts may also predispose the respiratory tract to infection and malnutrition inhibits the natural response to it.

EPIGLOTTITIS

This is an acute bacterial infection particularly prevalent during the second, third and fourth years of life. It is principally caused by the bacteria *Haemophilus influenzae*, type B. It is an acute and severe infection which is often associated with simultaneous spread to the bloodstream. There is a rapid onset of severe illness with high fever, sore throat, stridor and generalized toxicity. The stridor worsens quickly and within a few hours there is the development of acute upper airway obstruction. This results in hypoxia and the child becomes restless with increased difficulty in breathing. Airway size at this time is critical and even mild disturbance can produce acute airway obstruction which can be fatal.

It is extremely dangerous and can be life threatening to attempt to examine the throat directly in this situation; such activity may result in acute, complete airway obstruction and death. If the diagnosis is suspected the child should be admitted to hospital immediately and inspection of the airway should occur in the presence of an anaesthetist who can intubate the child (Mitchell and Thomas, 1980). In addition preparations must be made to undertake a tracheostomy should intubation fail. This is rare in modern day practice and most children can be satisfactorily managed with an airway at this time. There is an increasing trend to allow the child to be fully awake and mobile once the airway is placed providing that the arms are splinted so that the tube cannot be removed. Within 48 to 72 hours, in most cases, the swelling has subsided sufficiently for the artificial airway to be removed.

It is important to give intravenous antibiotics, usually a third generation cephalosporin, and general support with intravenous fluids and hydration until the child recovers. Physiotherapy is not usually helpful in this situation unless there is complicating lower respiratory tract infection. Steroids such as dexamethasone are used acutely to reduce the airway obstruction.

LARYNGOTRACHEOBRONCHITIS

Laryngotracheobronchitis (croup) is a form of acute airway infection, most frequently due to viruses such as parainfluenza or respiratory syncytial virus (RSV). It can also be caused by bacteria such as *Staphylococcus aureus* or *Streptococcus pneumoniae*. The onset is more gradual than that of acute epiglottitis but the clinical features are similar. It is unusual for the child to require intubation and airway support but this will be necessary for those with the most severe form of the illness. Treatment is otherwise symptomatic with oxygen and fluid support and also systemic steroids for the most severe cases (Tibballs *et al.*, 1992).

Lateral X-ray of the neck in this situation can be helpful in determining airway obstruction, but this should not be carried out in those where there is any suspicion that the disease may be due to acute epiglottitis, since this procedure can also precipitate major airway obstruction. Recurrent episodes of croup occur in some children who either have intrinsic airway narrowing from congenital or acquired abnormalities or those who are highly allergic.

PERTUSSIS

This is a major lower respiratory tract infection usually caused by *Bordetella pertussis*. It can be seen at any age although it is most common in younger children who are unimmunized. It previously occurred in major epidemics but since the immunization rate has increased recently the number of cases has fallen significantly. It can still be fatal, particularly in children under one year of age, where it can cause an overwhelming bronchopneumonia. The onset of the typical cough is preceded by cold-like symptoms for a week to ten days; thereafter the acute coughing spasms commence and occur repeatedly, terminating in a 'whoop' as air is drawn into the lungs. In severe cases subconjunctural haemorrhage and even hypoxic convulsions can occur during coughing spasms. The airway is acutely irritable and the cough reflex is initiated by minimal triggering factors such as cold air, excitement or even laughter. The coughing spells will continue for an average of three months although they will gradually lessen in severity towards the end of this period. Lower respiratory tract infection resulting in bronchopneumonia is not uncommon at this stage (Dinwiddie, 1990).

Treatment is by general supportive measures and antibiotics; although these do not influence the length of the illness, they will shorten the infectivity of the patient in the acute phase. Salbutamol has been shown to have some effect on the frequency of the coughing spasms. Physiotherapy is very difficult to perform in cases where there are retained lung secretions because any stimulus often produces further coughing spasms. However, if the child requires ventilation physiotherapy is often important to assist with the removal of secretions and once the acute stage of the disease is over it may be indicated in cases where there is persistent lobar collapse. Active immunization is the most important form of prevention and should be given to all children except for those who have had significant previous adverse reactions to the vaccine or those who are acutely ill at the time of proposed immunization. Children with previous neurological damage or a history of nonfebrile convulsion need special consideration in each case. Most children who are otherwise well do not have long term pulmonary sequelae from pertussis (Johnson *et al.*, 1983), although this is seen in those who have underlying immune deficiency or malnutrition at the time of infection.

BRONCHIOLITIS

Bronchiolitis is by far the most common serious respiratory tract infection in the first year of life. It is caused in the majority of cases by respiratory syncytial virus (RSV). Other viruses are, however, responsible and these include parainfluenza, influenza and adenovirus. Bronchiolitis occurs annually in epidemics during the late autumn, winter and early spring. It not only affects the small airways but frequently causes pneumonia as well. There is an acute inflammatory response to infection with the virus and this leads to marked airway obstruction with air trapping, wheezing and hyperinflation. In severe cases these will result in respiratory failure. A number of infants with underlying diseases such as cystic fibrosis (Abman *et al.*, 1988) or immune deficiency may in fact present with acute bronchiolitis which fails to improve in the normal time period. Those with other problems such as bronchopulmonary dysplasia (BPD) are also at increased risk during this time (Smith *et al.*, 1991). Rapid diagnostic techniques including immunofluorescence allow the diagnosis to be made on pharyngeal secretions very early in the illness.

Treatment is supportive with added oxygen and humidity. Those with severe illness or underlying lung problems should be treated with ribavirin by special nebulizer (small particle aerosol generator – SPAG) (Hall *et al.*, 1983). Bronchodilators are often used especially after the fist six months of life although it is difficult to prove their efficacy. Systemic steroids have not proved to be of immediate benefit, although studies are underway at present to assess the use of inhaled steroids in this situation. Antibiotics are not indicated unless there is secondary bacterial infection. Physiotherapy may be helpful once the acute stage is passed in clearing lower airway secretions but can make wheezing and bronchospasm worse, which could lead to further air trapping and impaired clearance of lung secretions. Infants who have acute bronchiolitis have a high incidence of wheezing after recovery (Mallory *et al.*, 1989) but this gradually decreases over the next four or five years of life.

Those with infection due to adenovirus may suffer much more severe lung damage with destruction of the small airways and the accompanying blood vessels resulting in obliterative bronchiolitis (Sly *et al.*, 1984). These children tend to have permanent sequelae with persistent overinflation and airway obstruction leading to wheezing which may be poorly responsive to bronchodilators. There is a significant incidence of impaired immunity in these children.

PNEUMONIA

Infants and young children are particularly prone to generalized lung infection and as has already been mentioned, RSV is the principal pathogen in the younger age group. Bacteria such as staphylococci, streptococci and pneumococci can also cause major problems. In the older child viruses are coped with much better and bacterial infections become more prevalent. These include *Streptococcus pneumoniae* and other bacteria such as *Staphylococcus aureus*, haemolytic streptococcus and *Haemophilus influenzae*. Mycoplasma pneumonia is seen in the older child and adolescent. Less common organisms such as *Pseudomonas aeruginosa* or *Pneumocystis carinii* are seen in those with underlying disease such as cystic fibrosis or AIDS. In the young child the infection tends to be generalized with bilateral involvement of the lungs usually confirmed by chest X-ray whereas in the older child the infection tends to be more confined to single lobes. The possibility of inhalation of a foreign body resulting in lobar pneumonia should never be forgotten, especially when there is no previous history of chronic respiratory illness and if there is any suggestion that foreign body aspiration may have occurred.

Viral pneumonia is most prevalent in the community and may occur in epidemics particularly due to RSV in the winter months. In this case treatment is supportive with adequate fluids, humidity and general supportive measures. If oxygen therapy is required then admission to hospital should be arranged as increased respiratory support may be necessary for several days. Apart from recurrent wheeze those who are previously healthy will usually make a complete recovery. In some cases mild immune deficiency such as low immunoglobulin subclasses may lead to more serious infections and potential complications such as bronchiectasis.

In bacterial pneumonia, *Streptococcus pneumoniae* is the commonest cause of pneumonia in the community and usually responds very rapidly to antibiotic treatment. In the otherwise healthy child complete recovery is the rule. Pneumonia due to other pathogens such as staphylococci, the beta haemolytic streptococcus or Gram negative organisms is more serious and requires more intensive treatment, frequently in hospital. These children are more likely to develop complications such as lung abscess, persistent consolidation and ultimately bronchiectasis. When these situations arise it is important to evaluate the child for underlying problems such as cystic fibrosis or primary or secondary immune deficiency. Some children suffer from recurrent pneumonia due to uncommon organisms such as fungi or *Pneumocystis carinii* and these children have a high incidence of underlying major immune deficiency. Specific treatment for them will include antifungal agents such as amphotericin or flucytosine for fungi, or co-trimoxazole or pentamidine for *Pneumocystis carinii*.

Physiotherapy plays an important role in the treatment of serious pneumonia in facilitating the clearance of lung secretions, but only when the consolidation phase of the illness is resolving and the inflammatory response is very active in returning the lung to its previous normal condition.

BRONCHIECTASIS

This is due to persistent damage and dilatation of the bronchi which results in mucus collection with or without secondary infection. It may occur secondary to congenital abnormalities of the lung, cystic fibrosis or functional defects such as cilia dyskinesia. Children with immune deficiency are also especially prone to this condition. It may, however, occur in those who are otherwise entirely normal if they have had a particularly severe pneumonic illness. Causes of bronchiectasis are listed in Table 10.1.

Table 10.1 Causes of bronchiectasis

Causes
Cystic fibrosis
Postpneumonic, e.g. pertussis, measles, adenovirus, tuberculosis
Recurrent aspiration
Foreign body
Immune deficiency
Immotile cilia syndrome
Congenital abnormality, e.g. lung cyst, pulmonary sequestration

Investigation will include ventilation/perfusion lung scan and high resolution CT scan of the lungs (Figure 10.1). Bronchography is rarely used nowadays as the modern imaging techniques are safer and can be more specific in outlining the distribution of the underlying abnormalities. Predisposing conditions such as recurrent aspiration or immune deficiency should be

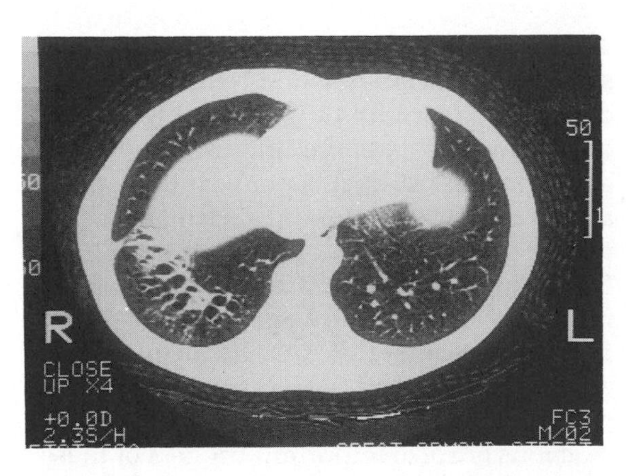

Figure 10.1 Thoracic CT showing bronchiectasis

sought by investigation with barium swallow, pH studies, radioisotope milk scans and particularly evaluation of immunoglobulins and immunoglobulin subclasses. Treatment is primarily aimed at clearing lung secretions and allowing the underlying lung to recover if at all possible. Physiotherapy is of prime importance in this situation. It should be accompanied by exercise and if necessary prophylactic antibiotics, along with immunoglobulin infusions should there be an underlying immunoglobulin deficiency of significance. Segmental or lobar surgery is indicated where there is localized disease and can produce excellent results. Where the disease is bilateral then surgery is usually contraindicated unless there is one very severely affected lobe.

RECURRENT ASPIRATION

Recurrent aspiration of gastric secretions into the lungs is being increasingly recognized as a cause of significant severe acute or recurrent disease. Gastro-oesophageal reflux is particularly prevalent in the ex-preterm infant and those with underlying congenital abnormalities of swallowing such as CHARGE syndrome (Blake *et al.*, 1990) or previous oesophageal atresia. It can, however, occur in those who have no other obvious underlying abnormality. Although many children display symptoms such as difficulty in swallowing or recurrent vomiting, in some cases this can be quite subtle without such predisposing factors present. Those who have neurological disease are at special risk. The possibility of direct communication between the oesophagus and trachea, such as a tracheo-oesophageal fistula, should also be considered.

Investigation includes barium swallow to exclude obvious reflux, hiatus hernia, pyloric stenosis or malrotation of the gut. Attention should also be paid to the sucking and swallowing mechanism to ensure that this is occurring normally. More specific tests including pH studies or radioisotope milk scan can be very helpful in evaluating these symptoms over a longer period than during a barium swallow.

Treatment consists of a medical approach including thickening feeds, propping up to an angle of 30°, removal of drugs such as theophylline which may predispose to gastro-oesophageal sphincter relaxation and the administration of other agents which improve gastro-oesophageal motility such as domperidone or cisapride. Reduction of gastric acidity with the use of ranitidine is also helpful. Those who have persistent symptoms despite this treatment will require Nissen's fundoplication which in skilled surgical hands has an excellent outcome (Kiely, 1990). It is often accompanied by the placement of a gastrostomy for those with major feeding difficulties.

Acute foreign body inhalation should be considered in any child who suddenly becomes symptomatic with coughing or wheezing where there is no previous history of such symptoms. There may or may not have been an incident where the child obviously aspirated since many episodes are unrecognized initially (Cohen *et al.*, 1980). If there is any suspicion of such a history then a bronchoscopy is indicated. If the foreign body remains in the lung for more than a few days secondary collapse and infection occur with the risk of long term bronchiectasis. Supportive treatment includes antibiotics and fluid therapy. Physiotherapy to facilitate clearance of lung secretions from the affected area is only indicated following bronchoscopic removal of the foreign body. If the acute aspiration is dealt with appropriately then the long term outlook is excellent.

ASTHMA

Asthma is a common disease in children now thought to affect some 15% to 20% during the childhood period. The aetiology is complex and it is also increasingly recognized that recurrent wheezing in the young child may not be due to classic asthma as such. Other factors which are important include maternal smoking in pregnancy which may affect the airway growth before birth, passive smoking from other household members which in the UK affects nearly 50% of children and the effects of acute virus infection such as bronchiolitis in the early months of life. All of these conditions can predispose to recurrent wheezy episodes which will improve with time if the precipitating factors are removed. Those with an underlying atopic predisposition, often manifested by eczema or food allergy in the early months of life, are more at risk of prolonged recurrent wheezy episodes, especially if there is also a strong family history of atopic disease.

Asthma appears to be increasing in children and this may be due to a number of reasons. There is no doubt that asthma was under-recognized in the past and this is an important factor in the apparent increased frequency. Other influences include changing aeroallergens such as increased pollen due to altered agricultural practice in the last decade and increases in atmospheric pollution as traffic levels rise in urban areas. Asthma mortality has not significantly decreased and remains a major cause of concern for those with this disease in middle or late childhood. There are approximately 45 deaths per year in England and Wales from asthma (Silverman, 1985).

The underlying pathophysiology is increasingly recognized to be due to acute inflammation of the airway. This is mediated through a number of inflammatory factors especially related to infiltration with polymorphonuclear neutrophils. Allergic reactions are also important triggers of these responses but are thought to be less important than they were previously. Eighty percent of children with asthma will wheeze on exercise and this is an important limiting factor in their day-to-day lifestyle. This can be prevented with the use of bronchodilating agents or cromoglycate (Intal) before exercise begins.

The overall evaluation of children with asthma consists of a careful history to assess the age of onset, frequency and severity of attacks and especially precipitating factors. These can be induced by a wide variety of problems shown in Table 10.2. It is important to exclude other causes of wheezing in those who have apparent asthma, since conditions such as cystic fibrosis, chronic immune deficiency, gastro-oesophageal reflux, obliterative bronchiolitis or congenital malformations of the respiratory tract may present in this way.

Table 10.2 Precipitants of asthma

Respiratory tract infection
Inhaled or ingested allergens
Atmospheric pollution
Exercise
Cold air
Tobacco smoke
Emotional upset
Excitement
Psychogenic factors
Drugs – propranolol

Treatment of asthma consists of an understanding of precipitating factors and their avoidance if at all possible, education of the family and the child in the disease process itself, elimination of environmental factors or their reduction with particular attention to dust, dust mites, pets and other inhaled allergens and, if necessary, exclusion of precipitating food stuffs if these can be identified. Drug treatment is extremely effective these days and should follow the pattern outlined by the British Thoracic Society (*Thorax*, 1993). Intermittent bronchodilators are given to those who have occasional symptoms but if these are occurring at more frequent intervals, at least weekly, then prophylaxis with inhaled agents should be given commencing with cromoglycate in the younger child and moving to inhaled steroids if the wheezing is even more frequent or if there is not an early response to the initial prophylaxis. Inhaled steroids are extremely important in inhibiting the underlying inflammatory process and it is important that these are continued on a regular basis. Parents should be educated in their advantages and should understand that the side effects are minimal when these are given in appropriate dosage. Short courses of oral steroids are often indicated for acute episodes and do not cause any long term problems when given in this way. Prophylaxis with oral steroids is now uncommon and usually indicates that the asthma has some other basis either related to immune deficiency, other underlying structural defects of the lung such as chronic bronchopulmonary dysplasia or major psychosocial factors. Physiotherapy plays a vital role in one of the most important aspects of the management of this condition - education. Teaching children and parents how to use inhaled drug delivery devices may be the physiotherapist's responsibility in some centres and encouragement and advice on exercise, teaching techniques of breathing control for episodes of respiratory embarassment and awareness of posture are essential in the overall management of the disease.

Acute asthma requires intensive treatment in hospital principally with steroids either oral or intravenous and acute bronchodilator therapy with nebulized agents such as salbutamol, terbutaline or atrovent and the use of intravenous theophylline if bronchospasm is severe. Supportive measures such as adequate fluid balance and oxygen are also important. Physiotherapy is not helpful in the acute state as it can make bronchospasm worse, but in those who require ventilation, once paralysed and appropriately sedated, this can be very helpful in the clearance of lung secretions and mucus plugging.

HIV/AIDS

Increasing numbers of infants and children are seen principally with vertical transmission of HIV infection who develop AIDS in the first year or two of life (Editorial, 1988). The major presenting features are opportunistic infections, principally with organisms such as *Pneumocystis carinii*. These children often develop unremitting pneumonia which is not responsive to the usual supportive treatment and antibiotic therapy. Diagnosis can be facilitated by the use of bronchoalveolar lavage (see Chapter 6, pp. 88–9) where other opportunistic organisms such as fungi, adenovirus, RSV, cytomegalovirus or tuberculosis can be carefully searched for utilizing special techniques including immunofluorescence. The possibility of AIDS should be considered in any child who has persistent pneumonia when other predisposing factors such as cystic fibrosis or primary immune deficiency have been excluded. Treatment will centre on intensive therapy of the underlying organism if this can be identified and general supportive measures including oxygen, humidification, adequate nutrition and ventilation if necessary.

A significant proportion of AIDS infants present with *Pneumocystis carinii* infection in the first few months of life and unfortunately these infants have a very poor prognosis as 60% to 70% of them will die during the acute infection and the remainder frequently develop AIDS encephalopathy within the next year. These factors need to be borne in mind when discussing treatment plans and the prognosis with the parents.

Respiratory infections in children vary in their frequency and severity not only in relation to the child's development and underlying lung problems, but also in relation to changes in the disease process such as the onset of HIV/AIDS in recent years and the relative diminution in pertussis with the increase in effective immunization. Attention to general supportive measures particularly related to nutrition and the exclusion of predisposing factors such as gastro-oesophageal reflux or congenital anomalies is important in the prevention of long term lung damage.

REFERENCES

Abman, S.H., Ogle, S.W., Butler-Simon, N. *et al*. (1988) Role of respiratory syncytial virus in early hospitalisations for respiratory distress of young patients with cystic fibrosis, *Journal of Pediatrics*, **113**, 826–30.

Blake, K.D., Russel-Eggit, I.M., Morgan, D.W. *et al*. (1990) Who's in CHARGE? Multidisciplinary management of patients with CHARGE association. *Archives of Disease in Childhood*. **65**, 217–23.

Cohen, S.R., Herbert, W.I., Lewis, G.B. *et al*. (1980) Foreign bodies in the airways. Five year retrospective study with special reference to management. *Annals of Otology, Rhinology and Laryngology*, **89**, 437–42.

Dinwiddie, R. (1990) Respiratory tract infection, in *Diagnosis and Management of Paediatric Respiratory Disease*, (ed. R. Dinwiddie), Churchill Livingstone, London, pp. 101–26.

Editorial (1985) Acute respiratory infections in under fives: 15 million deaths a year. *Lancet*, **2**, 699–701.

Editorial (1988) Vertical transmission of HIV. *Lancet*, **2**, 1057–8.

Hall, C.B., McBride, J.T., Walsh, E.E. *et al*. (1983) Aerosolized ribavirin treatment of infants with respiratory syncytial virus infection. *New England Journal of Medicine*, **308**, 1443–7.

Johnson, I.D.A., Anderson, H.R., Lambert, H.P. *et al*. (1983) Pertussis long term morbidity. *Lancet*, **2**, 1104–8.

Kiely, E.M. (1990) Surgery for gastro-oesophageal reflux. *Archives of Disease in Childhood*, **65**, 1291–2.

Mallory, G.B., Motoyama, E.K., Koumbourlis, A.C. *et al*. (1989) Bronchial reactivity in infants in acute respiratory failure with viral bronchiolitis. *Pediatric Pulmonology*, **6**, 253–9.

Mitchell, D.P. and Thomas, R.L. (1980) Secondary airway support in the management of croup. *Journal of Otolaryngology*, **9**, 419–22.

Silverman, M. (1985) Asthma in childhood. *Current Medical Literature*, 3–36.

Sly, P.D., Soto-Quiros, D., Landau, L.I. *et al*. (1984) Factors predisposing to abnormal pulmonary function after adenovirus type 7 pneumonia. *Archives of Disease in Childhood*, **59**, 935–9.

Smith, D.W., Frankel, L.R., Mathers, L.H. *et al*. (1991) A controlled trial of aerosolized ribavirin in infants receiving mechanical ventilation for severe respiratory syncytial virus infection. *New England Journal of Medicine*, **352**, 24–9.

Thorax (1993) Guidelines on the management of asthma. *Thorax*, **48** (suppl), S1–S24.

Tibballs, J., Shann, F.A. and Landau, L.I. (1992) Placebo-controlled trial of prednisolone in children intubated for croup. *Lancet*, **340**, 745–8.

CYSTIC FIBROSIS

11

Robert Dinwiddie and S. Ammani Prasad

INTRODUCTION

Cystic fibrosis (CF) is the commonest serious inherited chest disorder in caucasian people. There are estimated to be around 6000 cases in the UK at present and it is thought to affect about one in 2500 live born infants (Dodge *et al.*, 1993) The illness is inherited as an autosomal recessive with a one in four chance of recurrence in further children by the same parents. The genetic abnormalities of CF have now been specifically identified (Rommens *et al.*, 1989). The abnormal gene lies on the long arm of chromosome number 7 and in each clinical case two cystic fibrosis genes combine to produce the illness. The most commmon gene is known as delta F508, which results in a deletion of the phenylalanine residue at position 508 on the CF protein. Since its initial discovery a very large number of other genes, currently over 400, have been described which can result in CF. The abnormal genes code for a protein which is called the cystic fibrosis transmembrane regulating protein (CFTR) (Gregory *et al.*, 1991). Intensive studies continue in order to relate the genetic defect to the specific protein abnormality.

The CFTR protein lies within the epithelial cells but is attached to the cell surface by specific channels which are important in the transfer of ions acoss the cell membrane. This principally results in a defect of chloride transport (Cuthbert, 1992) but carries with it an associated sodium and water defect as well. These abnormalities result in the classic elevation of sodium and chloride which are used in the diagnostic sweat test and in the salty taste which these patients often demonstrate when kissed. The principal clinical abnormalities in CF are shown in Table 11.1

Table 11.1 Principal clinical abnormalities in CF

Cause	*Effect*
Neonatal intestinal obstruction	Meconium ileus
Bronchial obstruction/ infection	Bronchiectasis
Pancreatic deficiency	Nutritional deficiency
Intestinal obstruction	Distal intestinal obstruction syndrome
Bile duct obstruction	Hepatic cirrhosis/ hypersplenism
Agenesis of the vas deferens	Male sterility
Sweat electrolyte abnormality	Elevated sodium and chloride

GENETIC FACTORS

The discovery of the CF genes has led to the possibility of heterozygote screening tests since the carrier rate is about one in 20 of the UK population. As there are many different types of CF gene, only the most common can be included in a screening programme. By far the most common gene type is delta F508 and preliminary studies have shown that it is possible to carry out population screening for selected individuals, such as those attending prenatal clinics or women of reproductive age attending for family planning advice (Watson *et al.*, 1991). There are various practical and ethical problems to be overcome before this process can be applied on a generalized basis.

Prenatal diagnosis is now, however, very reliable. At present this is carried out by chorion villus sampling (CVS) at 8–10 weeks gestation in families known to be at high risk of an affected fetus. Genetic markers are also available for tracking the abnormal CF genes within a family even where the gene itself cannot be specifically identified. The fetal loss rate after CVS is about 2%, so it is only appropriate to carry out this test where the parents intend to have a termination if the pregnancy is abnormal.

Neonatal screening for CF is also possible utilizing the fact that the pancreatic abnormality leads to elevated levels of trypsin in the neonate. This can be used as an initial screen and followed up by gene analysis for those who show initially elevated levels. This allows for a low retest rate thus decreasing parental anxiety about a false positive test. Screening tests are only of value if they can be shown to be of benefit both in the immediate treatment and in long term survival. Infants who are detected by neonatal screening spend less time in hospital during the first two years of life and may have an improved growth rate initially. There is no conclusive evidence that this improves their long term survival or the complications of the disease itself. Further studies are taking place to elucidate this approach in more detail (Weller and West , 1991). The advantages of screening are that early treatment, particularly of a preventative nature, can be undertaken and this may be important as new therapies such as gene replacement become available. Other disadvantages of screening include the fact that it may interfere with parent–child bonding in the early years of life particularly when the child is relatively asymptomtic and the parents may not be compliant with treatment because they deny the existence of the illness and want to disprove the diagnosis in an apparently healthy infant.

GENE THERAPY

The understanding of the basic defect in CF has led to the possibility of replacement of the faulty gene and clinical trials to assess this are now underway. The DNA which codes for normal CFTR can be introduced either through virus vectors such as adenovirus (Rosenfeld *et al.*, 1992) or by intracellular components such as liposomes which can carry the DNA into the cells. The assessment of this new treatment has been facilitated by the production of CF mice (Dorin *et al.*, 1992). These animals have been bred with the human CF gene in their genetic make-up so that they too produce abnormal CFTR and successful gene therapy has alrady been reported in them (Hyde *et al.*, 1993). Presently gene therapy is targeted towards the respiratory system where nebulized treatment, which is the only technique so far available, has direct application. The exact timing of introduction of this therapy remains to be investigated. The long term safety and efficacy are also unknown and careful clincial trials will be necessary before it can be generally applied.

PULMONARY COMPLICATIONS

Although the CF infant has normal lungs at birth, these soon acquire various defects secondary to the abnormal secretions through which the lung pathology begins during intercurrent respiratory tract infections. Recurrent infections lead to inflammation of the small airways and changes of the lining including mucus plugging, oedema, inflammation and squamous metaplasia. Further disease results in microabscess

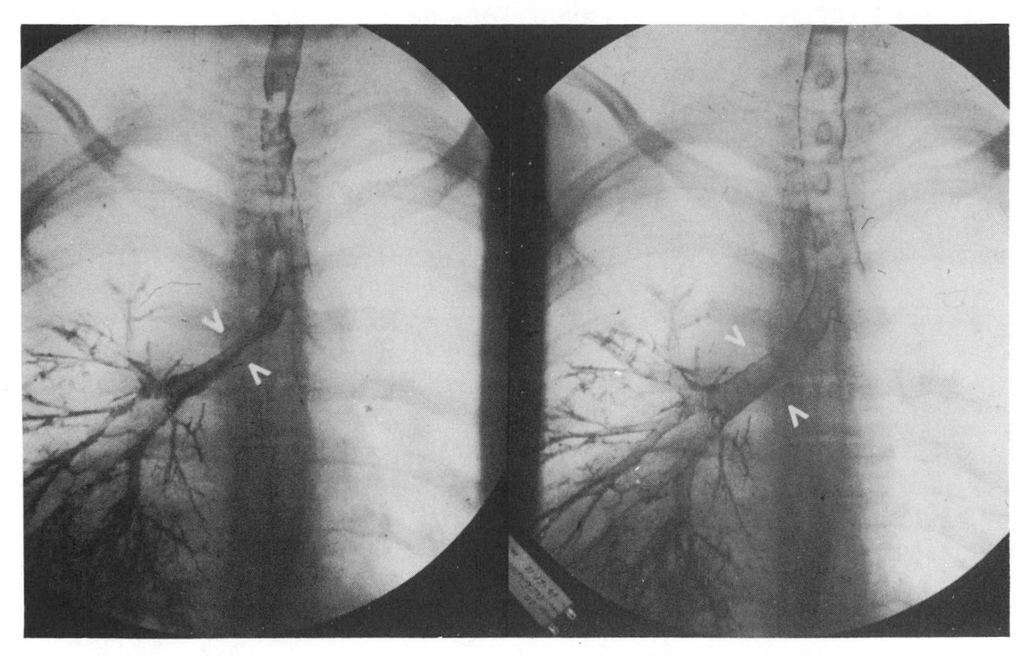

Figure 11.1 Bronchography demonstrating airway dilation at full inspiration (right) and airway collapse during forced expiration (left). Reproduced with permission from Professor M. Zach.

formation and leads on to bronchiectasis. There is distortion of the peripheral airways which results in abnormal tone leading to bronchospasm and airway collapse (Figure 11.1). These changes may be exacerbated by allergic reactions which may be facilitated by the abnormal lining of the airway and the underlying inflammatory process which occurs due to the persistent infection. The pathophysiology of the CF Lung is well reviewed by Zach (1990).

The major problems in the CF lung result from invasion by pathogenic bacteria, particularly *Staphylococcus aureus, Haemophilus influenzae* and *Pseudomonas aeruginosa*. The entry of these bacteria may be facilitated by intercurrent viral infections which are extremely common in CF children. A number of CF patients present with respiratory syncytial virus (RSV) bronchiolitis and CF should always be considered in those with persistent symptoms after intercurrent RSV infection.

Wheezing is a common symptom of CF. This frequently occurs after RSV but as the underlying disease progresses it also becomes a common feature in the older child. This happens for two reasons: firstly because of the underlying inflammatory process with oedema, mucus plugging and airway obstruction, and secondly due to bronchial hyper-reactivity. As many as 50% of CF children have wheezing as a frequent symptom. Asthma, however, is probably no more common in CF than in the child population generally, occurring in approximately 15% of cases. It is important, if possible, to distinguish the two entities since this can affect the response to bronchodilator therapy as those who do not have asthma may bronchoconstrict. It is always important to monitor the response by peak flow rate or respiratory function tests if at all possible.

RESPIRATORY CARE IN CYSTIC FIBROSIS

The principal treatments are shown in Table 11.2.

Table 11.2 Treatment of cystic fibrosis

Chest physiotherapy
Active cycle of breathing techniques (ACBT)
Positive expiratory pressure (PEP)
High pressure PEP
Autogenic drainage (AD)
Flutter VRP1
Physical exercise
Antibiotics
Bronchodilators
Steroids
Mucolytics

PHYSIOTHERAPY

Appropriate physiotherapy with postural drainage is the most important part of treatment to prevent progression of the lung disease and should be carried out in virtually all cases on a regular daily basis. This is discussed in detail later in the chapter.

PHYSICAL EXERCISE

There is no doubt that regular physical exercise is helpful to all patients with CF and a number of studies have shown significant benefit from this (Zach *et al.*, 1981). Although exercise does result in increased clearance of lung secretions it is not a substitute for other treatments, since it will not be effective in the long term unless the patient performs it on a regular basis throughout the year. Exercise should always be encouraged as much as possible and there is no doubt that it improves patients' well-being and general fitness which is of itself beneficial in the longer term.

ANTIBIOTICS

The administration of antibiotics is a major factor in the control of lung infection in CF. These need to be given both acutely and frequently long term in order to suppress the activity of various organisms which are active in the lungs. The principal bacteria involved are *Staphylococcus aureus, Haemophilus influenzae, Psuedomonas aeruginosa* and *Pseudomonas cepacia*. Viral infections are also particularly common in CF patients and may exacerbate underlying bacterial colonization. Antibiotics are usually indicated to cover these episodes. Fungi, such as *Aspergillus fumigatus*, are also pathogenic although the exact role of these organisms is not yet clearly understood (Hiller, 1992).

Antibiotic regimes remain controversial (Govan and Nelson, 1993); they should be given in high dose because of the difficulty in penetrating the sputum and for longer courses than usual, a minimum of at least two weeks in most cases. Continuous antibiotic administration is used by some clinics in an effort to prevent staphylococcal colonization, particularly during the early years of life. An alternative approach is to give these intermittently during intercurrent infections or if the patient is persistently symptomatic. Many older children do require continuous antibiotics in order to control symptoms of chronic sputum production and persistently purulent secretions. There is as yet no conclusive evidence that either continuous prophylaxis in the early years or intermittent use successfully prevents long term lung damage or improves prognosis. It is particularly important always to take bacterial cultures of throat or sputum at each clinic attendance in order to monitor the background of colonization in the respiratory tract.

PSEUDOMONAS

Pseudomonas is a particular organism which is seen with increasing age in CF patients.

The prevalence is up to 90% among CF adults and although it is uncommon in the early years of life the colonization rate rises steadily throughout middle childhood and adolescence. Once established it is very difficult indeed to eradicate it from the lungs. Recent studies have shown that treatment with nebulized colistin (one million units twice daily) and oral ciprofloxacin (250 mg twice daily) for three weeks can prevent longer term colonization with *Pseudomonas aeruginosa* (Valerius *et al.*, 1991).

Once the organism has colonized the lungs the treatment regime should be tailored to the individual's needs. Some clinics believe that a structured programme of aggressive three monthly preventative intravenous treatment should be given whether or not there is clinical deterioration. Others give intravenous therapy only during acute exacerbations manifested by increased purulent sputum production, weight loss, impaired lung function and patient well-being in association with anorexia. There are no good controlled trials to show that one type of regime is preferable to another. If intravenous therapy is being given it is important to support the patient with aggressive nutritional therapy, either by calorie counting or, in the chronically affected patient, with the use of supplementation frequently by gastrostomy.

For those who require regular treatments 3–4 times per year, the placement of a portable cannula, such as a Portacath, subcutaneously can be particularly helpful. It also facilitates home therapy which improves the patient's quality of life. Nebulized antibiotics are also used as prophylaxis, particularly colomycin since this is not used intravenously. Other antibiotics including gentamicin and tobramycin are also used in this way and may be particularly helpful during acute intercurrent respiratory infections which are not severe enough to require intravenous antibiotics. The use of mucolytic agents such as acetylcysteine (Parvolex) may be helpful in individual cases where there is particularly viscid sputum present. These agents should be used with caution and started at quarter or half strength dilution since they may induce bronchospasm and in a few cases result in haemoptysis. Wheezing or blood-streaked sputum are contraindications to their use. Occasionally large haemoptyses occur in CF patients and may require acute treatment such as embolization or possibly lobectomy.

PSEUDOMONAS CEPACIA

Recently another pseudomonad, *Pseudomonas cepacia*, has emerged as a major pathogen in CF. At present the colonization rate is about 7% in the UK (Govan and Nelson, 1993). It is usually multiresistant to antibiotics and therefore very difficult to treat. It is transmitted directly between patients, especially siblings and those who have intimate physical contact. *Psueudomonas cepacia* infected CF patients should be seen and treated separately from the others.

The clinical course after colonization is variable, some carrying it for years with little change in the gradual rate of decline of lung function, while others rapidly succumb to overwhelming pneumonia within a few weeks or months of acquisition of the organism. Some patients have severe lung disease confined to one lobe, particularly early in life, and in this situation elective lobectomy may be helpful before the disease spreads to other parts of the lung.

There is considerable interest in the underlying pathophysiology of CF lung disease and recent studies have indicated that there may well be an excessive inflammatory response on the part of the host. This has led to the use of immunosuppressive drugs such as oral or inhaled steroids, although there is as yet no conclusive evidence that their use alters the disease progress in any major way.

DNase

The inflammatory response in the lungs also leads to a vast influx of neutrophils. As these are destroyed in fighting the infection they release large quantities of DNA from within their nuclei. DNA in this form is extremely viscid and adds to the stickiness of the sputum. The natural human enzyme DNase which destroys this has been genetically produced and is currently being used as a nebulized solution to liquify the sputum in CF. Initial studies (Aitken *et al.*, 1992) have shown encouraging results in those with moderately severe disease. Further studies are necessary to demonstrate its efficacy in those with severe lung involvement.

PNEUMOTHORAX

Pneumothorax is a particularly serious complication of CF and occurs in as many as 19% of adult patients although it is much less common in children. It is usually unilateral but can occur on either side and be very acute in onset. There are various methods of treatment including increased oxygen therapy to facilitate absorption of gas within the pneumothorax, the placement of a chest drain and the possibility of pleurodesis. Pleurectomy was previously undertaken for this complication, but as it precludes later heart/lung transplantation, this has become a less preferable treatment unless other therapies are unsuccessful.

Haemoptysis is another relatively frequent complication but is usually only manifested as small amounts of blood with blood-streaking in the sputum or a relatively minor bleed which resolves spontaneously. Some patients have major episodes which result in anaemia and hypotension, although this is rare. It is important to exclude concomitant liver disease by checking the clotting studies as part of the liver function screen. If the haemoptysis is small then reassurance and an anxiolytic agent may be all that are required. Physiotherapy should be continued but less intensively until the bleeding stops and treatment of the acute lung infection should be increased. The vast majority of cases resolve spontaneously, but for those who have major haemoptysis then bronchial artery embolization or lobectomy may be indicated.

COR PULMONALE

Heart failure secondary to severe disease is a late complication in CF. Most patients who develop this complication have severe and very advanced lung disease and its onset usually heralds a more rapid deterioration to terminal respiratory failure. Treatment consists of diuretics such as frusemide and spironolactone and the use of oxygen therapy to decrease pulmonary hypertension.

HEART/LUNG TRANSPLANTATION

Heart/lung transplantation is a relatively new treatment for end stage CF and should be considered for those with chronic respiratory failure and an FEV1 of about 25% predicted (Whitehead *et al.*, 1991). It is utilized in those whose prognosis is thought to be less than two years and who have severe impairment of quality of life because of the lung disease. Contraindications are few but include major liver disease with cirrhosis and clotting abnormalities, previous extensive pleurodesis or pleurectomy and psychosocial problems which would indicate non-compliance with treatment. Donor organs are becoming increasingly difficult to find since other patients who require single lung transplant now have a better outcome and gain preference in donor selection.

Heart/lung transplantation in CF should be carried out in centres which are expert in this procedure and have developed a special experience (Scott *et al.*, 1993).

Intensive support is required from many health care professionals including nurse specialists, physiotherapists and psychologists. Less than 50% of those who require heart/lung transplantation are likely to obtain organs and the current outcome after transplantation is a survival rate of 78% in first year and 65% in the second (Higgenbottam and Whitehead, 1991). The longer term results show persisting mortality and morbidity from the complications of chronic rejection, especially obliterative bronchiolitis. Heart/lung transplantation is thus a potential treatment for some CF patients but only in a relatively small number is a really good outcome achieved. Further advances in our knowledge and understanding of the many problems associated with this procedure will undoubtedly improve the results in times to come.

LIFE EXPECTANCY

There have been many advances in the care of CF patients in the last 30 years and this has led to a steadily improving outcome for long term survival. At present median life expectancy is of the order of 29 years in the best centres but it is estimated that for a newly born infant of today this should be at least 40 years (Elborn *et al.*, 1991). New treatments such as gene therapy promise an even greater improvement in the future.

PHYSIOTHERAPY MANAGEMENT OF CYSTIC FIBROSIS

Chest physiotherapy is an integral part of the multidisciplinary approach to the management of cystic fibrosis. Its principal aim is to clear bronchopulmonary secretions which may cause airway obstruction and lead to atelectasis and hyperinflation (Zach, 1990). Lung clearance improves ventilation and reduces airway resistance in the short term and in the long term may slow the progression of elastase mediated damage to the airways and mucociliary transport system (Zach, 1991).

TREATMENT OF INFANTS AND SMALL CHILDREN

On confirmation of diagnosis the implementation of a daily physiotherapy regime is usually advised. This involves spending time with the parents and child to explain in detail the necessity and importance of the treatment and requires considerable sympathy and understanding at a time when the parents are trying to come to terms with the diagnosis and its implications. In an infant or small child treatment is initially passive, typically involving postural drainage and percussion. In the asymptomatic patient, treatment is usually advised once or twice per day and in the presence of clinical signs, up to four times per day. Postural drainage positions include alternate side lying and prone with a head down tip, supine lying flat and sitting to drain the apical regions (Parker and Young, 1991). In the presence of localized signs, confirmed radiologically, more specific drainage positions will be necessary (see Chapter 6, p. 72). If diagnosis is made in a specialist centre, it is important that the local hospital and community services are kept fully informed so that local follow-up and treatment may be instituted if appropriate.

The routine use of chest physiotherapy in cystic fibrosis before the onset of clinical stigmata (Parker and Young, 1991) is seldom questioned. Traditionally the argument made for the institution of therapy at the time of diagnosis is that clearance of pulmonary secretions can prevent or delay the onset of respiratory complications. It is generally considered that early incorporation of therapy into the daily routine may make it more readily acceptable to the child and thereby improve compliance. Although its efficacy in preventing/delaying the progress

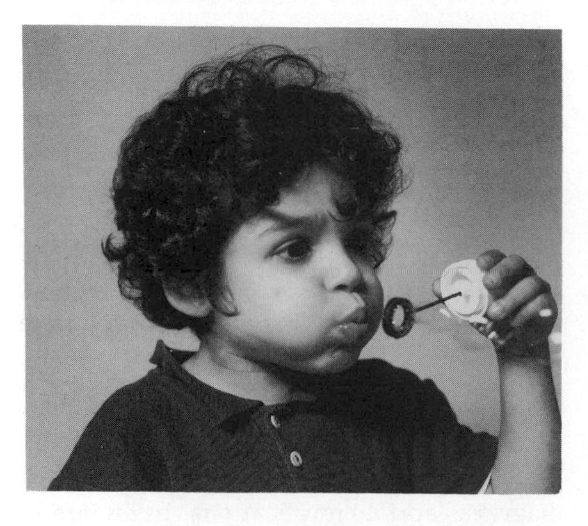

Figure 11.2 Breathing exercises in the form of play.

of lung disease has not been well substantiated some studies suggest that even asymptomatic infants have evidence of active inflammation (Khan *et al.*, 1989). In addition studies involving bronchoalveolar lavage have provided some evidence of airway obstruction in the form of macroscopic bronchial mucus casts (Wood, 1989). The use of chest physiotherapy in all patients with CF is now so well established that it may prove impossible, and perhaps unethical, to conduct a study in which early treatment of the condition is withheld in the asymptomatic group.

From approximately two years of age, breathing exercises may be introduced, usually in the form of play (Figure 11.2). As the child grows these can be instituted more formally into the treatment programme. By the age of four children are able to perform breathing control and forced expiratory manoeuvres (huffing) and begin to play a more active role in their treatment.

INDEPENDENTLY PERFORMED TREATMENT MODALITIES

In recent years the life expectancy of patients with CF has increased considerably; the majority of patients now live well into adulthood and should be able to lead as full and independent a life as possible. Most would agree that physiotherapy is a tedious and time consuming chore and it is essential, therefore, that treatment is efficient and effective but causes minimal disruption to the patient's lifestyle. In an attempt to achieve this aim, several chest physiotherapy techniques have been developed which allow the patient to perform his or her treatment without assistance (Prasad, 1993). During the transition to independent treatment the role of the community therapy services may be particularly important in helping to provide suitable support and continuing education.

The active cycle of breathing techniques

The active cycle of breathing techniques (ACBT) comprises thoracic expansion exercises, breathing control and forced expiration techniques (FET). It has been shown to improve the clearance of bronchopulmonary secretions and lung function (Pryor and Webber, 1979; Webber *et al.*, 1986). Thoracic expansion exercises are deep breaths which emphasize inspiration, based on the concept of interdependence whereby alveoli exert expanding forces on collapsed adjacent alveoli. The increase in lung volume also promotes collateral ventilatory flow (Chapter 2, p. 16), allowing pressure to build up behind bronchial secretions and assist in their mobilization. Breathing control is used between the more active components of the cycle and these periods of gentle breathing are performed at the patient's preferred rate. This avoids any potential increase in air flow obstruction which may be caused by forced expiratory manoeuvres. The FET is based on the physiological concept of the equal pressure point (West, 1987). If a huff is continued from mid to low lung volume the equal pressure point is shifted more peripherally, thereby allowing secretions to be mobilized from these areas. Breathing control is an integral part of the FET (Partridge *et al.*, 1989).

Percussion may be performed during the thoracic expansion exercises. It has been suggested that percussion may reduce FEV1 and have a detrimental effect on oxygenation (Campbell *et al.*, 1975; Wollmer *et al.*, 1985; Falk *et al.*, 1984). However, Pryor *et al.*, (1990) demonstrated no fall in oxygen saturation when percussion was performed during thoracic expansion exercises and for short periods of time only. Some patients may find self-percussion (Figure 11.3) difficult and of little value and it has been demonstrated that percussion is not an essential part of treatment provided the other techniques are performed effectively (Webber *et al.*, 1985).

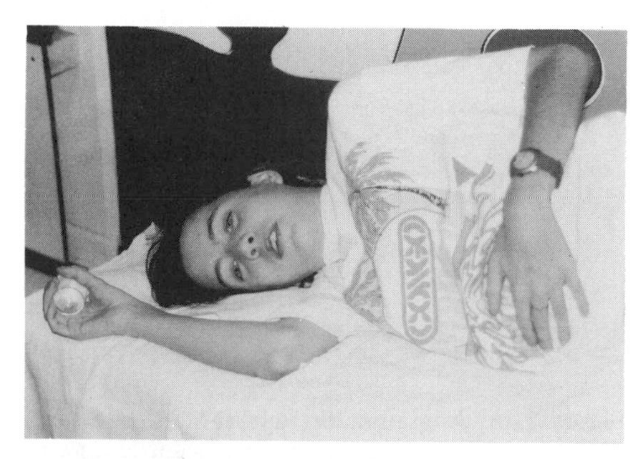

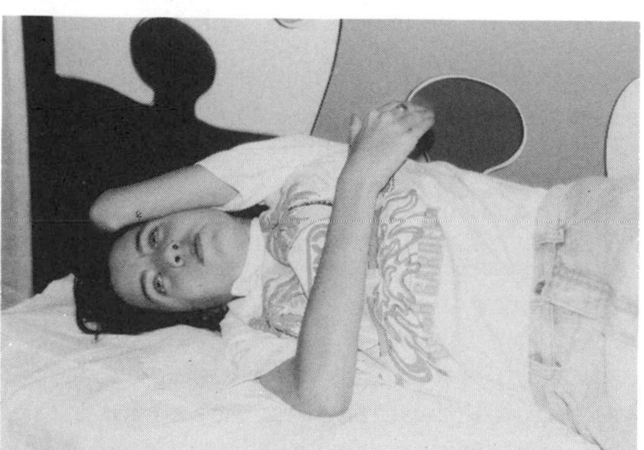

Figure 11.3 ACBT with postural drainage, relaxation and breathing control (top) and thoracic expansion exercises accompanied by percussion (bottom).

Positive expiratory pressure

Positive expiratory pressure (PEP) improves lung clearance by its effect on peripheral airways and collateral ventilatory channels. It is an effective treatment modality and may be applied via a face mask or mouthpiece (Falk *et al.*, 1984). The system consists of a mask, a one-way valve with an inspiratory and expiratory port and resistors of varying internal diameter which are inserted into the expiratory port to achieve PEP (Figure 11.4). The level of PEP is measured using a pressure manometer inserted between the expiratory port and resistance. To select the appropriate resistance the patient is required to breathe through the mask and the correct resistance is that which achieves a steady PEP of 10–20 cmH_2O during the mid expiratory phase. This pressure should be sustainable for two minutes of tidal volume breathing with only slightly active expiration.

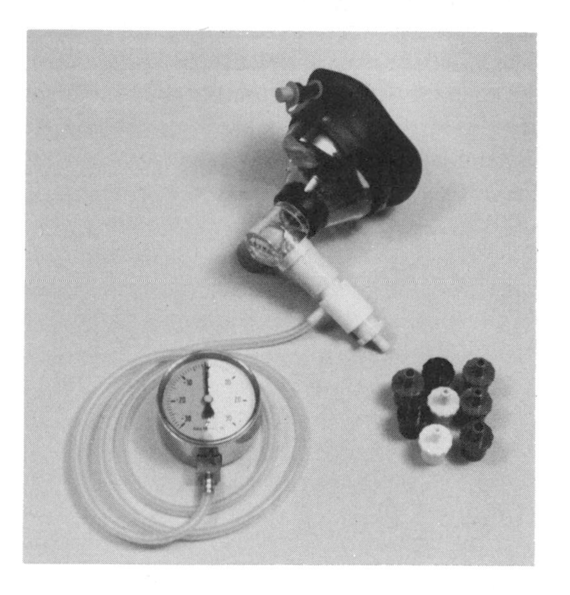

Figure 11.4 The PEP mask system.

Having selected the correct resistance the patient is trained in the treatment technique which is performed in the sitting position, elbows supported and the mask held tightly to the face (Figure 11.5). Ten to 12 breaths with slightly active (not forced) expiration are performed through the mask and followed by a period of huffing, breathing control and coughing. This cycle is then repeated until maximal clearance is achieved; treatment may last between 20–40 minutes. The reported beneficial effects of PEP include an improvement of sputum clearance and arterial oxygen tension (Falk *et al.*, 1984), an increase in FRC and a reduction in the volume of trapped gas (Groth *et al.*, 1985).

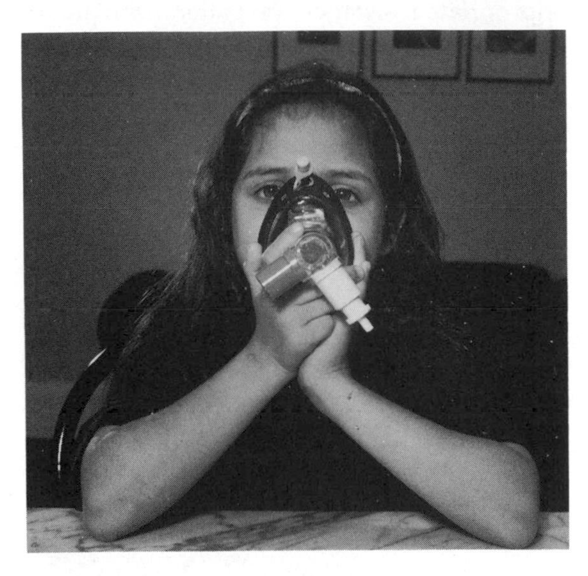

Figure 11.5 Treatment in the sitting position using PEP.

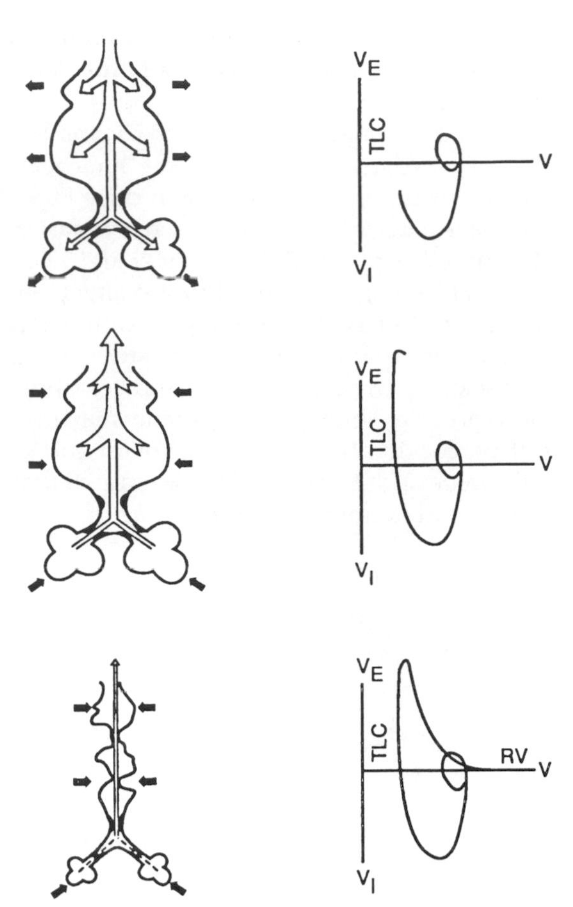

Figure 11.6 Diagrammatic representation of lung disease in CF as a combination of central airway instability and peripheral airway obstruction: deep inspiration (top), early forced expiration (centre), late forced expiration (bottom). Corresponding maximum inspiratory/expiratory flow–volume-curve tracing: V = volume; V_E, V_1 = expiratory and inspiratory flow, TLC = total lung capacity, RV = residual volume. Reproduced with permission from M. Zach, *Lung Disease in Cystic Fibrosis*, Excerpta Medica, 1988.

High pressure PEP

It has been suggested that the increase in positive transthoracic pressure during forced expirations may have a negative effect on clearing secretions by inducing bronchial collapse (Figure 11.6) in the unstable airways of advanced disease (Zach, 1990). If a forced expiration is performed through an external mechanical resistance, such as a PEP mask, a constant flow rate is produced during the early and middle part of expiration. This is due to the balance between muscular effort and the limitation to flow offered by the external resistor and results in the airway remaining dilated. As the manoeuvre is continued into low lung volume the respiratory muscles encounter a mechanical disadvantage and the driving pressure and expiratory flow will fall. An equal pressure point now develops, but at low lung volume and at a point much further downstream when compared to a normal full forced expiration. This results in the evacuation of trapped gas and the dilatory effect of positive pressure on the airway may enhance mucus clearance (Oberwaldner *et al.*, 1986).

The assessment of patients for high pressure PEP requires the patient to perform full forced vital capacity manoeuvres through the range of expiratory resistances with the mask connected to a pneumotachograph or rolling spirometer. This produces a series of flow volume curves (Figure 11.7) and the appropriate resistor is that which produces a curve showing a maximal FVC, good plateau and in which there is no curvilinearity. Treatment is performed in the sitting position; following 8–10 tidal breaths with an end inspiratory pause and slight emphasis on expiration, a full forced expiratory manoeuvre is performed through the mask. After coughing and expectoration at low lung volume the cycle is repeated until maximal clearance is achieved. Meticulous individual assessment and regular follow-up are essential to ensure maximal therapeutic value. High pressure PEP has been shown to be of benefit in both the long and short term with improved sputum clearance, lung function and a reduction in hyperinflation (Oberwaldner *et al.*, 1986, 1991; Pffleger *et al.*, 1992).

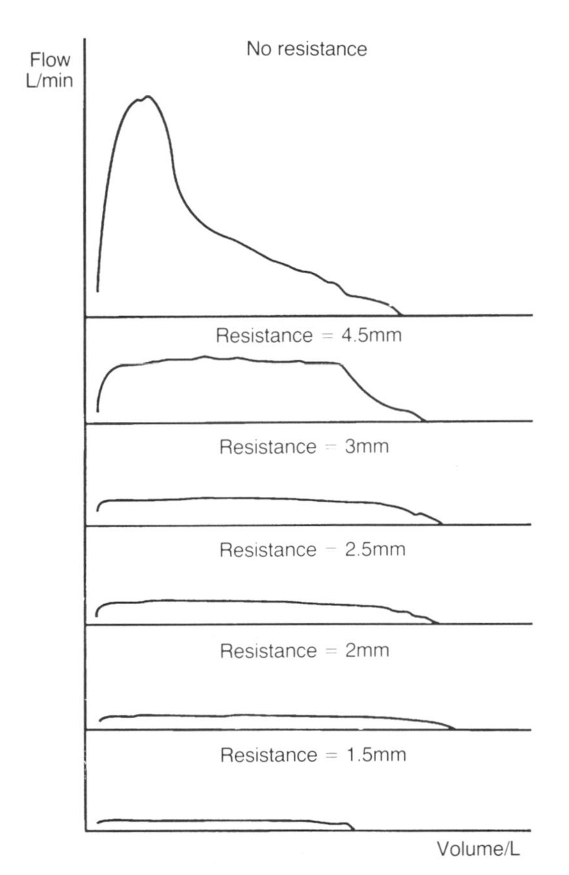

Figure 11.7 A series of maximum expiratory flow volume curves. There is an increase in FVC with the 2.0 mm internal diameter resistance, good plateau formation and elimination of any curvilinearity. Note the decrease below normal FVC with the 1.5 mm internal diameter resistance. Reproduced with permission from S.A. Prasad, Current concepts in physiotherapy, *Journal of the Royal Society of Medicine*, 1993.

Autogenic drainage

In its original form AD comprises a three-phase breathing regime performed in the sitting position. Controlled breathing is used to achieve the highest possible airflows without causing airway closure (Chevaillier, 1984; Schoni, 1989). Inspiration is performed through the nose with a slight pause prior to expiration which is performed through the mouth with an open glottis. The initial phase is performed at low lung volume (Figure 11.8) and is aimed at clearing peripheral lung regions. Secretions are collected centrally during the second phase which is performed at mid lung volume and finally expectorated in phase three at high lung volume. Flow velocity is carefully controlled to avoid high

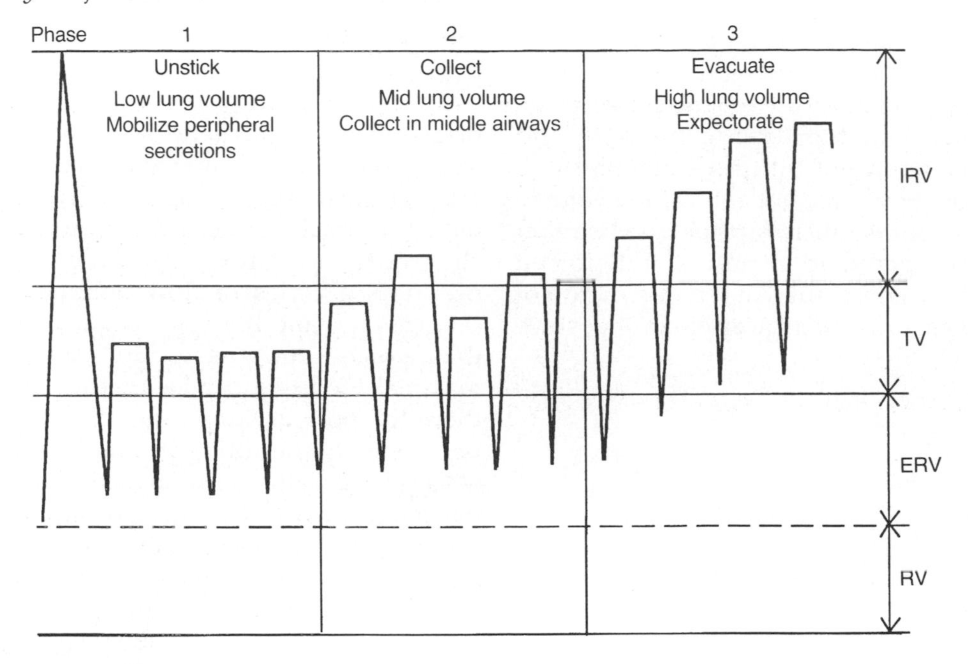

Figure 11.8 Phases of autogenic drainage: TV = tidal volume, ERV – expiratory reserve volume, IRV = inspiratory reserve volume, RV = residual volume. Reproduced with permission from S.A. Prasad, Current concepts in physiotherapy, *Journal of the Royal Society of Medicine*, 1993.

flow peaks and the emergence of an equal pressure point with collapse of the airway. Forced and unproductive coughing is avoided. This original technique has been modified because of difficulties encountered in performing the first phase at very low lung volume. The procedure has been simplified by varying mid tidal volume to suit the individual patient's needs and ability (David, 1991). Inhalation therapies, PEP and chest wall exercises may also be used in conjunction with this technique.

AD requires skilled tuition and careful follow-up by a trained therapist and full patient co-operation and discipline are essential in both the learning and treatment phase. Treatment may take up to 45 minutes per session and is usually required at least twice daily. There are few reported studies investigating AD in CF, but the beneficial effects reported include an improvement in oxygen saturation and sputum clearance (McIlwaine *et al.*, 1988; Leister *et al.*, 1993).

The flutter VRP1

This simple device produces oscillatory endobronchial pressure pulses during expiration thereby increasing airway patency and expiratory flow. In addition the vibratory effect is claimed to enhance mucus clearance (Althaus *et al.*, 1989; Schibbler *et al.*, 1992). The device is pipe shaped (Figure 11.9) and contains a cone and a steel ball. Prior to expiration the steel ball prevents air passing through the cone, but as expiratory pressure increases behind the ball, it is eventually displaced. The pressure is released as air escapes and the ball then falls back into the cone, thereby applying a cyclic oscillation during expiration. Treatment is performed in sitting and periods of flutter breathing

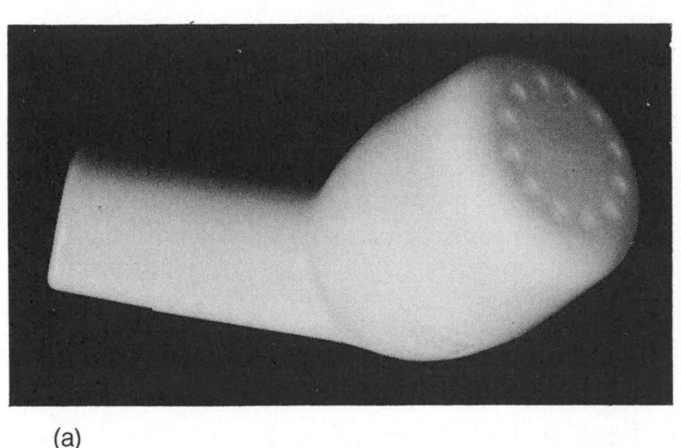

(a)

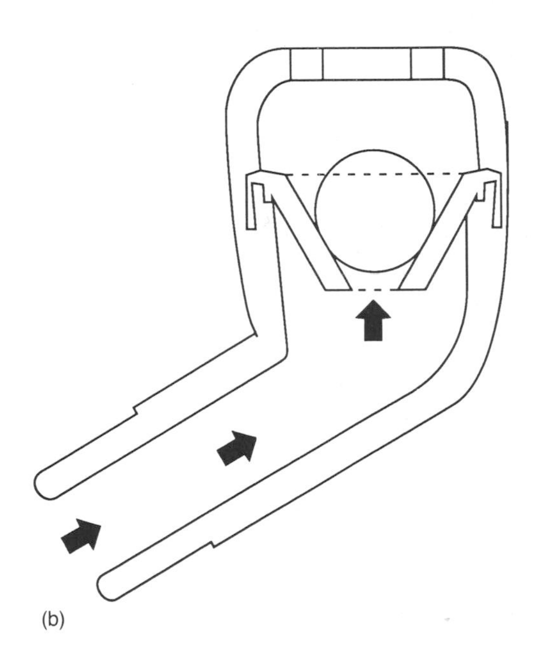

(b)

Figure 11.9 The flutter VRP1 (a), diagrammatic representation (b).

are interspersed with huffing, breathing control and coughing. As yet only a few studies have investigated the use of this device in CF but two have suggested that it adds little to other physiotherapy techniques such as the ACBT (Pryor *et al.*, 1992; Lyons *et al.*, 1992).

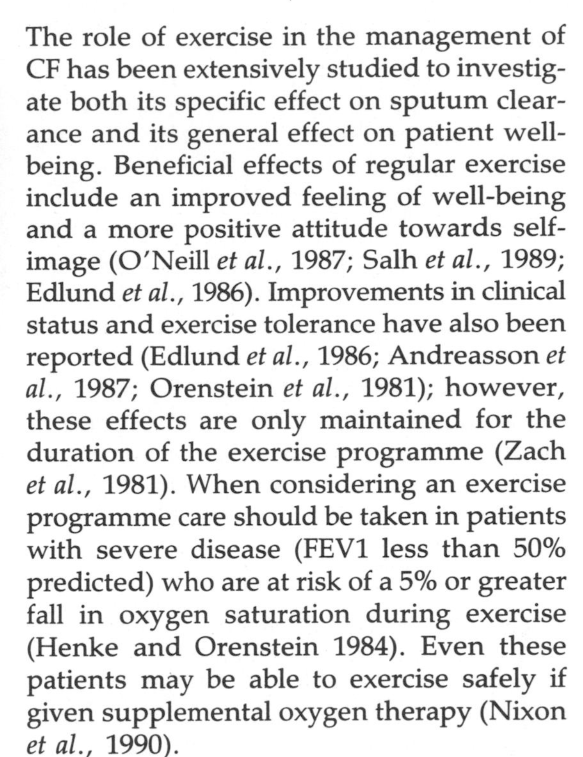

EXERCISE

The role of exercise in the management of CF has been extensively studied to investigate both its specific effect on sputum clearance and its general effect on patient well-being. Beneficial effects of regular exercise include an improved feeling of well-being and a more positive attitude towards self-image (O'Neill *et al.*, 1987; Salh *et al.*, 1989; Edlund *et al.*, 1986). Improvements in clinical status and exercise tolerance have also been reported (Edlund *et al.*, 1986; Andreasson *et al.*, 1987; Orenstein *et al.*, 1981); however, these effects are only maintained for the duration of the exercise programme (Zach *et al.*, 1981). When considering an exercise programme care should be taken in patients with severe disease (FEV1 less than 50% predicted) who are at risk of a 5% or greater fall in oxygen saturation during exercise (Henke and Orenstein 1984). Even these patients may be able to exercise safely if given supplemental oxygen therapy (Nixon *et al.*, 1990).

Exercise has also been reported to have a beneficial effect on sputum clearance and it has been suggested that it could replace conventional physiotherapy of postural drainage, percussion, vibration, forced expiration and coughing (Andreasson *et al.*, 1987; Blomquist *et al.*, 1986; Zach *et al.*, 1981). This effect may result from an increase in circulating catecholamines, stimulating mucus production and ciliary beat frequency, and from the increase in expiratory airflow during exercise (Kollberg *et al.*, 1988; Geddes, 1984). However most studies advocate that exercise should be used to complement physiotherapy rather than replace it (Sahl *et al.*, 1989). A recent study comparing combinations of chest physiotherapy (ACBT) and exercise versus exercise alone reported significantly higher sputum weights in patient treatments which included physiotherapy (Bilton *et al.*, 1992). Interspersing periods of exercise to mobilize secretions with a technique such as FET or PEP may prove to be an effective means of treatment, although this requires further investigation. Exercise involving the upper body or activities such as trampolining and swimming should be encouraged and may be more effective than lower body exercise such as bicycle ergometry.

The wide range of treatment modalities presents the dilemma of choosing an appropriate technique. Many of the existing comparative studies show conflicting results and there are several problems in interpreting and comparing these. For example, some use the term 'conventional' physiotherapy which may describe a variety of combinations of postural drainage, percussion and coughing performed in differing orders and for varying lengths of time (Falk *et al.*, 1984; Bain *et al.*, 1988; McIlwaine *et al.*, 1988). The ambiguous nature of this term renders it inappropriate in current comparative clinical studies. Similarly, well defined techniques such as the FET are frequently misinterpreted or modified and this may be responsible for the contradictory results documented. Few studies address the long term effects of a specific treatment modality (Oberwaldner *et al.*, 1986; McIlwaine *et al.*, 1988; Reisman *et al.*, 1988). The difficulties associated with such studies include patient compliance, variability of an individual's disease progression and patient withdrawal. Existing evidence would suggest that there is no one 'best' method of treatment. Each patient must be considered individually, paying particular attention to their respiratory status, social circumstances, age and personality. A plan of management may then be formed which will provide maximal therapeutic value.

REFERENCES

Aitken, M.L., Burke, W., McDonald, G. *et al.* (1992) Recombinant human DNase inhalation in normal subjects with cystic fibrosis. A phase 1 study. *Journal of the American Medical Association*, **267**, 1947–51.

Althaus, P., Bovay, F., Cao, P. *et al.* (1989) The bronchial hygiene assisted by the flutter VRP1. Congress Proceedings of the 16th European Working Group for CF, Prague, pp. 118.

Andreasson, B., Jonson, B., Kornfalt, R. *et al.* (1987) Long term effects of physical exercise on working capacity and pulmonary function in cystic fibrosis. *Acta Paediatrica Scandinavica*, **76**, 70–5.

Bain, J., Bishop, J. and Olinski, A. (1988) Evaluation of directed coughing in cystic fibrosis. *British Journal of Disease of the Chest*, **82**, 138–48.

Bilton, D., Dodd, M.E., Abbott, J.V. and Webb, A.K. (1992) The benefits of exercise combined with physiotherapy in the treatment of adults with cystic fibrosis. *Respiratory Medicine*, **86**, 507–11.

Blomquist, M., Freyschuss, U., Wyman, L.G. and Strandvik, B. (1986) Physical activity and self-treatment in cystic fibrosis. *Archives of Disease in Childhood*, **61**, 362–7.

Campbell, A.H., O'Connell, J.M. and Wilson, F. (1975) The effect of chest physiotherapy upon the FEV1 in chronic bronchitis. *Medical Journal of Australia*, **1**, 33.

Chevaillier, J. (1984) Autogenic drainage (AD) in, *Cystic Fibrosis Horizons*, (ed. D. Lawson), John Wiley, Chichester, pp. 235.

Cuthbert, A.W. (1992) The biochemical defect in cystic fibrosis. *Journal of the Royal Society of Medicine* (suppl. 19), **85**, 2–5.

David, A. (1991) Autogenic drainage – the German approach, in *Respiratory Care* (ed. J.A. Pryor), Churchill Livingstone, London, pp. 65–78.

Dodge, J.A., Morison, S., Lewis, P.A. *et al.* (1993) Cystic fibrosis in the United Kingdom, 1968–1988: incidence, population and survival. *Paediatric and Perinatal Epidemiology*, **7**, 157–66.

Dorin, J.R., Dickinson, P., Alton, E.W. *et al.* (1992) Cystic fibrosis in the mouse by targeted insertional mutagenesis. *Nature*, **359**, 211–15.

Edlund, L.D., French, R.W., Herbst, J.J. *et al.* (1986) Effects of a swimming programme on children with cystic fibrosis. *American Journal of Disease in Childhood*, **140**, 80–3.

Elborn, J.S., Shale, S.J. and Britton, J.R. (1991) Cystic fibrosis: current survival and population estimates to the year 2000. *Thorax*, **46**, 881–5.

Falk, M., Kelstrup, M., Anderson, J.B. *et al.* (1984) Improving the ketchup bottle method with positive expiratory pressure, PEP, in cystic fibrosis. *European Journal of Respiratory Disease*, **65**, 423–32.

Geddes, D.M. (1984) Physical exercise in cystic fibrosis, in *Cystic Fibrosis Horizons*, (ed. D. Lawson), John Wiley, Chichester, pp. 117–38.

Govan, J.R.W. and Nelson, J.W. (1993) Microbiology of lung infections; themes and issues. *Journal of the Royal Society of Medicine* (suppl 20), **86** 11–18.

Gregory, R.J., Rich, D.P., Cheng, S.H. *et al.* (1991) Maturation and function of CFTR variants bearing mutations in putative nucleotide binding domains 1 & 2. *Molecular Cell Biology*, **11**, 3886–93.

Groth, S., Stafangel, G. Dirksen, H. *et al.* (1985) Positive expiratory pressure (PEP mask) physiotherapy improves ventilation and reduces volume of trapped gas in cystic fibrosis. *Bulletin of European Physiopathology and Respiration*, **21**, 339–43.

Henke, K.G. and Orenstein, D.M. (1984) Oxygen saturation during exercise in cystic fibrosis. *American Review of Respiratory Disease*, **129**, 708–11.

Higgenbottam, T.W. and Whitehead, B. (1991) Heart–lung transplantation for cystic fibrosis. *Journal of the Royal Society of Medicine* (suppl 18), **84**, 18–21.

Hiller, E.J. (1992) Aspergillus. *Journal of the Royal Society of Medicine* (suppl 19), **85**, 33–5.

Hyde, S.C., Gill, D.R., Higgins, C.F. *et al.* (1993) Correction of the ion transport defect in cystic fibrosis transgenic mice by gene therapy. *Nature*, **362**, 250–5.

Khan, T.Z., Wagener, J.S., Riches, D.W.H. and Accurso, F.J. (1993) Increased interleukin-8 levels and gene expression by pulmonary macrophages in bronchoalveolar lavage fluid from infants with cystic fibrosis. *American Review of Respiratory Disease*, **147**, A463.

Kollberg, H., Schoni, M., Turler, K. *et al.* (1988) Dopamine and catecholamines in cystic fibrosis in response to a marathon race. *International Journal of Sports Medicine*, **9**, 56–9.

Leister, E., de Boer, P. and Schoni, M.H. (1993) Short term effect of physiotherapy on lung function and DLCO. 18th European Cystic Fibrosis Conference, Madrid, pp. 96–7.

Lyons, E., Chatham, K., Campbell, I.A. and Presott, R.J. (1992) The evaluation of the flutter VRP1 device in young adults with cystic fibrosis. Proceedings of the 11th International CF Congress, Dublin, AHP 30.

McIlwaine, M., Davidson, A.G.F., Wong, L.T.K. *et al.* (1988) Comparison of positive expiratory pressure and autogenic drainage with conventional percussion and drainage therapy in the treatment of CF. 10th International CF Congress. Excerpta Medica, Asia Pacific Congress Series, Sydney, pp. 120.

Nixon, P.A., Orenstein, D.M., Curtis, S.E. and Ross, E.A. (1990) Oxygen supplementation during exercise in cystic fibrosis. *American Review of Respiratory Disease*, **142**, 807–11.

Oberwaldner, B., Evans, J.C. and Zach, M.S. (1986) Forced expirations against a variable resistance: a new chest physiotherapy method in cystic fibrosis. *Pediatric Pulmonology*, **2**, 358–67.

Oberwaldner, B., Theissl, B., Rucker, A. and Zach, M.S. (1991) Chest physiotherapy in hospitalised patients with cystic fibrosis: a study of lung function effects and sputum clearance. *European Respiratory Journal*, **4**, 152–8.

O'Neill, P.A., Dodds, M., Phillips, B. *et al.* (1987) Regular exercise and reduction of breathlessness in patients with cystic fibrosis. *British Journal of Disease of the Chest*, **81**, 62–9.

Orenstein, D.M., Franklin, B.A., Doershuk, C.F. *et al.* (1981) Exercise conditioning and cardiopulmonary fitness in cystic fibrosis. *Chest*, **80**, 392–8.

Parker, A.E. and Young, C.S. (1991) The physiotherapy management of cystic fibrosis in children. *Physiotherapy*, **77**, 584–6.

Partridge, C., Pryor, J.A. and Webber, B.A. (1989) Characteristics of the forced expiration technique. *Physiotherapy*, **75**, 193–4.

Pfleger, A., Theissl, B., Oberwaldner, B. and Zach, M.S. (1992) Self-administered chest physiotherapy in cystic fibrosis: a comparative study of high pressure PEP and autogenic drainage. *Lung*, **170**, 323–30.

Prasad, S.A. (1993) Current concepts in physiotherapy. *Journal of the Royal Society of Medicine*, **86** (suppl 20), 23–9.

Pryor, J.A. and Webber, B.A. (1979) An evaluation of the forced expiratory technique as an adjunct to postural drainage. *Physiotherapy*, **65**, 304–7.

Pryor, J.A., Webber, B.A. and Hodson, M.E. (1990) Effect of chest physiotherapy on oxygen saturation in patients with cystic fibrosis. *Thorax*, **45**, 77.

Pryor, J.A., Webber, B.A. Hodson, M.E. and Warner, J.O. (1992) The flutter VRP1 as an adjunct to chest physiotherapy in cystic fibrosis. Proceedings of 11th International CF Congress, Dublin, WP102.

Reissman, J.J., Rivington-Law, B., Corey, M. *et al*. (1988) Role of conventional physiotherapy in cystic fibrosis. *Journal of Pediatrics*, **113**, 632–6.

Rommens, J.M. Iannuzi, M.C., Kerem, B.S. *et al*. (1989) Identification of the cystic fibrosis gene: chromosome walking and jumping. *Science*, **245**, 1059–65.

Rosenfeld, M.A., Yoshimura, K., Trapnell, B.C. *et al*. (1992) In vivo transfer of human cystic fibrosis transmembrane conductance regulator gene to the airway eithelium. *Cell*, **68**, 143–55.

Salh, W,. Bilton, D., Dodd, M. and Webb, A.K. (1989) Effect of exercise and physiotherapy in aiding sputum expectoration in adults with cystic fibrosis. *Thorax*, **44**, 1006–8.

Schibbler, A., Casaulta, C. and Kraemer, R. (1992) Rationale of oscillatory breathing as chest physiotherapy performed by the flutter in patient with cystic fibrosis. *Pediatric Pulmonology*, **4** (suppl 8), 301.

Schoni, M.H. (1989) Autogenic drainage: a modern approach to chest physiotherapy in cystic fibrosis. *Journal of the Royal Society of Medicine*, **82** (suppl 16), 32–7.

Scott, J.P., Dennis, C. and Mullins, P. (1993) Heart-lung transplantation for end-stage respiratory disease in cystic fibrosis patients. *Journal of the Royal Society of Medicine* (suppl 20), **86**, 19–22.

Valerius, N.H., Koch, C. and Hoiby, N. (1991) Early treatment of *Pseudomonas aeruginosa* colonisation in cystic fibrosis. *Lancet*, **338**, 725–6.

Watson, E.K., Mayall, E., Chapple J. *et al*. (1991) Screening for carriers of cystic fibrosis through primary health care services. *British Medical Journal*, **303**, 504–7.

Webber, B.A., Parker, R.A., Hofmeyer, J.L. and Hodson, M.E. (1985) Evaluation of self-percussion during postural drainage using the forced expiration technique. *Physiotherapy Practice*, **1**, 42.

Webber, B.A., Hofmeyer, J.L., Morgan, M.D.L. and Hodson, M.E. (1986) Effects of postural drainage, incorporating the forced expiration technique, on pulmonary function in cystic fibrosis. *British Journal of Disease of the Chest*, **80**, 353–9.

Weller, P.H. and West, J.V. (1991) Neonatal screening – should we or shouldn't we? *Journal of the Royal Society of Medicine* (suppl 18), **84**, 7–9.

West, J.B. (1987) *Pulmonary Pathophysiology*, Williams and Wilkins, Baltimore.

Whitehead, B., Helms, P., Goodwin, M. *et al*. (1991) Heart–lung transplantation for cystic fibrosis. 2: Outcome. *Archives of Disease in Childhood*, **66**, 1022–6.

Wollmer, P., Ursing, K., Midgrem, B. and Eriksson, L. (1985) Inefficiency of chest percussion in the physical therapy of chronic bronchitis. *European Journal of Respiratory Disease*, **66**, 233.

Wood, R.E. (1989) Treatment of CF lung disease in the first two years. *Pediatric Pulmonology*, **4**, 68–70.

Zach, M.S. (1990) Lung disease in cystic fibrosis – an updated concept. *Pediatric Pulmonology*, **8**, 188–202.

Zach, M.S. (1991) Can we improve airway clearance? in *Cystic Fibrosis, Basic and Clinical Research*, (eds N. Hoiby and S.S. Pedersen), Excerpta Medica, Amsterdam, pp. 71–7.

Zach, M.S., Purrer, B. and Oberwaldner, B. (1981) Effect of swimming on forced expiration and sputum clearance in cystic fibrosis. *Lancet*, **2**, 1201–3.

INDEX

Page numbers in *italics* refer to tables; those in **bold** type to figures